SURGICAL CONDITIONS IN INFANCY AND CHILDHOOD

MARK M. RAVITCH, M.D., *Series Editor*

HIRSCHSPRUNG'S DISEASE

THEODOR EHRENPREIS, M.D., F.A.A.P.

Associate Professor of Pediatric Surgery, Karolinska Institutet;
Head, Department of Pediatric Surgery,
Karolinska Sjukhuset, Stockholm, Sweden

ANO-RECTAL MALFORMATIONS IN CHILDREN

F. DOUGLAS STEPHENS, M.S.

Director, Surgical Research Unit, Royal Children's
Hospital Research Foundation, Melbourne, Victoria, Australia

AND

E. DURHAM SMITH, M.D.

Senior Surgical Research Fellow, Royal Children's
Hospital Research Foundation, Melbourne, Victoria, Australia

ANO-RECTAL MALFORMATIONS IN CHILDREN

Ano-Rectal Malformations in Children

by

F. DOUGLAS STEPHENS, D.S.O., M.S. (Melb.), F.R.A.C.S.

Director, Department of Surgical Research, Royal Children's Hospital Research Foundation; Pediatric Surgeon, Royal Children's Hospital, Melbourne, and Royal Children's Hospital Clinical School, University of Melbourne; Honorary Pediatric Surgeon, Royal Women's Hospital, Melbourne, Australia

and

E. DURHAM SMITH, M.D. (Melb.), F.R.A.C.S., F.A.C.S.

Senior Surgical Research Fellow, Royal Children's Hospital Research Foundation; Pediatric Surgeon, Royal Children's Hospital, Melbourne, and Royal Children's Hospital Clinical School, University of Melbourne, Australia

YEAR BOOK MEDICAL PUBLISHERS, INC.

35 EAST WACKER DRIVE • CHICAGO

Library of Congress Catalog Card Number: 75-125805

International Standard Book Number: 0-8151-8200-7

DEDICATION

To children everywhere, deformed anywhere

Preface

THE AUTHORS present an up-to-the-moment survey of work published in the English language in the past one hundred and fifty years on malformations of the rectum and anus, an account of the pathological anatomy of most of the regularly occurring deformities, their embryological classification and the detailed management of each type. Also presented are the results of much original work of the authors, as well as of Robert Fowler, J. H. Kelly and Ruth Magnus, all of whom have devoted time intermittently in the past twenty years to this subject, as members of the Surgical Research Unit of the Royal Children's Hospital Research Foundation. Most of the research work published in a previous book entitled, *Congenital Malformations of Rectum, Anus and Genito-Urinary Tracts* (Edinburgh and London: E. & S. Livingstone, Ltd.; 1963), is included in this book, together with reports of subsequent work, embracing management, results of treatment and a coverage of recent research of other authors.

The original descriptions based on autopsy dissections and microscopical studies of serial sections of the pelvic and perineal organs and muscles by F. D. Stephens have been considerably augmented by the work of J. H. Kelly and R. Magnus. J. H. Kelly's invaluable diagnostic and functional studies of the levator ani musculature by radiographic techniques, including defecography, have provided much meaningful data which are included in the appropriate chapters.

In the composition of this book, E. D. Smith has been responsible for most of the manuscript in its original form, the analysis of the results of treatment, the tables which show them and for the survey of the vast array of references and the bibliography. Dr. Reginald Webster, Burton Research Fellow, compiled the historical chapter. Dr. Mark Ravitch's experience as author of many journal articles and books, and as editor of this series, has been of inestimable value to us.

This subject is complex, in part because of the thirty-three regularly occurring types of ano-rectal deformities described, in part because of the male and female counterparts of each deformity and in part because of the confusion created by the multiplicity of terms ascribed by different authors to the same deformity. We have tried to clarify our descriptions by adding to the text a profusion of illustrations, using not only figures numbered in orthodox manner, but also diagrams denoting each type of deformity. These diagrams appear in Appendix C, which is inside the back cover of this book. They are ready *aides-mémoires* for the mind's eye of the reader. We have purposely separated the male and female deformities in classification, description and in management throughout the book, and we have given each deformity a descriptive title which incorporates the terms ano- or recto- (or the words anus and rectum), which denote the embryological segment which is chiefly involved. Anal deformities are referable to pit, membrane and perineal aberrations, whereas rectal deformities refer to defective subdivision of the internal cloaca in the pelvis.

One of the most unsatisfactory aspects of the subject has been lack of agreement in the world literature on a common classification. After completing our manuscript, a major breakthrough may have come on a proposal for an internationally agreed classification, during the course of a symposium on Anorectal Anomalies in a Paediatric Surgical Congress at our Hospital in March, 1970. Over 200 pediatric surgeons from 27 countries attended this symposium on terminology and a "Proposed International Classification (1970)" was formulated. In addition to this main symposium, a smaller working group continued the discussions to formulate details; this group included Doctors T. V. Santulli; W. B. Kiesewetter; A. H. Bill, Jr.; and S. Gans (U.S.A.); Professor J. H. Louw and Associate Professor S. Cywes (South Africa); Mr. H. H. Nixon (U.K.); Professor F. Rehbein (Germany); Dr. D. Vervat (Netherlands); Dr. G. Grotte (Sweden); Miss R. Magnus, and the present two authors (Australia). The classification is described in detail in Chapter 6. So important was the new agreement, however, that we rearranged our textual layout and order of descriptions to follow the new scheme and prevailed upon our patient Publisher to incorporate the changes. We are most grateful to Year Book Medical Publishers for this, for the book is now the first to be published in the new form and expresses the coordinated views of the principal writers on the subject from many countries.

It would be presumptuous to regard the descriptions in this book as all embracing, but for the commonly recurring types a section will be found which will help the management of most babies so afflicted. However, there is a rare group of cloacal deformities comprising complicated ectopia vesicae, absence of the cloaca and other monstrosities of the pelvi-perineum, which receive less detailed description, mainly because of their rarity, incompatibility with life and paucity of study on our part. It is hoped that in time a greater coverage of the super rarities will be added.

The book is a reference work for all those involved in the care of cloacal and rectal deformities, and such include pediatric surgeons, radiologists and neonatologists for the immediate crises, and proctologists and obstetricians when the patients grow to adulthood and sometimes to motherhood. Others intimately concerned in the early days are urologists and, behind the scenes, embryologists, anatomists and pathologists.

The authors hope that this detailed presentation of the state of our knowledge today provides a solid base upon which to mount a springboard for further research, and a basis for surgical improvements in the management of these tangles of the human cloacal derivatives.

Acknowledgments

The Royal Children's Hospital, Melbourne, is currently celebrating its centenary year.

Most of the authors referred to in the References have made their contributions to this mass of published work during the same period. Their pioneering achievements along the road of surgical endeavor most certainly deserve pride of place in Chapter 1.

We also recognize the help of former surgeons and members of the medical staff of the Royal Children's Hospital and its Research Foundation, as well as our contemporaries who have actively taken part in the management of the patients and in the research work on these anomalies.

One of us (F. D. Stephens) had the good fortune to study and work at the Hospital for Sick Children, Great Ormond Street, in the early postwar years, with the late Sir Denis Browne, K.C.V.O., F.R.C.S., F.R.A.-C.S. (Hon.), who, through his great interest in ano-recto-genital deformities, attracted a multitude of patients and stimulated colleagues to conduct research into these deformities.

Dr. Reginald Webster, M.D. (Melb.), D.Sc. (Melb.), F.R.A.C.P., F.C.P.A. (Hon.) and Burton Research Fellow, Royal Children's Hospital Research Foundation, and Pathologist to the Royal Children's Hospital from 1914–1948, wrote the historical section which appears in this book as Chapter 1. We are grateful to him for this contribution and for his grammatical refinements elsewhere in the manuscript.

In the composition of this book, material has been gathered from previously published and unpublished works of both authors and former members of the Surgical Research Unit of the Royal Children's Hospital Research Foundation and from the writings of a host of authors whose names are listed in the references.

We wish to thank authors, editors and publishers for their permission to reproduce illustrations and extracts from books and articles published elsewhere. These have been acknowledged in the preface, in the text and in the appropriate legends to illustrations.

We are indebted to the Royal Australasian College of Surgeons, in whose journal many of the illustrations first appeared, and also the *Australian and New Zealand Journal of Obstetrics and Gynaecology* for allowing us to reproduce illustrations previously published in their respective journals.

It is not possible to acknowledge in full our indebtedness to the Medical and Nursing Staff of the Royal Children's Hospital, Melbourne, who cared for the children, to all those members of the ancillary services who helped in one way or another, to all the medical practitioners who looked after the families; to Dr. H. Hiller, Director of the Department of Radiology and his staff; Dr. A. Williams, Director of the Department of Pathology, and Dr. P. Campbell, Morbid Anatomist, and their staff; and Mr. A. Daniel, Head of the Department of Medical Illustration, and Mrs. Cottril and other members of his staff, all of whom have advised and actively shared in the compilation of the information contained herein; and to the parents, whose assistance is so essential at all times in the day-to-day care of the children.

We are grateful to Dr. Hans Bettinger, formerly the Director, and Dr. D. W. Fortune, the present Director of the Department of Pathology of the Royal Women's Hospital, Melbourne, for the opportunities they have provided for us to study untouched malformations of stillborn babies or neonates who died from multiple deformities shortly after birth.

Most of the diagrams and art work have been accomplished by Mr. Eric Thake of the Department of Audio-Visual Aids of the University of Melbourne. Other diagrams were drawn by Mrs. D. James, who is a member of the Department of Medical Illustration of the Royal Children's Hospital.

Mr. John Komissarov has maintained the collections of specimens and has carried out the tedious, time-consuming cutting of serial sections which are the basis of many of our studies.

Miss Hitchcock, the senior secretary of the Surgical Research Unit, Miss J. Biggin and Miss G. Clarke typed the manuscript and retyped and typed again parts of it and attended to the arrangement of the illustrations and the tedious compilation of the References. Mrs. J. Ball and Mrs. W. Morris, members of the Volunteer Service of the Royal Children's Hospital, helped with the documentation of the legends, diagrams, references, etc. To all, we owe much for their accurate, conscientious work in putting the manuscript together.

F. Douglas Stephens

E. Durham Smith

Table of Contents

CHAPTER 1

Historical Review

IN THE STORY of the evolution of modern surgical technique as applied to occlusion of the rectum and/or anus, surgeons of the French school were pre-eminent. The operation of proctoplasty, a simple procedure devised by Amussat in 1835, notable as a landmark along the tedious route to surgical perfection, soon superseded the earlier procedures of blind groping with trochar or bistoury and relegated these efforts of proved futility to the limbo of forgotten things. These involved for the infant the travail inseparable from repeated dilatations following incision, achieving nothing better than a semicicatrized fistula.

The earliest account of surgical intervention as a lifesaving measure in the management of imperforate rectum appears in the writings of Paul of Aegina (A.D. 625–690), who maintained by dilatation with bougies the opening in the rectum made by a blind plunge with a bistoury. Records are scarce after this annotation in the 7th century, and it has been possible to trace but few between the 7th and the 18th centuries. Among the few are to be numbered those of Scultet (1660), who is cited by Bradham (1958) as having successfully dilated anal stenosis with gentian roots, and Cooke (1676), described by J. H. Cule (1965) as a Cromwellian army surgeon of taciturn optimism. Cooke recounted in 1676 his treatment of an imperforate anus for which he had made a small incision and afterwards "dilated with an Elder-Pith, and the child did very well." Cooke exhorted care of the sphincter muscles by any who sought to repeat his success.

Saviord, in 1693, as recorded by Crowell and Dulin (1940) also treated a bulging membranous closure of the rectum in a newborn infant by incision and dilatation, but 94 years elapsed before Benjamin Bell (1787) of England conceived and ventured on the first perineal dissection in 1787. Bell's innovation was noted by Bodenhammer (1860), perhaps the foremost writer of his time on congenital malformations of the rectum and anus, and consisted of perineal incision in the midline, followed by dilatation of the wound with the finger; if the rectal ampulla was not thus located, it was to be sought for in the hollow of the sacrum with a trochar. Copeland Hutchinson (1822) slightly modified Bell's operation by limiting the incision from 1½ to 2 inches, beyond this limit, trusting to the trochar only. John Campbell (1860) was the first surgeon in the United States to accomplish successfully the operation of incision and dilatation.

On June 1, 1789, a surgeon of Dover named Mantell, in the course of a letter to Dr. J. C. Lettsom, after stating his belief that where there was no perceptible mark or vestige of the anus relief was not to be accomplished "by the efforts of nature or art" proceeded to recount his procedure in dealing with complete absence of the anus and an associated recto-vaginal fistula in a child of a few days old. He made an incision in the perineum at the usual site of the anus onto the tip of a probe which he had passed into the rectum through the vaginal opening. This operation was performed in September 1786, and within 2 years, in the spring of 1788, it was found necessary to operate again to enlarge the resultant stricture. Nearly a year after the second operation, Mantell had the satisfaction of finding that the child continued perfectly well, but her subsequent history and probably recurrent dilatations are not related.

In March, 1800, William Kennedy, likewise claimed to have operated successfully on a male infant with congenitally absent anus, dissecting upwards from the perineum until he found "the end of the gut, round and pointed like a cone, quite tense." The incision made into the gut was kept open by means of a sponge, and the child was reported as having "ever since discharged faeces naturally . . . and thriving in every respect."

It is evident that by the end of the 18th century puncture and blind groping with trochar or bistoury had been superseded by a midline incision in the perineum and visual search for the imperforate rectal cul-de-sac and that other surgeons were moving haltingly towards the exploitation of perineal incision, upon which depended the notable advance of proctoplasty devised by Amussat (1835).

On May 15, 1833, prior to Amussat's "break-through," an operation by J-N. Roux de Brignolles carried dissection from a perineal incision a stage further. The infant was afflicted with an imperforate urethral meatus as well as an imperforate anus. By the time he had been relieved of the former he had become very ill, and Roux's procedure was to have the child held in the lithotomy position in order that he might dissect from the midline of the perineum, through the middle of the elliptical muscles of the sphincter ani and the levatores ani, until his finger felt the lower end of the intestine. After he had incised the gut, lint dressings were used to prevent occlusion of the opening and continued for the first 2 weeks, but some bougienage became necessary.

Roux was aware that if the perineal approach to very high imperforations was used the access was inadequate and resulted in serious complications of stricture.

Shortly after this, in September 1835, Amussat operated on the female child of an Englishwoman resident in Paris.

The operation devised by Amussat for the relief of imperforate rectum in the infant proved an advance in surgical technique, which was soon appreciated and adopted; in those infants in whom the terminal end of the rectum could be reached readily through the perineum, the method of Amussat, with but trivial changes, maintained its pre-eminence until well beyond the turn of the century.

In this infant, Amussat was of opinion "that the rectum was obturated at the depth of about two inches, and that it communicated with the vagina . . . that the septum by which the rectum and vagina were parted was deficient for a considerable extent." He attributed his failure in two earlier cases "to the resorption of bile, infiltration and the formation of abscesses along the artificial opening . . ." and reasoned that the fatal termination which almost always took place in a short time when the rectum had been opened with a trochar, bistoury or lancet might be accounted for "by the want of protection which a mucous surface would afford the new passage." Therefore, having found the blind termination of the rectum by dissection upwards from the perineum, limited strictly to the midline in the interest of the sphincters, he drew the gut down and sutured the mucosa accurately to the skin margin, without undue tension.

Thus was conceived and practiced the operation of proctoplasty, indissolubly linked with the name of Amussat, fulfilling the purpose of obviating the contraction of the opening in the bowel, which in earlier methods always narrowed into a simple fecal fistula and necessitated constant dilatation to permit discharge of the content of the colon.

The methods described illustrate the practice that prevailed up to the middle of the 19th century. The period 1800–1850 witnessed the gradual abandonment of blind groping for the rectal ampulla by cut and thrust. Midline dissection from a perineal incision gradually acquired the status of accepted practice. In the operation of Roux de Brignolles, as he used it in May 1833, 2 years before Amussat's advance, strict adherence to the midline and care of the sphincters were cardinal points.

The history of transplantation of the anus backwards from the site of a recto-vaginal fistula dates from the first performance by Dieffenbach in 1826, and included the resuture of the divided sphincter muscles in front of the anus. Almost 50 years passed before further transplantation operations were described for this lesion. Rizzoli

(1874) divided the posterior vaginal wall, fourchette and perineum, detached the anus and resutured the perineal structures in front. Similarly, Pierre Delbet and Kirmisson all used a racquet incision and continued the incision backwards to the coccyx. Ombredanne pointed out that the anus sometimes moved back to its original site and suggested two separate transverse incisions. There was little change in approach until Stone (1936) described a method in which the anus was transplanted by separate incisions, but in which the perineal body and anal sphincter muscles were not severed.

Extensions of the Operative Field.—With a view to the more facile accomplishment of his object, the suture of the rectal mucosa to the skin, Amussat recommended that if necessary the field of operation be enlarged by excision of the coccyx, or part of it. This first hesitant step towards the application of the principle underlying the Kraske operation was advised and practiced by Amussat towards the end of 1835 to meet objections of his contemporaries, who argued with some force that when the rectum was very much underdeveloped and remained high in the pelvis it would not be feasible to bring it down to the level of the perineal opening. Amussat met this objection by bringing the incision up to the rectal ampulla, if necessary removing a portion of the coccyx to do so.

For some obscure reason, the practice of excision of the coccyx unaccountably lost favor with the surgeons of the period and lapsed until 1873, when it was recalled by Verneuil (1873), to whom in consequence it was erroneously ascribed by many authors, and particularly by compatriots of the two surgeons with whom the technique had become identified. Other surgeons who strove to obtain more room in the neonatal pelvis were Delens (1874), who resorted to dislocation of the coccyx backwards instead of removing it, and Polaillon (1875), who advocated and practiced median division of the semicartilaginous bone and forcing the two halves asunder, thus gaining more room for deeper dissection. Byrd (1882) of Quincy, Illinois, was the first surgeon in the United States to perform coccygectomy to facilitate the approach to rectal anomalies.

Two years after Polaillon's communication, Vincent of Lyons (1887) applied the sacral route to two infants with congenital imperforation of the rectum, availing himself of the principle of sacral resection, the feasibility and advantages for which in the surgical extirpation of the rectum had been proclaimed and demonstrated by Kraske in his papers of 1885, 1886 and 1887. But within a short time, he discarded the operation of median coccygo-sacrotomy for an approach by an incision which became widely known and practiced as Vincent's parasacral incision. It commenced in the perineum at the posterior edge of the proctodeum, if this were present, and passed backwards to the tip of the sacro-sciatic notch. Vincent maintained that by means of his parasacral incision the anomalous and elusive rectum could be reached easily, and brought to the surface.

With his pupil Maitre, Vincent contended that the rectum could be reached even when it lay as much as 3 or 4 cm. above the level of the perineum and that as the promontory of the sacrum was at most only 5 cm. above the anal site (more often only 3 cm. in the deformed pelvis of the neonate) it was feasible to bring the bowel down to the level of the wound; with the access provided by his parasacral incision, Vincent, indeed, claimed that he had been able to explore the iliac fossa, from which situation he was enabled to bring down the rectal pouch to the sacrum in one infant upon whom he had operated by his adaptation of the sacral method.

Matas (1897) has expressed himself as of the opinion that notwithstanding the simplicity of Vincent's parasacral operation, a simple median incision through the coccyx and sacrum was a preferable operation as a preliminary exploratory procedure on the grounds that this greatly reduced the risk of injuring the levators and the coccygeus, or the 3d and 4th pair of sacral nerves, which supply the sphincters, levators and bladder. Other considerations were that a median incision was less likely to be followed by serious hemorrhage or to interfere with the lateral blood supply, a point of some importance in relation to osteoplastic operations.

Heinecke, in 1888, seems to have been the first to modify Vincent's sacral technique, antedating Morestin's exhaustive thesis (1894) on Kraske's operation. Heinecke devoted a short chapter to the possible application of the sacral approach to the surgical management of congenital imperforations and defects but failed to mention the pioneer work of Vincent.

Heinecke's operation involved a T-shaped external incision and division of the sacrum and coccyx along the lines of this incision, thus producing two triangular osteointegumentary flaps, designed to be replaced and sutured after the rectal operation was finished.

Heinecke's operation was in turn modified by Kocher, with the object of enabling the surgeon to divide the sacrum above the 3d sacral foramen, without injury to the 3d and 4th anterior sacral nerves.

In Roux's modification of Vincent's sacral technique, the horizontal limb of the incision crossed the midline below the 3d sacral foramen; the resulting osteoplastic flap was turned to the left.

Morestin's thesis (1894) and a communication by Sieur (1896) are regarded by Mastin as important documents from the historical point of view.

During the 10 years which followed the publication in 1887 of a thesis by J. Maitre, of Lyons, who worked in the clinic of Professor Vincent, and the appearance of Professor Vincent's own report to the Société de Médicine of Lyons, in March of the same year, reports of varying degrees of merit and importance emanated from many authors, among whom are Chaput (1896), Matas (1897), Burnell (1896), Ceci (1890), Czerny (1893), Keen (1897) and Elliot (1896).

As both Mastin and Matas emphasize, the sacrifice of any portion of the sacrum reduces the strength and support of the pelvic floor and frequently involves injury to muscular attachments and impairment of blood supply. Much weight was attached to these considerations by Matas (1897), who showed that in the majority of instances the rectal infundibulum can be located and drawn down through either the simple parasacral incision of Vincent or some one of the forms of osteoplastic resection of the sacrum. Preference was to be given at all times to sagittal division of the sacrum, and the bone was not to be divided at a higher level than the lower border of the 3d sacral foramen.

The experience of the pioneers in the surgery of congenital anorectal defects proved that nothing was to be gained by transverse incision of the perineum as a means of enlarging the operative field (even in the extreme but uncommon degree of contraction of the pelvis, which brought the ischial tuberosities almost into apposition). Such attempt to gain more space for intrapelvic dissection and manipulation was discouraged as fraught with danger to the fibers of the external sphincter and, more importantly, risk of irreparable damage to the fibers of the levator ani, *which muscle was properly considered the mainstay of the future control of the rectal outlet.* Even Amussat's original T-shaped incision was abandoned, and Anders (1892), whose authority in this matter is described by Matas as indisputable, expressed himself as of the opinion that while an abnormal contracture of the pelvis is unfortunate, and not to be lightly disregarded, it must not be permitted to influence the choice of operation.

The middle of the 19th century is an appropriate juncture in the history of the surgical treatment of congenital imperforation of the rectum and/or anus at which to note the interesting and informative biographical sketch of one John Pughe, by Cule (1965). In this delightful vignette, Cule describes Pughe as a stern Baptist and scholar surgeon, who practiced in Aberdovey for 30 years and as one of the 12 Fellows of the Royal College of Surgeons at that time domiciled in Wales. Pughe is revealed as both courageous and skillful enough to have ventured on and successfully accomplished on March 10, 1854, the operation devised by Amussat for the urgent relief of congenital rectal imperforation. Pughe was impressed by Amussat's classification of the several types of imperforate rectum, which he listed as five, and the clarity of his exposition of the appropriate operative procedure for each type. In the first of Amussat's types, he described the anus as "preternaturally narrowed" and recommended treatment by incision and dilatation; in the second type, the anus was "closed up by membrane," and dilatation with tents after incision was the treatment advocated; in the third type, the rectum was "intercepted by a simple septum" at a variable distance from the anal opening, and, in dealing with this type, Amussat advised suture of the lower portion of the supraseptal gut to the skin, rather than simple incision of the membrane; in the fourth type, the anus was imperforate and the rectum deficient to a greater or less extent, and, for this, the largest group, as for the fifth type, in which the rectum opened into some other organ, such as the bladder, urethra or vagina, Amussat prescribed the operation which he had himself introduced, the purpose of which was to bring the rectum down to its natural position between the sphincters.

Eleven months after he had operated, Pughe visited his little patient and found him a "fine thriving boy," with control which was on the whole good but "not quite equal to the emergencies occasioned by undue relaxation of the bowels."

Stromeyer's Suggestion.—Until some years after the introduction of the technique of proctoplasty by Amussat, surgeons eschewed opening the peritoneum in perineal dissection and viewed its accidental breaching with great trepidation; hence the insistence in the older literature on following the curve of the hollow of the sacrum in directing exploring instruments, such emphasis being based on fear of damaging the pelvic peritoneum, rather than the desire to avoid injury to other pelvic viscera such as the bladder.

Stromeyer was the first to suggest that if the rectal pouch could not be found after careful subperitoneal dissection in the perineal wound, it was proper to open the peritoneum in the pelvic floor. It is a strange irony that although Stromeyer's claim to priority in advancing the suggestion which has figured ever since in the literature of the surgery of imperforate rectum as Stromeyer's suggestion has never been questioned, the operation embodying its principle was never performed by Stromeyer himself. Leiserink (1872) is credited with having applied the idea, with brilliant results. It was not long before the universal application of Listerian principles removed the restraining factor on incision of the peritoneum of the pelvic floor, i.e., the fear of infection, with ensuing peritonitis and pelvic cellulitis.

In 1879, Krönlein reported an operation in which he deliberately opened the peritoneal cavity through a perineal incision, and the authoritative Anders (1892) availed himself of Stromeyer's suggestion to perform a proctoplasty successfully by pulling down to the perineal incision the blind rectal pouch, which he had found high in the pelvis.

Vincent, of Lyons (1887), reported successfully opening the peritoneum through the perineal wound in two cases. A. Mayo Robson, of Leeds (1886–1887), in reporting the case of an infant in whom the peritoneum was deliberately opened and the cul-de-sac of the colon thus recognized and safely sutured to the peritoneum, suggested that a uniform principle or plan, which recognized the advantages of perineal exploration, be adopted in operating for imperforate anus—a procedure made more universally applicable by the aseptic opening of the peritoneum.

Iliac Colostomy.—The operation of iliac colostomy, proposed by Littré, in 1710, was performed for the first time in the surgical management of imperforate rectum by Duboise (1783), whose case report was soon followed by those of Dinet and of Desault.

The idea of utilizing a colostomy opening for the introduction of a guide distally to locate the blind end of the rectum and fashion an anus in the normal position in the perineum seems to have originated with the younger Martin, of Lyons (1798), but it was not until 1856 that Chassaignac (1856) applied the suggestion in the surgical treatment of congenital imperforation of the rectum. Chassaignac advised that a preliminary iliac anus be constructed with a view to the passage of a probe along the colon at some later date; with the probe, the terminus of the colon was to be pushed down against the perineum and the perineal body incised against the impinging tip. The iliac anus was then to be closed.

Martin's suggestion was amplified in 1863 by Demarcquay, who advocated the passage of a sonde gardé, a guarded stylet, through the colostomy opening and along the distal segment of the colon; by its means, the rectal cul-de-sac could be forced against the perineum and held in position by the stylet driven through the intestinal wall. The blind end of the rectum would thus be effectively located prior to making the perineal incision.

Chassaignac's conception of this then modern operation was clearly stated at a meeting of the Société de Chirurgie de Paris, in February (1856). His claim to priority in the performance of the operation appears to be definitely established, although French writers have often attributed the original conception and operation to Lannelongue (1884), who was apparently unaware of its prior performance by Chassaignac.

Chassaignac's technique was given effect for the second time by Haynes (1884), who operated upon a newly born infant for the relief of congenital imperforation 23 days after a preliminary Littré inguinal colostomy. On September 30, 1883, a sound was passed through the iliac opening to the distal end of the colon in such a way as to push the rectal cul-de-sac against the perineal anus, which was made to bulge. A cruciform incision was then made over the guide and a permanent ano-rectal communication established.

Lannelongue's patient (1884) was handled by a technique identical with that adopted by Chassaignac and by Haynes.

Sir William McCormac (1886), with no knowledge of the previous reports of Chassaignac and Lannelongue, advocated the Littré colostomy in those patients in whom the imperforate bowel terminated at an unknown distance from the anus, holding that from the opening in the groin the condition of the bowel could be ascertained with tolerable accuracy. When practicable, the natural channel could be reestablished with the unquestionable advantage of having an exact guide to the position of the extremity of the gut.

Following McCormac's report, and in similar vein, there appeared those of Demelin (1895), Maylard (1896) and Stuart and Bierworth (1897). The procedure, which began with Chassaignac's patient, appears from the records to have been well supported by clinical evidence, as in seven instances in which it was reasonably well carried out (Chassaignac, Krönlein, Haynes, Lannelongue, Demelin, Maylard, and Stuart and Bierworth), there were seven operative recoveries.

An unquestionable advantage was that urgent symptoms could be relieved by evacuation of meconium, and a reasonable delay afforded, allowing the infant an opportunity to recover from shock and be restored to better condition to withstand the complete perineal operation. It was also held possible that the rectal ampulla might descend spontaneously and later be found at an accessible site. Possible disadvantages of such a preliminary colostomy were (1) the risk of puncture of the rectal ampulla by injudicious use of the guide and (2) the possibility that the preliminary anchorage of the colon might limit its subsequent mobility and preclude a spontaneous descensus.

With the advent of colostomy, however, surgeons had an alternative procedure to offer for high imperforations in which perineal exploration was fraught with complications. Robson (1887), for example, suggested exploring the perineum in the midline from the coccyx and dissecting in until either the rectum was located or the peritoneum opened. If no rectum was found, he advocated sigmoid colostomy.

The Abdomino-Perineal Operation.—Although abdominal section had been practiced since the advocacy and inception of preliminary colostomy by Chassaignac in 1856, no intraperitoneal exploration was involved until Neil McLeod (1880) suggested combining abdominal exploration with perineal section. McLeod advised that after failure to locate accessible bowel by perineal dissection the abdomen be opened in the midline and the position of the gut determined; then, with the finger in the abdomen as a guide, the perineal incision be deepened until it opened into the peritoneal cavity; the next step was to seize the rectum, pull it down and fasten it in the perineum. The abdominal wound was then to be closed.

McLeod's article appeared in the *British Medical Journal,* in 1880, but the first recorded operation in which his suggestion was adopted was that of Hadra, reporting from Germany, in 1886. An interval of 7 years elapsed before Conant (1893) reported in the *Boston Medical and Surgical Journal,* March 24, 1893, the further application of McLeod's suggestion. Chaput, in 1896, used the abdomino-perineal route.

Delagenière (1894) achieved the same object as McLeod, but by a reversed procedure. He performed an initial or primary lateral celiotomy and, after locating the rectal cul-de-sac, incised the perineum through into the peritoneal cavity; guided by a finger within the pelvis, the surgeon was enabled to draw the rectum down to the surface of the perineal incision.

Further support for the abdomino-perineal technique was forthcoming in an article by Brenner, who, in 1915, advocated celiotomy as enabling the rectum to be pushed down into the pelvis and maneuvered to the anal site for the performance of proctoplasty.

Cave (1934) described a 7-hour-old baby with blind imperforate rectum, in whom, after the abdomen was open, blunt dissection was made from the perineum up to the pelvis and the rectum pulled down on a catheter. The infant died from a cardiac defect on the 8th day. Mixter (1934) also described an abdominal approach in which a sound was passed into the sigmoid colon from above, and the rectum pushed into the perineum.

The contributions show that by the end of the century the merit of the abdomino-perineal operation devised originally by McLeod in 1880 to cope with an imperforate rectum situated high in the pelvis and inaccessible by perineal incision alone had been widely conceded. The operation was generally practiced as a two-stage procedure, the first stage being a colostomy designed to be temporary. In 1948, a communication by Rhoads *et al.* (1948) marked the introduction of a one-stage abdomino-perineal operation in the neonatal period for infants adjudged by their vigor and general clinical state not to need the respite afforded by a preliminary colostomy. Successful results attending such operative management were reported by Rhoads in 1948 and by Norris in 1949. Actually, Norris had first performed the one-stage operation in 1943, and Rhoads in 1944, and, although the one-stage abdomino-perineal operation gained in favor after the publication of the work of the surgical teams headed by Rhoads and Norris in 1948 and 1949, respectively, presumably no surgeon would deny the benefit and "breathing space" of a preliminary colostomy to a debilitated and exhausted newly born infant.

The one-stage abdomino-perineal operation ushered in the modern procedure for rectal deformities. The subsequent modifications and alternatives since that time are current practice.

A landmark to be noted in traversing the steps by which the surgical procedure for imperforate rectum and/or anus has advanced is the introduction by Wangensteen and Rice (1930) of their original and ingenious application of radiography to the determination of the position of the blind rectal pouch; it was the essentially simple expedient of holding the infant with his head down while a plain x-ray was taken of the abdomen and pelvis. In the infant's inverted state, the gas in the intestine would rise and outline the rectal pouch, thus indicating its position with relation to the anal membrane.

The inversion radiography of Wangensteen and Rice has been for years accepted routine in the preoperative examination of infants afflicted with the distressing malformation of congenitally imperforate rectum, and it, and its more recent extensions, will be the subject of more detailed discussion in the ensuing pages.

In a review of the history of the treatment of ano-rectal deformities and the views maintained by contemporary writers on this important question, it is apparent that surgeons have differed in their opinions and practice regarding preliminary colostomy and the two-stage operation which it entails. For the first half of the current century, two-stage operations with an abdomino-perineal approach, as exemplified by the writings of Helwig (1929), Ladd and Gross (1934), Berman (1938) and others, were accepted as routine practice, but, since the articles by Rhoads *et al.* (1948) and Norris *et al.* (1949), several authors have urged the adoption of a one-stage abdomino-perineal procedure.

In view of the anatomical and functional results now within reach of competent surgeons, iliac colostomy with a permanent artificial anus should be regarded as a last-ditch operation, only to be resorted to in extreme conditions of malformation in which the rectum is totally absent or is situated so high as to preclude the possibility of bringing it down to the surface by even the most extensive perineal and sacral dissection or its sphincter muscles or their nerves are deficient.

MORTALITY.—Although progress has not been spectacular, the mortality rate attending the surgical management of congenital ano-rectal malformations, the majority of which pose an urgent problem, has shown a steady decline since Amussat's operation of proctoplasty superseded incision and dilatation. Methodical plastic surgery, first applied by Amussat in 1835, has acquired over the years a progressively improving technique.

In his comprehensive review, Matas (1897) included statistics relating to perineal incision with coccygectomy, covering the period 1842–1897, which showed a primary mortality of 37.5%, reduced to 12.5% by the exclusion of 4 infants who died from conditions not believed to have had any direct bearing on the operative result. Matas' review of the records of 14 infants in whom an inaccessible rectal ampulla rendered sacro-coccygectomy advisable showed an immediate or operative mortality of 21.42% but a secondary and actual mortality of 64.27%.

In the last decade of the 19th century, the mortality rate in the surgery of ano-rectal malformations, according to Cripps (1892), stood at 40%.

In drawing conclusions from over-all statistical tables, it is to be remembered that very often they have included a significantly large number of patients in whom the ano-rectal deformities have been of a relatively minor, even trivial, character, such as those of types I and II of Ladd and Gross. Obviously, the operative risk in dealing with either of these types, which include anal stenosis and imperforate anal membrane, is or should be relatively low, and, to the extent to which they occur in any given series, their inclusion determines a relatively low mortality rate.

Hence, the method of presentation of results by Ladd and Gross (1934) has much to commend it. In a report covering 162 cases of ano-rectal deformities, these authors recorded 43 deaths, of which at least 12 were due to associated congenital abnormalities, such as cardiac malformations, tracheo-esophageal fistula, and others. Ladd and Gross' corrected mortality rate for ano-rectal deformities and their complications was 19%, the fatalities being classified as follows, according to the deformities: type I, 9.5%; type II, 16.6%; type III, in which occur 85% of the anomalies and virtually all of the fistulas, 24.8%; type IV, 61.6%.

A notable further decrease in the mortality rate attending correction of ano-rectal deformities occurred in the 18 years which elapsed between 1934 and 1952. A report by Norris, Brophy and Brayton (1949) on the surgical management and results achieved in a series of 59 infants born with deformities of the anus and/or rectum recorded an operative mortality of 9.1%, whereas the hospital deaths in a series of 165 similarly afflicted infants in the care of Mayo and Rice (1950) were 15, which included 3 infants with tracheo-esophageal fistulae, 1 with congenital heart disease and 1 with atelectasis. If the last mentioned 5 babies are excluded as having died from causes unrelated to the ano-rectal malformation, the operative mortality is reduced to 6.1%. Two years later, Santulli (1952), in a review of the results attending surgery in 62 consecutive infants with congenital ano-rectal deformities, of which the fistula-prone type III accounted for 85%, reported the striking figure of 3.1% operative mortality rate and total case fatality rate of 6.4%.

It is important to note that all the deaths in Santulli's series were due to associated malformations. It would appear that surgical judgment and ingenuity can overcome all but the most formidable obstacles in dealing with ano-rectal anomalies.

NOTE ON THE BIBLIOGRAPHY OF HISTORICAL REVIEW.—Some of the references included have not been accessible to me. Generally speaking, I have been able to consult articles by British and American writers in the majority of instances, but the references to French and German literature have been culled from the article by Rudolf Matas in the *Transactions of the American Surgical Association* (vol. 15, p. 453, 1897), a truly heroic exposition of the history and bibliography of reconstructive surgery of congenital ano-rectal defects.

In any instance in which a reference in the text does not appear in the bibliography, it may be taken to have been derived from Matas' article, from which I have drawn heavily; I have also availed myself freely of articles referred to by Mastin in his contribution to *Surgery, Gynecology and Obstetrics* (vol. 7, p. 316, 1908), not omitting the delightful historical essay by J. H. Cule, published in *Annals of the Royal College of Surgeons of England* (vol. 37, p. 247, 1965).

REGINALD WEBSTER

CHAPTER 2

Anatomy and Function of the Normal Rectum and Anus

SPHINCTERIC CONTROL, either actual or potential, is the prime consideration in dealing with malformations of the ano-rectum. The management depends upon the predicted capacity of the sphincter muscles to maintain an adequate measure of cleanliness. It is important to understand not only the function of the muscles governing the normal sphincters but also the potential function of the muscles which are found in the standard visceral malformations.

Sphincters of the rectum and anus are controlled both consciously and unconsciously in order to be entirely effective at all times of the day and night. The receptors which provide knowledge of the content of the anal canal lie in the bowel wall and the surrounding pelvic and perineal muscles. The muscles which govern the flow of flatus, feces and mucus are the internal and external sphincters and specialized parts of the levator ani muscles. The 2d, 3d and 4th sacral segments of the spinal cord link the sensory and motor sides of the nervous arc with the higher centers of the central nervous system. Defects of development of the distal spinal segments, which often accompany malformations of the rectum, may also impair continence.

The social conventions unique to humans demand an extreme degree of efficiency of the function of continence, and this applies as much to control of flatus as to feces. To ensure such control, tail and pelvic muscles of lower animals have been adapted to the human rectum and anus, both as additional sphincters and as warning devices.

Comparative Anatomy

The "tail" muscles are adapted in the human to form the pelvic diaphragm and rectal sphincters. Magnus (1968) considers that the ano-coccygeal raphe of the human is phylogenetically the tail of lower animals and that some of the tail muscles of the lower animals are rearranged around the raphe in humans. In man, these muscles form the pelvic diaphragm and its raphe and are composed of the ilio- and pubo-coccygeus muscles. The remainder of the pubo-coccygeus muscle becomes an extrinsic muscle of the rectum, and acts as a suspender, elevator, compressor, and sensor.

The pubo-rectalis muscle, which is grouped anatomically with the levator ani muscle, is not found in lower animals. It appears to be a modification of the external or cloacal sphincter (Fig. 1). It is intimately related functionally to the pubo-coccygeus in its action on the rectum and in structure and function is unique to the human species. This muscle is very closely aligned with the deep external sphincter muscle and shares its nerve supply, but its fibers of origin deviate from the external sphincter, ascending to the back of the pubis, where they are in contact with the origins of the pubo-coccygeus muscles. Hence in man, it is betwixt and between the cloacal sphincter and the levator complex of muscles. By contraction, the pubo-rectalis muscle sling compresses that zone of the anal canal which lies cranial to the external and internal sphincters, effectively occludes the rectum, and elongates the span of the effective sphincter, thus improving the functional security demanded of man in his social environment.

The anal canal, embryologically, may be defined as that part of the proctodeum lying between the anal valves (or pectinate line) and the anal orifice (Jones, 1904). The surgeon's definition is based on the functional length of the anal canal as determined by digital examination of the subject in the conscious state. The anal canal is that part which extends from the ano-rectal ring, or cranial margin of the pubo-rectalis muscle in the contractile state, to the orifice (see Fig. 8) (Milligan and Morgan, 1934). (Throughout this book the term anal canal refers to the surgical definition, unless otherwise qualified.)

The anal canal is lined by skin and mucous membrane and clothed in sphincters and muscles forming the pelvic floor.

Epithelial Lining

The epithelium of the anal canal changes abruptly at the pectinate line, from skin of the anus to mucosa of the rectum. This line also demarcates the level of the deep part of the external sphincter, the lowermost limit of the pubo-rectalis sling, and the junction of the upper third with the lower two thirds of the internal sphincter. It is

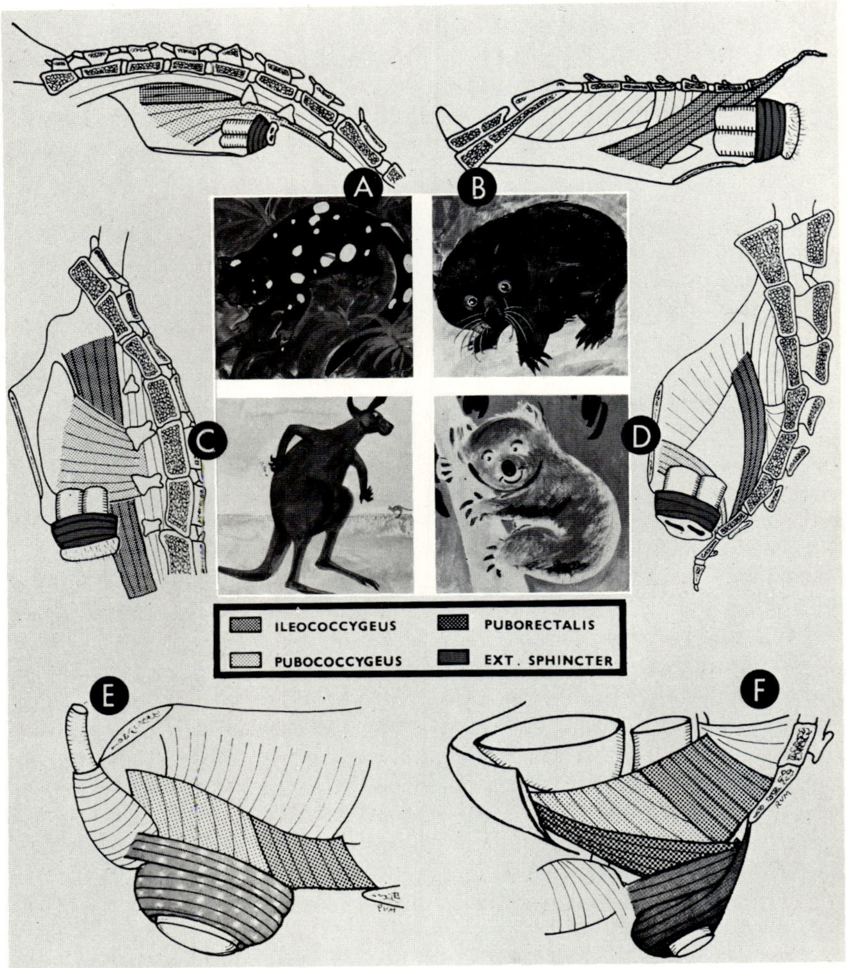

Fig. 1.—Phylogeny of the levator ani muscles, external sphincter, and puborectalis. From a study (R. Magnus, 1968) of examples of 17 species of tailed and nontailed pronograde and orthograde animals, including the marsupials tiger cat, **A;** wombat, **B;** kangaroo, **C;** koala bear, **D,** the chimpanzee **E** and man **F.** Levator ani group of muscles: In tailed pronograde and orthograde animals, ilio- and pubo-coccygeus are strong tail muscles, e.g., tiger cat (**A**) and kangaroo (**C**). In the nontailed pronograde animal, the ilio-coccygeus is the tail muscle and the pubo-coccygeus is absent, e.g., wombat (**B**). In the nontailed orthograde animal, the ilio- and pubo-coccygeus are both present but partly membranous, acting on the buried "tail" vertebrae, e.g., koala bear (**D**). In nontailed orthograde primates, the ilio- and pubo-coccygeal muscles converge on the ano-coccygeal raphe and

firmly tethered to the internal sphincter by the muscularis submucosae ani. It is, in fact, a fixed line about which to orient the descriptive anatomy (Fig. 2).

Epithelium Caudal to the Pectinate Line.—Adjoining the valves is the pecten, a smooth zone of pink shiny skin, lacking in hair or sebaceous glands, extending distally to the caudal margin of the internal sphincter, which is readily palpable as a firm ring at the orifice.

At the orifice, and in the surrounding skin, hair follicles and sebaceous glands appear. The skin is puckered by the pull of the coattails of the longitudinal muscle of the bowel wall, and in this puckered perianal area, the skin is brownish in color. This is the location of perianal abscesses.

At the valves, the epithelial change is abrupt from stratified squamous to stratified columnar.

Epithelium Cranial to the Valves.—Stratified columnar epithelium lines the zone of the anal columns to near the level of the ano-rectal ring. It was estimated to vary in length from 0.1 to 1.0 cm. in prepared specimens by Aldridge [1968], who examined the zone in premature, full-term babies, and in children up to 12 years. It lacks specialized structures, although, at its upper limit, it exhibits gradual addition of goblet cells.

At the level of the ano-rectal ring, the epithelium thickens and exhibits crypts, goblet cells and mucus-secreting glands typical of rectal mucosa.

---

rectum within the pelvis to form the levator diaphragm and levator ani in the chimpanzee (**E**) and man (**F**). External sphincters: Tailed and nontailed pronograde and orthograde marsupials all have similar cloacal-type external sphincters (**A–D**), and the chimpanzee and man have specialized sphincters (**E** and **F**), all being unrelated to posture or tail. In the nontailed orthograde primate animals, the deep external sphincter is attached anteriorly to the bulb (vagina) in the chimpanzee (**E**); in man (**F**), the superficial part is attached posteriorly to the coccyx, and the deep part is attached anteriorly to the perineal body—a fore and aft suspension. Pubo-rectalis. This muscle is peculiar to man and occupies a position external to the pubo-coccygeus and is arranged as a third ring tilted to the external sphincter but attached to the pubis. It may well evolve not so much from the levator muscle as from the external sphincter; it has the same nerve supply, is a key sphincter muscle and is in the column alignment with the external sphincter. Magnus (1968) considers that the ano-coccygeal raphe to be the vestigial tail in the tailless animals, that the "tail" muscles insert into it, that the pubo-coccygeus is changed to a levator of the anal canal in orthograde apes and man, that the pubo-rectalis muscle is added to achieve a greater degree of continence in man and that the external sphincter is typical of the order and not related to tail or posture. (Reproduced with permission from Dr. Ruth Magnus.)

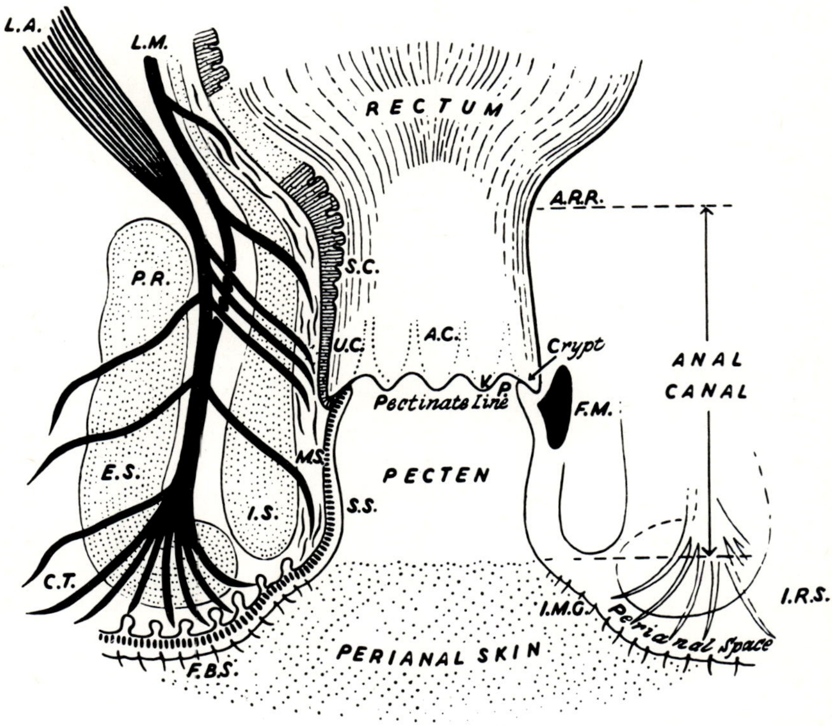

Fig. 2.—Composite diagram of anal canal to correlate epithelial, muscular and clinical landmarks. *A.C.* = anal columns; *A.R.R.* = ano-rectal ring; *C.T.* = "coat-tails" of the conjoined longitudinal coat; *E.S.* = external sphincter; *F.B.S.* = follicle-bearing skin; *F.M.* = zone of relatively fixed mucosa; *I.M.G.* = intermuscular groove; *I.R.S.* = ischio-rectal space; *I.S.* = internal sphincter; *L.A.* = iliococcygeus portion of levator ani; *L.M.* = longitudinal smooth muscle of bowel wall; *M.S.* = musculus submucosae ani; *P.* = anal papilla; *P.R.* = pubo-rectalis; *S.C.* = specialized columnar epithelium with goblet cells and intestinal glands; *S.S.* = smooth stratified squamous epithelium of pecten; *U.C.* = unspecialized stratified columnar epithelium lacking goblet cells or intestinal glands; *V.* = anal valve.

Sphincter Anatomy

The anal canal is well endowed with involuntary and voluntary muscles which comprise the sphincters. The smooth muscle of the internal sphincter is intrinsic to the bowel wall and spans the distal two thirds of the canal; the external sphincter clothes the distal half of the canal lying at and distal to the anal valves and outside the internal sphincter, and the levator ani complex operates in sling-and-sleeve fashion upon the cranial half of the canal.

THE INTERNAL SPHINCTER.—The internal sphincter is intrinsic to the bowel wall, and lies chiefly distal to the pectinate line. It is a thickening of the inner circular muscle coat of the bowel wall, supplemented and permeated by the dividing and permeating coattails of the longitudinal muscle coat. The caudal rim is palpable digitally as a prominent cushion around and external to the anal orifice. This cushion is separated from the lowermost fibers of the external sphincter muscle by a palpable circumferential groove called the anal intermuscular groove.

The tendrils or coattails of the longitudinal muscle of the rectum joined by contributions from tendinous fibers of the pubo-coccygeus muscle fan out caudally, some penetrating the circular smooth muscle sphincter and tethering the mucosa to the circular muscle a few millimeters cranial and caudal to the pectinate line. The coattails also penetrate the muscle bundles of the external sphincter, terminating in the ischio-rectal and perianal fat and on the deep aspect of the pigmented and puckered perianal skin (Fowler, 1957).

This complex network of coattails knits the mass of the sphincters

Fig. 3—External sphincter ani. Disposition of muscle fasciculi of two dissected representative specimens of the external sphincter, indicating the plexiform arrangement and spiraling course of some of the bundles. **A,** subcutaneous and, **B,** deeper groups of fibers. *B.C.* = bulbo-cavernosus; *T.P.* = transversus perinei.

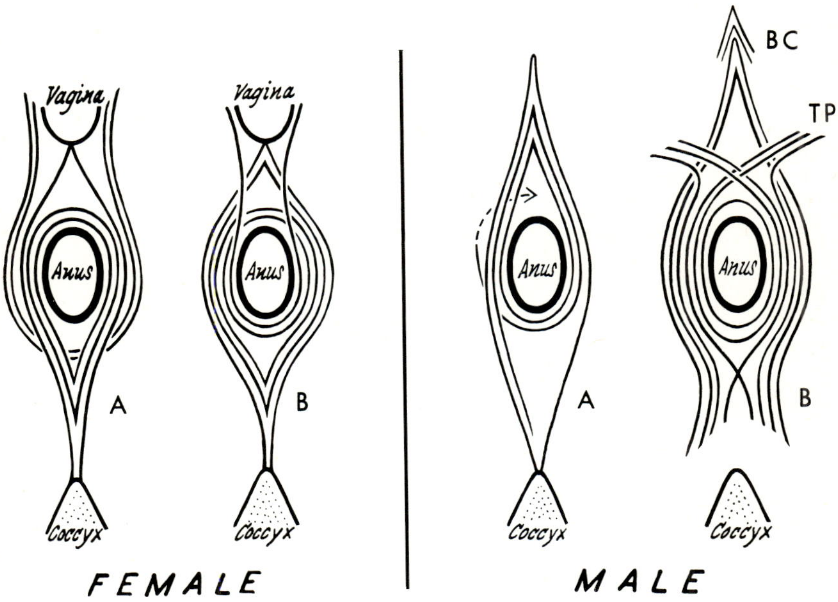

to the perineum, holds the canal firmly in its grasp, tethers the mucosa and skin above and below the pectinate line to the circular muscle of the internal sphincter, corrugates the perianal skin, and exerts an opening action on the internal and external sphincters during defecation.

THE EXTERNAL SPHINCTER.—This voluntary muscle is an elongated collar around the rectum and anus from the region of the anal valves to the anal orifice, suspended between the perineal body and the ano-coccygeal raphe (Fig. 3). It is a subcutaneous bundle which is cut into fasciculi and moored to the skin by the coattails of the longitudinal muscle coat of the rectum. This layer of muscle attaches to the perineal body or the superficial perinei muscles in front and to the ano-coccygeal raphe behind. The muscle forms an admixture of circular and elliptical fasciculi. The deeper and greater part of the external sphincter is penetrated sparsely by the coattails, which terminate in the surrounding ischio-rectal fat, and is composed of anteroposterior and circular fibers (Fowler, 1957). Its cranial extremity is contiguous with and cradles the caudal cuff of the sling of the pubo-rectalis muscle, thus ensuring a continuity of voluntary muscle throughout the length of the anal canal.

THE PELVIC DIAPHRAGM.—The outlet of the pelvis is a wide diamond-shaped area bounded in front by the inferior pubic and ischial rami and posteriorly by the sacro-tuberous and spinous ligaments and the coccyx. The floor of the front half is the thick, tough triangular ligament. In the posterior half, the floor is resilient and muscular.

The Ligamentous Diaphragm.—The triangular ligament (syn. perineal membrane, uro-genital diaphragm) spans the pubic arch, gaining strong attachment to the inferior rami of pubis and ischium. Its apex is anterior and its base posterior. The central point of the perineum of the male or the perineal body of the female lies at the midpoint of its base. In the male, the ligament is a strong sheet with a central perforation for the urethra. In the female, the ligament is cleft in two and weakened by the passageways for the urethra and vagina. The outer walls of the vagina and urethra are firmly attached to the ligament and reinforced, snugged and supported by the pubo-urethralis and pubo-vaginalis muscles.

The Muscular Diaphragm.—The levatores ani muscles arise directly or indirectly from the inside walls of the true pelvis and converge upon the midline to form a bipennate, laminated muscular hammock posteriorly and a funnel-shaped portal of exit from the anal canal. The muscle spans most of the pelvic outlet, but for two small gaps on the postero-lateral aspects which are filled by thin, fibro-muscular structures called the coccygei muscles.

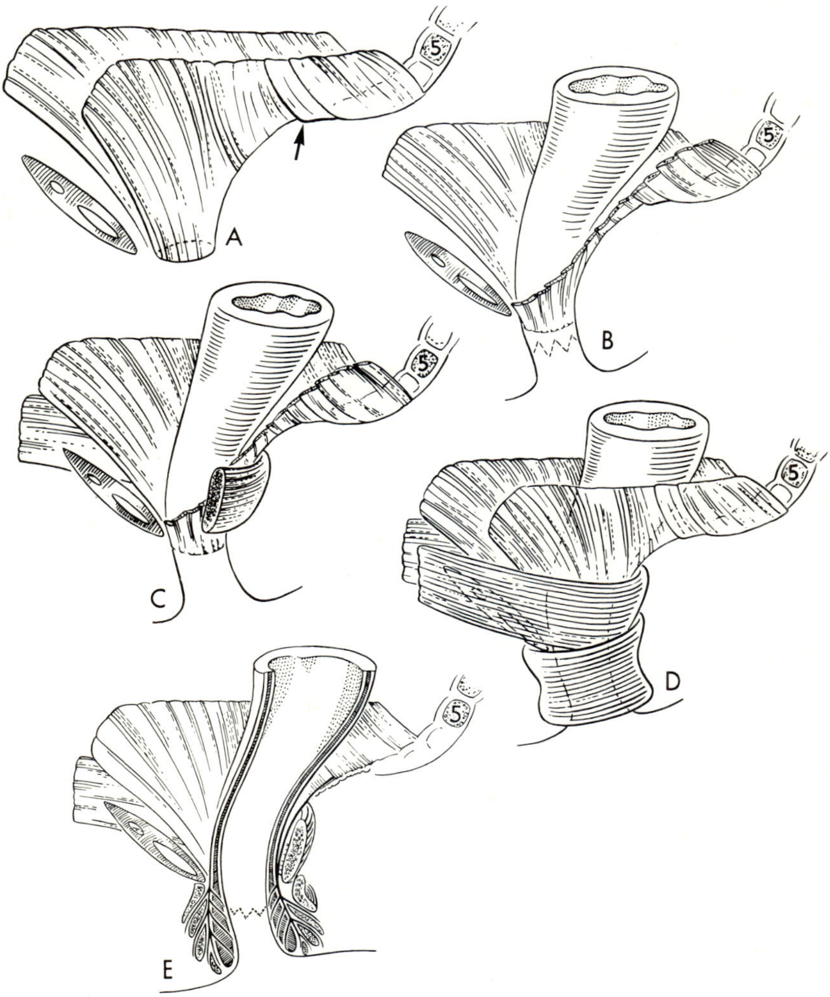

Fig. 4.—The normal levator ani muscle. **A,** pubo-coccygeus stripped of rectum; ileo-coccygeus posteriorly and on a slightly more caudal plane (*arrow*); perineal membrane anteriorly with urethral and vaginal openings. **B,** cutaway view of pubo-coccygeus attaching to longitudinal muscle of the rectum several millimeters cranial to the anal valve level. **C,** pubo-rectalis wrapping itself around the outside of the pubo-coccygeus, a little cranial to the valve line. **D,** external sphincter clothing the anal canal caudal to the pubo-rectalis. **E,** sagittal section through bowel and muscle, showing the conjoined insertion of the pubo-coccygeus and longitudinal coattails into the internal and external sphincters caudal to the anal valves.

The levator musculature comprises the ilio-coccygeus, pubo-coccygeus and the pubo-rectalis subdivisions (Fig. 4). The ilio-coccygeus muscle arises from the white line of the obturator fascia posterior to the obturator nerve, and unites with the muscle of the opposite side and with the sides of the coccyx to form the caudal lamina of the posterior half of the pelvic diaphragm. The pubo-coccygeus has a linear attachment to the back of the body of the pubis and the anterior part of the white line as far back as the obturator canal. The fibers take a posteromedial and medial course to attach to the perineal body, the walls of the rectum, and the muscle of the opposite side to form a lamina of the pelvic diaphragm more extensive than, and cranial to, that of the ilio-coccygeus. This muscle is funnel shaped, the distal fibers in the funnel forming a sleeve which joins the longitudinal muscle coat of the rectum to form a conjoined tendon which breaks up into the "coattails" of Fowler which permeate into all the layers of the anal canal and its sphincters. It elevates, straightens, steadies, suspends, and opens the anal canal. These intimate attachments to the rectum soundly seal the defect in the muscular floor created by the portal of exit of the rectum from the pelvis.

The pubo-rectalis muscle is the third component. It is a slinglike riband of muscle firmly anchored anteriorly to the bodies of the pubic bones and elsewhere attached to relatively mobile structures. The sling is set on an inclined plane from the pubis to the back of the rectal wall, is approximately 1–2 cm. deep, is attached to the rectum several millimeters above the valves, and hugs the back and sides of the terminal rectum and its funnel-like sheath of pubo-coccygeus muscle, to which it is delicately adherent. The caudal edge of the sling is cradled posteriorly by the upper extremity of the deep external voluntary sphincter at approximately the level of the pectinate line. By its action, the pubo-rectalis apposes the back and side walls of the rectum against the anterior wall and jams the rectum against the fixed structures of the triangular ligament; the anal canal is thereby tilted anteriorly, shut and elevated, and the rectum is angulated between the canal and the ampulla, which seats itself upon a muscular hammock posteriorly.

That part of the anal canal cranial to the pectinate line is intimately wrapped in the pubo-coccygeus and pubo-rectalis muscles – the sleeve-and-sling complex – while the part distal is clothed by the encircling internal and external sphincters. The narrow zone of the pectinate line is ringed by the deep part of the external sphincter muscle. Wilson (1967) considers that it is more correct and logical to call the pubo-rectalis muscle the pubo-recto-analis muscle, because of its intimate relationship to that part of the rectum which forms part of the anal canal.

THE SUSPENDING MECHANISM.—The rectum is held in place by suspending fascial ligaments and muscles which counterbalance the abdominal pressures exerted on it as by coughing or the erect posture.

Wilson (1967) has demonstrated the direct suspender effect of the fascia of Waldeyer where its fascial "claws" gain attachment to the rectum close to the site of junction of the pubo-coccygeal sleeve with the longitudinal muscle coat of the rectum. Indirectly, the parietal, visceral and other septal components of the pelvic fascia serve to stabilize the ano-rectum. The pubo-coccygeus, in which are found numerous membranous fibers, and pubo-rectalis are the chief pelvic muscular suspenders (see Fig. 4).

The external sphincter is attached directly or indirectly to the perineal body and to the coccyx. Other ligaments, condensations of the pelvic fascia, attach to the prostate, the vagina, and rectum, and all serve to take the strain and create a firm anchorage.

However, we consider that the fascial suspension, although important, is not the essential mechanism and that the perineal membrane, from which the perineal body gains fixation, and the muscular diaphragm are the chief supporters of the viscera.

Nerve Supply of the Normal Rectum and Sphincters

The 2d, 3d, and 4th sacral segments of the spinal cord are the nerve centers of the arcs which subserve the receptors and effectors of the rectum and anus, and the bladder and urethra, and together with higher centers in the brain are responsible for continence. These centers in the spinal cord also subserve cutaneous sensation in the anus and perianal region. The sympathetic supply, however, arises in the 2d, 3d, and 4th lumbar segments. Malformations of the spinal cord pertaining to the sacral segments involve all systems, but damage of nerves within the pelvis or perineum may have more localized effects.

PARASYMPATHETIC NERVES.—The parasympathetic nerves to the bowel arise on either side of the pelvis from the anterior divisions of the 3d and 4th sacral nerves, with twigs sometimes from the 2d. These preganglionic nerve fibers join to form usually two nervi erigentes which give short branches directly to the rectum at the level of the ischial spine (Figs. 5, *A*, and 6), and continue as longer trunks to the pelvic plexuses where they are redistributed to pelvic organs, directly or via blood vessels. In the wall of the rectum, these fibers relay in the ganglia of Auerbach's plexus. Other small parasympathetic nerves from the anterior divisions of the 3d and 4th sacral nerves join and ascend in the presacral sympathetic nerve, and then follow the ramifications of the inferior mesenteric artery.

These delicate tenuous nervi erigentes run lateral to the rectum in Waldeyer's fascia close to the ischial spine or in the newborn baby at

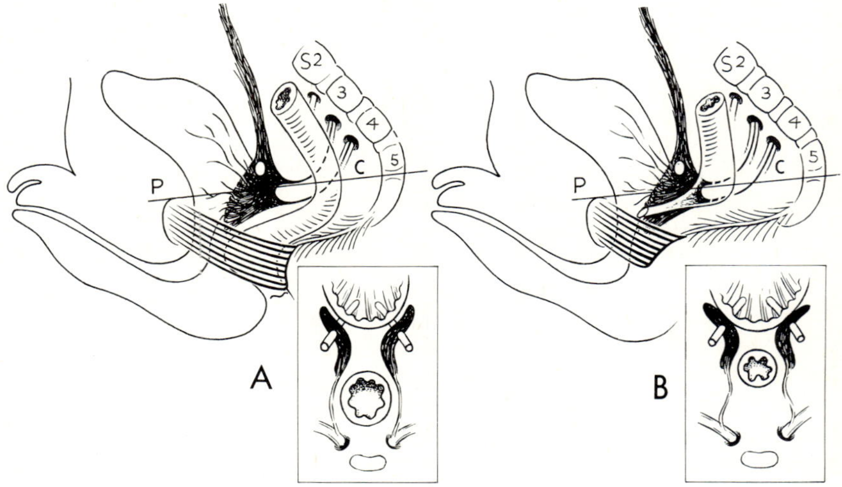

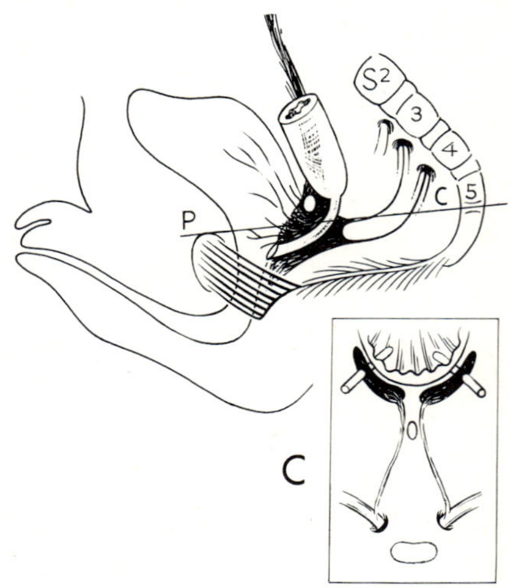

Fig. 5.—Course of nervi erigentes. **A,** normal course roughly parallel with *P/C* line; rectum separates the right and left nerves (*inset*). **B,** recto-urethral fistula issuing at level of *P/C* line; nervi erigentes separated by the rectum, which reaches to the *P/C* line (*inset*). **C,** recto-urethral fistula with rectum cranial to *P/C* line; nervi erigentes run a more medial course and are vulnerable in sacro-perineal dissection.

the level of the pubo-coccygeal line. The main trunks can be separated safely from the rectum because a natural plane of cleavage can be found between Waldeyer's fascia, which contains the nerves, and the visceral layer of pelvic fascia which invests the rectum. Hence bladder and urethral function is spared in excision of the rectum for nonmalignant conditions.

The nervi erigentes in rectal deformities are separated throughout their course by the rectum if it descends to the level of the pubo-coccygeal line (Fig. 5, *A* and *B*). When the rectum is located higher in the pelvis than the pubo-coccygeal line, these nerves run a more medial course in Waldeyer's fascia beneath the rectum to reach the region of the bladder base and neck (Scott and Swenson, 1959). In this situation, they are more vulnerable, especially if mobilization of the rectum is attempted from the sacro-coccygeal approach (Fig. 5, *C*).

Furthermore, in some patients, the nervi erigentes and nerve to levator ani have a common stem or origin before dividing and diverging in their different fascial investments; in which event, if the common trunk is damaged, both the function of the bladder and levator ani would be affected (Stelzner, 1957).

Sympathetic Nerves.—The sympathetic nerves arise in the 2d, 3d, and 4th lumbar ganglia and the preaortic plexus. They unite on either side and form the hypogastric plexus in front of the 5th lumbar vertebra, and then continue down the postero-lateral pelvic walls as the presacral nerves which join the pelvic ganglion on either side of the pelvis. Several fine sympathetic nerves from the 2d and 3d ganglia of the sacral sympathetic chain also join the pelvic ganglion in close company with the parasympathetic nervi erigentes.

The pelvic ganglion is a flat pannus which lies closely applied to the base of the bladder and prostate, the region of the uterine cervix, and the adjoining antero-lateral wall of the rectum. The ureter passes through it to get to the bladder. The ganglion has two posterior dog ears, one in the line of the presacral nerves and one adjacent to the 3d and 4th sacral segments, reaching backwards towards the contributions from the nervi erigentes. The pelvic ganglion is composed of multiple convoluted nerves and large clusters of ganglion cells packed into the tessellated pannus. It lies in the parietal layer of pelvic fascia, and can be separated from the rectum, which can be freed and resected without interference with function of the urinary or genital tracts (see Fig. 5).

The sympathetic and parasympathetic nerves to the rectum and anal canal are responsible through the ganglion plexuses of Auerbach and Meissner for organized peristalsis, and tone in the internal sphincter. The sympathetic fibers are said to be inhibitors of the bowel wall and motor to the involuntary internal sphincter, whereas the parasympathetic nerves are motor to the bowel and inhibitors to the sphincters.

The parasympathetic nerves carry, in addition, sensory fibers which convey knowledge of distention of the rectum (Nixon and Callaghan, 1964).

Nerves to the Levatores Ani Muscles and the External Sphincter.—Branches from the anterior roots of the 3d and 4th sacral nerves unite to form the main nerve pathway to the ilio- and pubo-coccygeus muscles. The trunk runs a lateral course on the

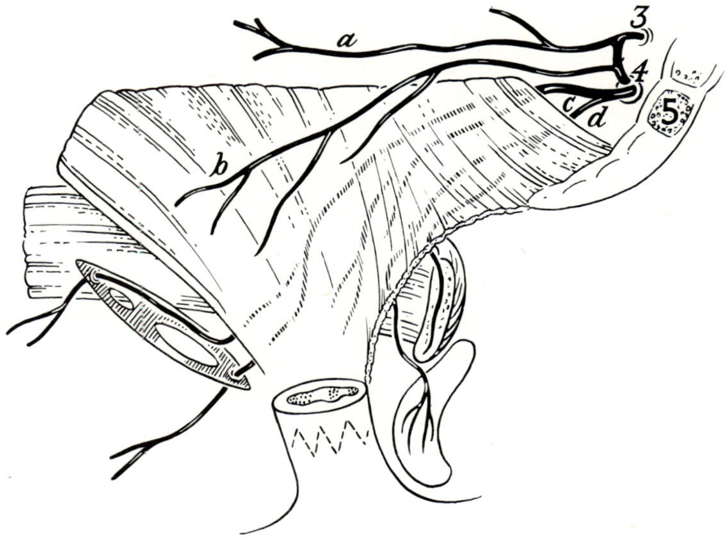

Fig. 6.—Nervi erigentes and nerves to levator ani. Right half of pelvis from within). (*a*) Right nervi erigentes arising from the roots of S3 and 4; (*b*) branch of S3 and 4 to cranial aspect of levator ani; (*c*) pudendal nerve giving branches to caudal aspect of levator ani and to the external sphincter; (*d*) perineal branch of S4 to pubo-rectalis and external sphincter.

cranial or pelvic surface of the levator ani muscle in Waldeyer's fascia, not far from and parallel with the white line of origin. Its branches run obliquely, anteriorly, and medially on these muscles (Fig. 6).

This nerve may be single with peripheral oblique branchings, a single stem with two main branches, or be represented by two separate nerves running parallel to each other, arising independently from the nerve roots of 3d and 4th sacral nerves (Stelzner, 1957).

The pudendal nerve, arising from the anterior divisions of the 2d, 3d, and 4th sacral nerves, clings to the lateral wall of the pelvis in Alcock's canal. It supplies branches to both the ilio- and pubo-coccygeus muscles and to the pubo-rectalis through its inferior hemorrhoidal and perineal branches which cross the ischio-rectal space to enter the muscles (Fig. 7).

The perineal branch of the 4th sacral nerve, a nerve which must be distinguished from the perineal branches of the pudendal nerve, enters the ischio-rectal fossa medial to the ischial spine on the caudal and lateral aspect of the coccygeus muscle, and its branches are directed medially to the posterior fibers of the pubo-rectalis sling and external sphincter (Wilson, 1967). This nerve is only at surgical risk when deep lateral cuts are directed from the vicinity of the coccyx and ano-coccygeal raphe.

The coccyx and the distal sacral vertebrae are absent in many patients exhibiting rectal deformities, and the coccygeal nerves and corresponding sacral nerves in some such patients are defective also. The levatores ani muscles may be devoid of contribution from the 4th sacral segment yet function satisfactorily with nerves of supply from the 2d and 3d or 2d sacral segment only.

Nerves to the External Sphincter.—The inferior hemorrhoidal and perineal branches of the pudendal nerve, and the perineal nerve arising from the 4th sacral segment supply fine nerves to the external sphincter mass in addition to the components of the levator muscles.

Fig. 7.—Pudendal nerves and perineal branch of S4. Course of pudendal nerve (*arrow*) with radial branches to pubo-coccygeus and pubo-rectalis. Perineal branch of S4 to pubo-rectalis and external sphincter. Note the midline zone around and in front of the coccyx is free from nerves and safe for dissection.

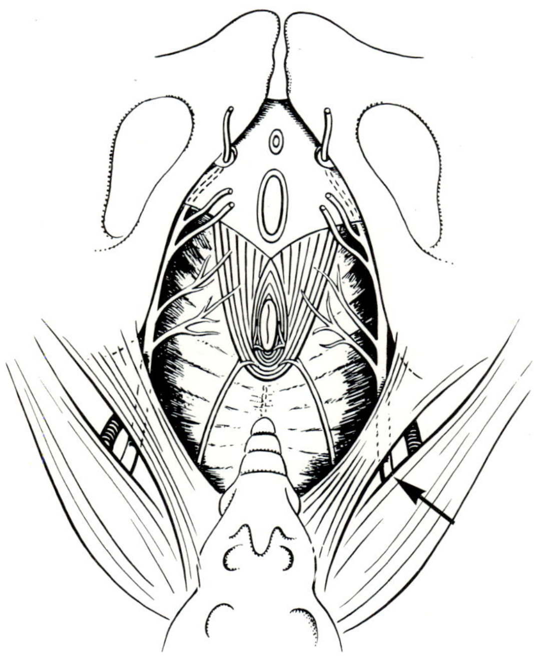

Rectal and Anal Sensation and Control

Efficient control of the rectum is effected only if the sensory afferent messages from the bowel and pelvis are correctly interpreted by the brain control mechanisms. There is still much to be learned concerning the location and nature of the afferent receptors, of the muscles which guard continence by day and night, and of the differential function of the sphincter muscles.

INTRINSIC SENSORY RECEPTORS OF THE ANAL CANAL.—Duthie and Gairns (1960) carefully plotted the sensory nerve ends in the anal canal. They found an abundance of conventional nerve endings, such as are presumed to denote pain (free intraepithelial), touch (Meissner's corpuscles), cold (Krauss end-bulbs), pressure or tension (corpuscles of Pacini and Golgi-Mazzoni), friction (genital corpuscles), together with unnamed unconventional receptors in the anal canal of adults, distal to the valves and to a point 0.5–1.5 cm. cranial to these valves. These receptors were responsible for acute and fine sensory discrimination, which in the skin beyond the pecten, was mediated through receptors around the hair follicles. There was a crescendo of free nerve endings and genital corpuscles on the valve line waning in the stratified columnar zone cranial to the valves. No receptors were found in the rectal mucosa, although myelinated and nonmyelinated nerve trunks were present under the epithelium and Meissner's plexus of ganglion cells was readily identified. The rectal mucosa of the anal canal did not appreciate any of the above stimuli when tested by the techniques used, and appeared to lack the appropriate receptors.

They considered that receptors may be present in the rectum to receive distention stimuli but that they were unable to demonstrate them by present staining methods.

In two other papers, Duthie and Bennett (1963) and Duthie and Watts (1965) suggested the effect of rectal distention (by balloons in these experiments) was to relax the internal sphincter and contract the external sphincter. They claimed that the relaxed internal sphincter allowed feces to contact the very sensitive and effective anal canal receptors which induced external sphincter contraction, which is thus important in the fine control of continence. We suggest in the following section that the initiating signal of distention of the rectum may not only be from the rectal mucosa. In the rectal deformities discussed, both the internal and external sphincters may be rudimentary, and yet a high degree of continence can be achieved.

EXTRINSIC SENSORY RECEPTORS.—Work and observations on malformations of the anus and rectum lead us to evaluate the absence of receptors in the rectal mucosa in a different way. We consider that coarse perception of distention of the rectum is in part a function of the parasympathetic nerves conveying impulses from the muscle spindles in the walls of the rectum and colon but that fine appreciation of distention, even of minor changes, is the function of the muscles surrounding the anal canal. Furthermore, the pubo-coccygeus and pubo-rectalis, with their intimate sleeve-and-sling relationship to the anal canal on the cranial aspect of the valves, provide the warning of impending peristaltic progress towards the anus. With the bowel empty and at rest, no sensation is registered, but gas or solid or liquid content moving into the sleeve-and-sling zone provides a stretch which is immediately and keenly appreciated. By deductive reasoning from evidence obtained from patients who have gained a large measure of control following surgical construction of an anal canal endowed with the sleeve-and-sling sphincter only, we consider that this extrinsic muscle has both fine sensory and motor functions essential to continence.

Goligher and Hughes (1951) in studies in adults using balloon distention of bowel brought down in pull-through operations also concluded that the response to distention probably arose in structures surrounding the bowel. Similarly, Parks *et al.* (1962) and Porter (1962) in studies on the pelvic floor muscles, in rectal prolapse, suggested that the receptors lay in the rectal wall and the surrounding pelvic floor muscles.

Kiesewetter and Nixon (1967) by their anatomical and physiological studies of rectal sensation in patients following surgical correction of ano-rectal malformations considered that the sensory receptors responsible for a measure of rectal sensation were probably present in the pubo-rectalis muscle.

Control of the Anal Canal.—The lumen of the anal canal in the normal resting state is occluded by the pubo-rectalis sling cranial to the valves and by the resting tone of the external and internal sphincters at and caudal to the valves. The first warning from the cranial end of the anal canal is picked up by the stretch receptors of the sleeve-and-sling complex. If this complex contracts to arrest a weak peristaltic wave, the event barely rises to consciousness. A stronger peristaltic drive creates a tension in the sleeve-and-sling, which calls for more urgent contraction aided by a conscious effort on the part of the subject to bring to bear a powerful contraction of the sling and possibly also of the external sphincter to arrest the peristaltic movement, as in resisting the passage of flatus. Further detrusor actions can be arrested similarly, although with greater effort and with accompanying colic as the calls become more insistent, until the time is convenient to permit the waves of smooth muscle to run through the canal unimpeded, and return to a resting phase of ease and comfort after evacuation of the content.

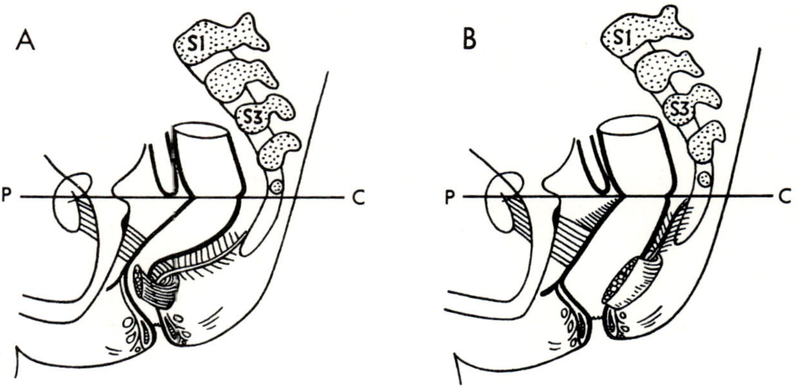

Fig. 8.—Sagittal diagram of rectum and anal canal showing different concepts of the anal canal. **A,** the anatomical or surgical concept of the canal extending from the apex of the prostate and ano-rectal ring to the orifice of the anus and surrounded by the sphincters, including the pubo-rectalis. **B,** the embryological concept of the canal extending from the level of the valves to the orifice of the anus, surrounded by the internal and external sphincters only and demonstrable when the pubo-rectalis is relaxed (e.g., under spinal anesthesia). *P/C* = pubo-coccygeal line.

It is considered further that the sleeve-and-sling can perceive the difference between the impending passage of flatus, solid or fluid feces, or even combinations, and has the ability to permit one to escape with or without the other. Furthermore, having assessed the content, the sleeve-and-sling moulds and shapes the bolus so that it can be accommodated in the narrowest skin-lined part of the anal canal (Figs. 8 and 9).

We regard the internal sphincter, that built-up and split-up circular muscle collar around the anus, as the end of the propelling muscle which actively discharges the feces or flatus from the orifice of the anus. Its combination of circular and longitudinal fibers is conducive to peristalsis throughout the anal canal to the anal orifice; its longitudinal coattails, being derived partly from the pubo-coccygeus muscle and partly from the involuntary muscle of the rectum, actively produce an "ectropion" of the anus during the peristaltic phase of expulsion of a bolus of feces, a function predisposing to cleanliness of the skin-lined part of the canal. Its sphincteric action is one of resting tone and coaptation of the walls of the anus relaxing in coordination with peristalsis but not in response to intra-abdominal pressure changes.

The external sphincter is a powerful muscle which is brought into action in moments of stress to supplement the sling action in arresting defecation or deflation. It, too, has a resting tone which mildly occludes the anus, and when forced open by flatus under high pressure it exhibits a flutter valve action with the accompanying characteristic noise. The tone of the internal and external sphincters which surround the skin-lined anal canal is probably responsible for prevention of wetting of this part of the canal with mucus secreted from the adjoining rectal mucosa, in the long intervals between the acts of defecation. Neither of these sphincters account for the minute-to-minute day and night fecal continence, which appears to be the function of the sleeve-and-sling.

Further observations of children who become chronically constipated indicate that the sleeve-and-sling become easily tired by impacting feces, become relaxed, and permit shortening of the anal canal to the length only of the skin lined anus. It is then found that the short passage, although encircled by external and internal sphincters, is barely sphincteric, permitting constant leakage which is momentarily arrested only at the time of conscious muscular contractions of the external sphincter surrounding the skin-lined anus.

Finally, the anal canal constructed in patients exhibiting a congenital recto-urethral fistula is endowed with a high degree of sensation, content discrimination, and muscular sphincteric function if the new canal is lodged within the sleeve-and-sling, which is then its only sphincter. If the canal is directed to the perineum through the muscular diaphragm posterior to the sling, the bowel lacks appreciation of its content and all power to control defecation (Stephens, 1963, 1965, Kiesewetter and Turner, 1963).

Fig. 9.—Defecogram in normal child. **A,** anal canal closed around a catheter and pubo-rectalis (*arrow*). (Note level of the inferior margin of obturator foramen in relation to upper level of resting anal canal.) **B,** catheter removed, anal canal is open and pubo-rectalis relaxed during defecation.

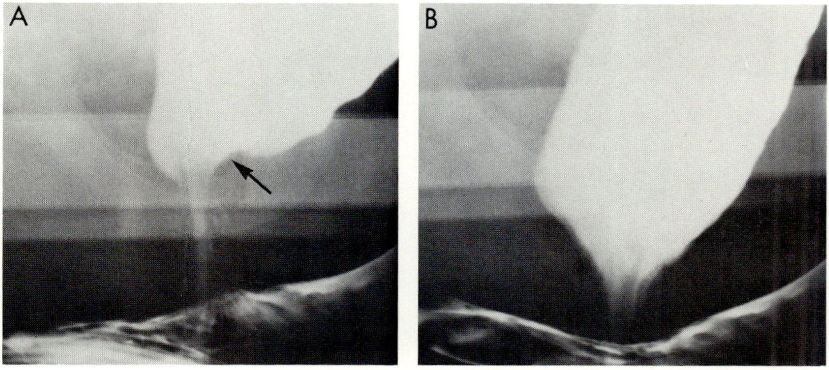

The observations of Duthie and Gairns, in our view, support this extrinsic theory of rectal sensitivity as far caudally as the anal valves, and we take cognizance of their findings of keen intrinsic receptiveness of the short, skin-lined anus to distention, temperature, friction, etc., but we believe that this short distal segment alone creates a warning which is too late and hence is ill-timed, and reaction to it is inexpedient.

The intrinsic receptors have a complementary function to that of the extrinsic receptors in an intact anal canal. The acute tactile discrimination of these intrinsic receptors is also of importance in the proper maintenance of anal cleanliness. All these receptors and all these sphincters account for perfect control.

It appears, however, that the sleeve-and-sling muscles of the levatores ani complex are the chief instruments of continence, the pelvic substation of the cerebral computer, the wind sentinel, and flow regulator. They are the keys of the lock, without which social embarrassments are inevitable.

CHAPTER 3

Individual Deformities in the Male

(Anatomy, Sphincters, Clinical Appearance, Investigations and Rationale of Management)

MAINTENANCE of the integrity of the available sphincters is essential for effective control of feces after operative repair. Both diagnosis and treatment therefore depend upon accurate knowledge of the anatomy of each defect and especially its relation to the surrounding sphincters. The descriptions which follow are based upon the clinical and operative experience of many surgeons but in particular on the detailed serial sections and dissections of autopsy material performed by one of us (F. D. S.) and by Magnus (1967).

The purpose of this and the next chapter is to provide a didactic description of the visceral and sphincteric anatomy, the clinical appearance, the pertinent investigations and general principles of treatment of each anomaly. Details of methods of diagnosis by special radiographic techniques are described in Chapter 8, Diagnosis and Investigations.

In the discussions of management in this chapter, the stress is on the *rationale* of treatment for each particular malformation and on the recommended choice of operative procedure for that lesion. Details of the reasons for choosing a one-stage rectoplasty or a colostomy and delayed rectoplasty for rectal anomalies, details of the various operative techniques and their advantages and disadvantages and of the pre- and postoperative care common to all these developmental defects are described in separate chapters on management—Chapters 9 and 10.

The order of description follows that of the "proposed International Classification (1970)," described in Chapter 6 (Table 1 [b]), the basis of which is the site of the bowel in relation to the chief muscle of continence, the pubo-rectalis sling of the levator ani muscle—arrested development above the sling, *high or supralevator*; at the sling, *intermediate*; and through the sling, *low or translevator*.

A. High Anomalies (Supralevator)

In these anomalies, the imperforate rectum, or its fistulous connection, lies above the pubo-rectalis sling of the levator ani muscle. In the principal group of high anomalies, ano-rectal agenesis, both anal canal and rectum fail to develop, in whole or in part; the less common group, rectal atresia, refers to an acquired secondary occlusion of the formed rectum, the anal canal remaining normal. Both groups are thus "rectal deformities."

1. Ano-rectal Agenesis

The most common variety of ano-rectal agenesis is the recto-urethral fistula, and the most detailed description is given to this lesion. However, in the classification, the blind rectum without fistula appears first, and the reader is advised to read its description in conjunction with that of recto-urethral fistula which follows.

Ano-Rectal Agenesis (No Fistula).—*Anatomy.*—Less commonly than a recto-urethral fistula, the rectum may end blindly. Sometimes a fibrous cord without a lumen or a nerve plexus of ganglia may connect with the urethra. The terminal bowel may be imperforate at any level in the pelvis but generally lies at or cranial to the pubo-coccygeal line (Fig. 10). No gas or meconium appears in the urine, but radiographically the appearances of the invertogram are similar to those in high recto-urethral fistula. The micturating cystourethrogram fails to show any fistulous communication or any disturbance to the shape of the urethra (Fig. 11).

Sphincters.—The muscle components in ano-rectal agenesis are identical with those that obtain in recto-urethral fistulae. Sacral agenesis sometimes accompanies ano-rectal agenesis, in which event, the nerves to the levator ani may be defective.

Perineum.—The perineal appearances are similar to those associated with recto-urethral fistulae.

Management.—The principles of investigation and treatment conform with those recommended for recto-urethral fistula, except that there is no risk of contamination of the urinary tract from the rectum. An abdominal exploration is required in addition to the sacro-perineal approach, if the bowel lies cranial to the pubo-coccygeal line.

Rare variants of ano-rectal agenesis are as follows:

1. *Vesico-intestinal Fissure.* The most frequently occurring of the rarer variants is ano-rectal agenesis combined with *vesico-intestinal fissure*, also called *ectopia cloacae* (Williams, 1958) or *exstrophy of*

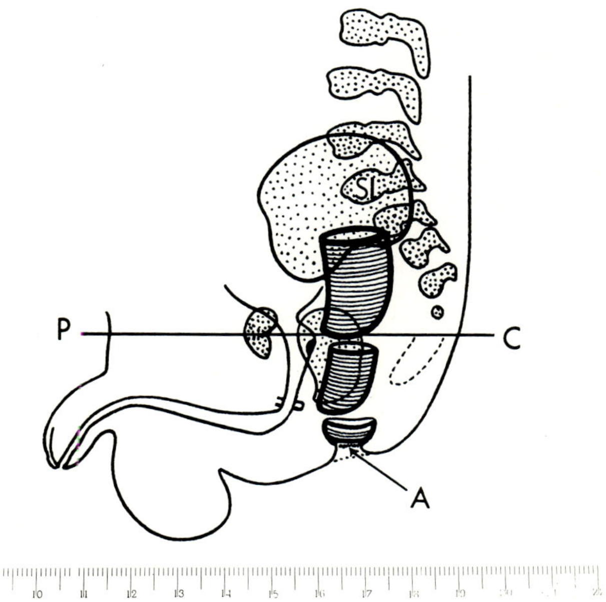

Fig. 10.—Ano-rectal and anal agenesis (no fistula). Occlusions of the rectum and anus occur at three levels—at the *P/C* line in ano-rectal agenesis, at the lower ischial margin (the I point) in anal agenesis and approximately 1–1.5 cm. caudal to this point in imperforate anal membrane. Rectal atresia, as distinct from agenesis, a rare entity, may occur at any level.

the cloaca (Johnston and Penn, 1966). The lesion is a complex one, involving many other organs, and is separately described in Chapter 13.

2. Isolated cases of total absence of the rectum and varying lengths of colon have been reported. Spriggs (1912) described a specimen in the London Hospital Museum with absence of the left half of the colon and rectum. Zaidi (1959) performed a colostomy (without survival) in an infant with no colon or rectum beyond the ascending colon. Trusler *et al.* (1959), in 271 cases of "imperforate anus" had no less than 7 with a colon deficiency as well—in all, the left half of the colon and rectum were absent, and there was a saccular dilatation of the proximal colon. In 3 patients the colon terminated in a colo-vesical fistula, in 2 patients in a colo-vaginal fistula and in 2 patients the colon ended blindly. Six of their patients were operated upon with three deaths (anuria, electrolyte disturbance and associated urinary abnormalities); in 2 of the 3 survivors the colostomy had to be revised because of poor motor function in the dilated terminal bowel. Dickin-

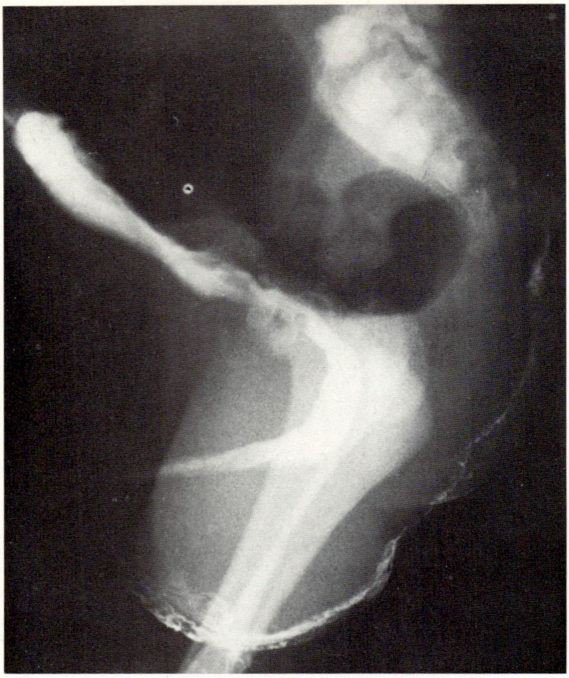

Fig. 11.—Ano-rectal agenesis (no fistula). Occlusion of gas at *P/C* line. The micturition cystourethrogram shows no leakage of iodide into rectum and no angulation of the urethra.

Fig. 12.—Recto-urethral and recto-vesical fistulae: levels in relations tc pubo-coccygeal line and pubo-rectalis muscle.

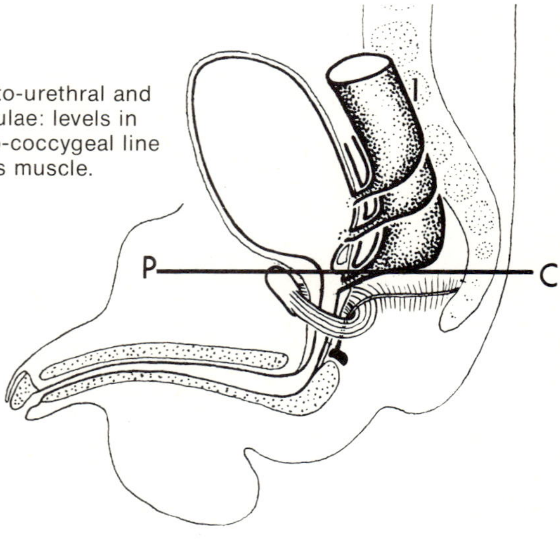

son (1967) described a further patient with no colon or rectum beyond the hepatic flexure, in whom the terminal ileum and appendix were duplicated.

Ano-Rectal Agenesis with Fistula

(i) Recto-Vesical Fistula.—*Anatomy.*—In many early papers the rectum was frequently described as entering the bladder. However, more careful dissections have shown that such a communication is rare. When it occurs, the fistula is usually at the bladder base, close to the urethra. Earlier descriptions were probably those of high recto-urethral fistulae (Figs. 12, 13, and 14). Vesical fistulae are generally associated with other serious and often lethal abnormalities of the urinary tract, the spine and other organs.

Gas or meconium appears in the urine and can always be recovered from a catheter; radiographs show the bowel gas shadow above the pubo-coccygeal line and frequently gas in the bladder.

The sphincter anatomy and perineal appearances are identical with those of recto-urethral fistula.

Fig. 13.—Recto-vesical fistula. Hemisection of pelvis showing rectum terminating in a long fistula issuing by a fine orifice in the trigone, which is thickened by prostatic tissue around the end of the fistula. Note absence of distal sacral vertebrae.

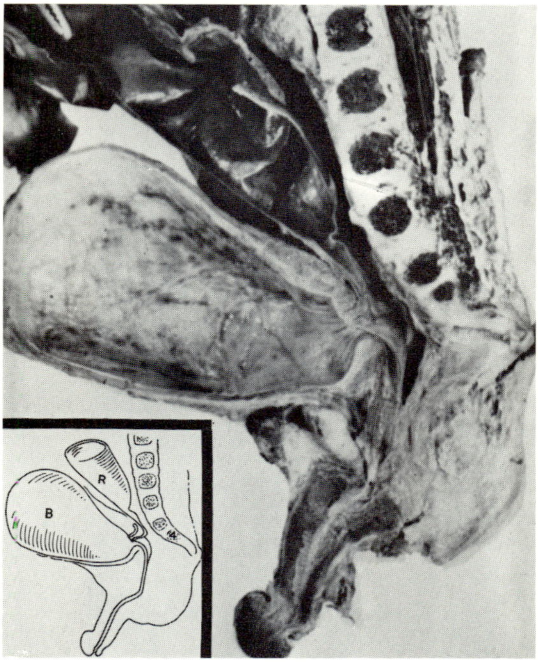

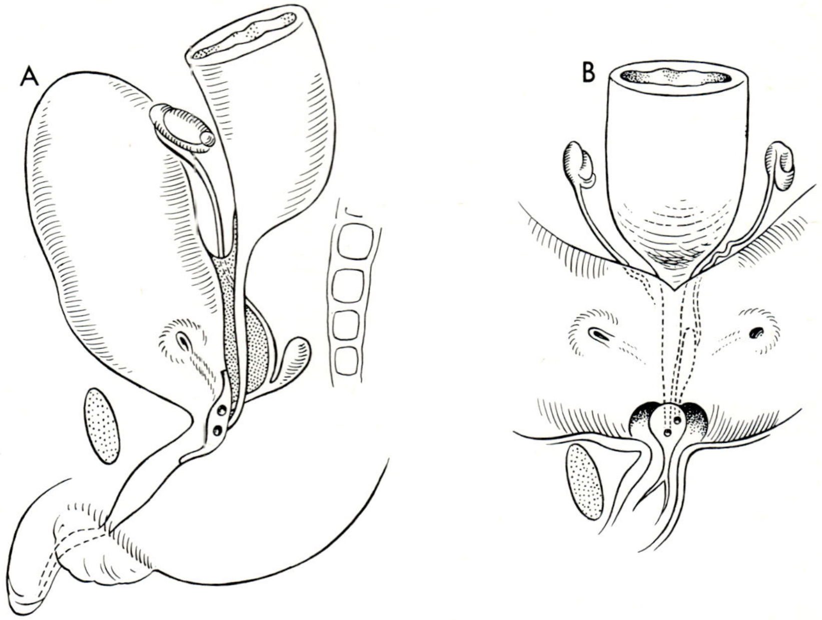

Fig. 14. — Recto-vesical fistula — fistula issuing at a bladder neck. Diagram of the anatomy of dissected specimen. **A,** sagittal section showing long rectal fistula issuing in midline in the internal urethral meatus distal to the vas. **B,** anteroposterior view showing the verumontanum lying in the opened out internal urethral meatus and the fistula issuing onto the verumontanum.

Micturition cystourethrography combined with colography and endoscopy, after colostomy, are invoked to define the site of the fistula.

Management. — Management and recommendations are similar to those described for recto-urethral fistula. However, the risk of urinary tract infection through the fistula is greater than in recto-urethral fistulae, because in the latter the closed bladder neck affords some protection to the retrograde flow of fecal material into the bladder. This situation may more frequently require division of the fistula as one stage, with completion of the rectoplasty later.

Further to be remembered in the approach to the fistula is that its level is so high that an abdominal exploration must always be combined with the sacro-perineal approach.

Rare variants of recto-vesical fistula are as follows:

1. Combined recto-vesical and recto-urethral fistulae in 2 patients (Swenson and Grana, 1962).

2. Combined recto-vesical and recto-perineal fistulae in 1 patient (Moore and Lawrence, 1952).

3. Recto-vesical fistula opening into ectopia vesicae in 2 patients (Moore and Lawrence, 1952), but without the other features of ectopia cloacae.

4. Trusler *et al.* (1959) describe 7 patients in a series of 271 cases of imperforate anus, who displayed absence of rectum and part absence of colon, and 3 of whom had colo-vesical fistulae.

5. Prasad (1970) depicted a patient with recto-vesical fistula, but in whom the rectum continued to a patent stenotic anus at the normal site.

6. Recto-vesical fistula plus vesico-intestinal fissure (Santulli, 1970).

(II) RECTO-URETHRAL FISTULA.—*Anatomy.*—This is a very common rectal anomaly in males and is more common than the corresponding recto-cloacal fistula and recto-vaginal deformity in females. The fistula is very fine, and the commonest site of entry into

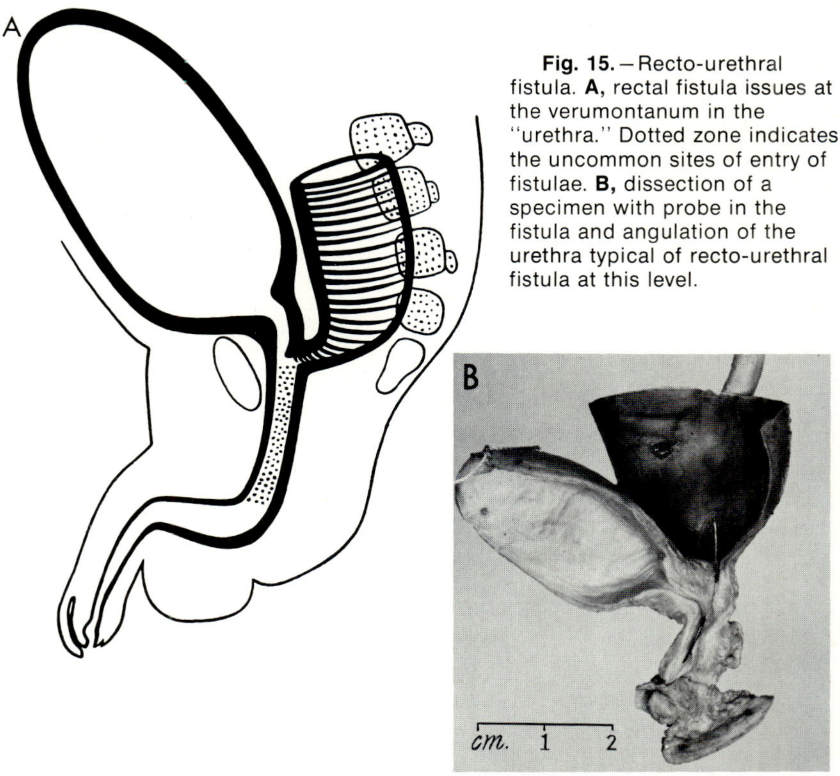

Fig. 15.—Recto-urethral fistula. **A,** rectal fistula issues at the verumontanum in the "urethra." Dotted zone indicates the uncommon sites of entry of fistulae. **B,** dissection of a specimen with probe in the fistula and angulation of the urethra typical of recto-urethral fistula at this level.

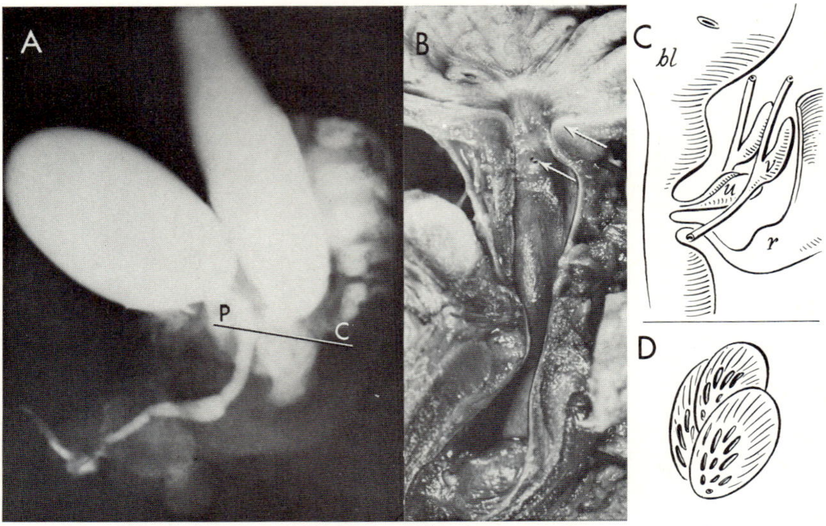

Fig. 16.—Recto-urethral fistula. **A,** cologram and cystourethrogram in a specimen. Fistula issues at verumontanum cranial to *P/C* line. **B,** view of opened out posterior urethra; bladder neck indicated by upper arrow and orifice of fistula in verumontanum by lower arrow. **C,** diagram of sagittal section through verumontanum, showing bifid utriculus and fistula between the vasa deferentia. *u* = utriculus, *r* = rectum, *bl* = bladder, *v* = vas. **D,** trilobulation of the prostate.

the urethra is the posterior urethra adjacent to the ejaculatory duct and utriculus masculinus. The urethra at this site is characteristically ballooned or angulated (Fig. 15).

The fistula permits the passage of small quantities of gas or meconium into the urethra but not to a degree sufficient to effectively decompress the gut. The baby thus presents with intestinal obstruction and gross distention of rectum and colon in the pelvis.

Less commonly the recto-urethral fistula opens at a higher level in the urethra, immediately adjacent to the bladder neck, and then the narrow fistulous tract may be long and tenuous (Fig. 16).

Very rarely, it may open lower into the urethra between verumontanum and bulb. In two such instances, the fistulous opening was very wide and occupied almost the whole of the membranous urethra as far as the bulb—on urethroscopy, the instrument preferentially entered the fistula rather than the proximal urethra. This wide fistula conveys meconium and gas freely through the urethra, thus postponing the obstructive crisis.

Whenever the fistula issues into the urethra cranial to the normal site of the verumontanum, the vasa and prostatic tissue ascend with it. In recto-vesical fistulae, these structures actually lie in the bladder. When the fistula is distal to the verumontanum, it departs from this structure and from the vasal and prostatic organs, opening independently at a more caudal level.

Sphincters.—(a) Levator Ani.—Reference should be made to the description in Chapter 2 of the normal muscle and to the vital importance of its pubo-rectalis section in anal control, which it effects by compressing the rectum and elevating and angulating it forwards at the ano-rectal ring.

When the sacrum is complete in its development, the levator is well developed, despite the rectal dysplasia. The innermost pubo-rectalis fibers lie caudal to the rectum and blend with the pubo-rectalis sling, surrounding the membranous urethra intimately, up to the precise level of the recto-urethral fistula (Fig. 17). This muscle sling is attached anteriorly to the pubis and caudally to the perineal

Fig. 17.—Diagram of recto-urethral fistula, showing the pubo-rectalis muscle and a rudimentary external sphincter composed of longitudinal muscle only, some of which may insert into the skin of the perineum.

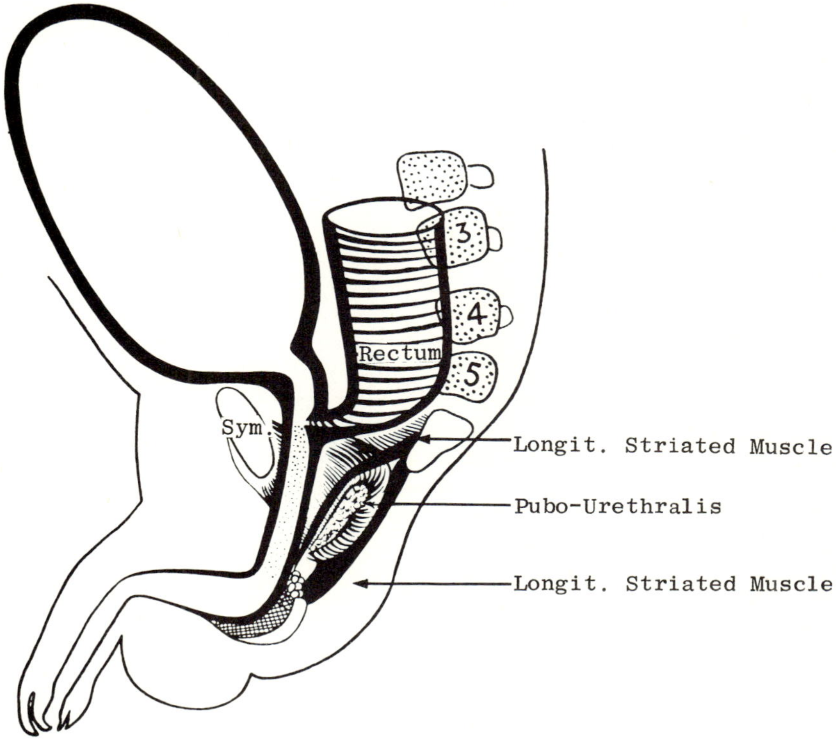

body. Lateral, posterior and at right angles to this combined collar of muscle around the urethra, the levator forms the pelvic diaphragm, which extends to the side walls of the pelvis and to the sacrum behind. The terminal portion of the rectum lies cranial and posterior to the collar of muscle and on the cranial aspect of the diaphragm. The collar of muscle surrounding the urethra and fistula is on a slightly higher plane than the normal pubo-rectalis, and, on contraction, the levator diaphragm is raised up to the level of the sling. The characteristic gas shadow at the pubo-coccygeal line in the inverted lateral radiograph lies a little cranial to the upper limits of the sling.

Scott and Swenson (1959) found that provided the sacrum was fully developed the pelvic and hypogastric nerves and their ganglia were essentially normal, except for displacement due to the rectal abnormality. However, in cases with associated sacral agenesis, both the levator ani and its nerve supply may be defective. Stephens (1953) found in autopsy dissections that in the absence of the 5th and 4th sacral segment the muscle was usually normal; in absence of the 5th, 4th and 3d segments, the muscle was thinly developed; in absence of segments including the 2d or 1st, the levator was totally deficient. Similarly, the nerve supply may be grossly affected.

The anatomy of the sacral nerves in sacral agenesis is discussed more fully in Chapter 8, including the clinical tests which may be applied to assess their integrity.

(b) Internal Anal Sphincter.—In rectal agenesis, no trace of this muscle is found by dissection, Stephens (1953), Scott (1959), Sommerschild *et al.* (1964).

(c) External Anal Sphincter.—The degree of development of the external sphincter appears to be variable. Considerable attention is paid to it in operative repairs described in many North American series. Bill (1958) claims it is always present because it develops independently of the bowel. This view is also held by Kiesewetter (1956, 1966), Scott (1959) and Sommerschild *et al.* (1964). Harken (1942) shows a photomicrograph of a recto-urethral fistula with part of the external sphincter present. Smith and Gross (1961) did serial sections on 16 randomly selected examples (of several types) of 31 autopsy specimens and found that, in all but one, voluntary muscle was present in the locality of the external sphincter. They stated that although the sphincter was proportionally small it "is not a fragmentary structure to be disregarded." Other authors (Nixon, 1961; Sommerschild *et al.*, 1964; and Swenson and Donnellan, 1967) report that although present, it may be poorly developed, and this has been our finding and our experience. In two dissected specimens of recto-urethral fistulae, longitudinal strands of voluntary muscle were found between the perineal body and coccyx, lying beneath the perineal

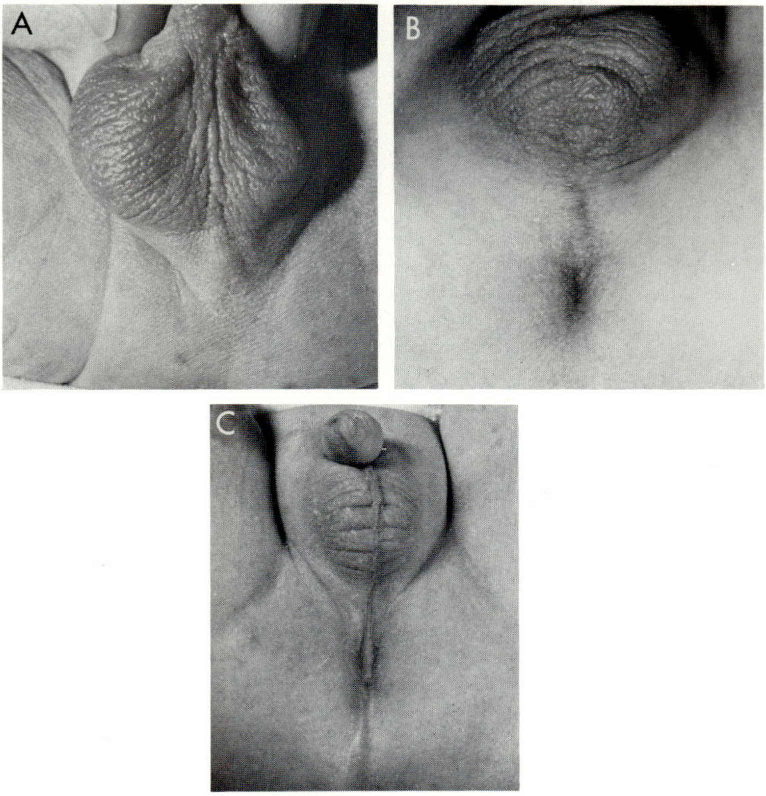

Fig. 18. – Perineums of recto-urethral fistula patients. **A,** absence of anal pit. **B,** small anal dimple only. **C,** raphe prominent across the perineum. There is no distinctive pattern of perineal appearance, and the internal anatomy cannot be predicted.

raphe. In one specimen, these fibers were inserted into the skin in the region of an anal dimple. This saillike sagittal muscle with its attachment may be responsible for the frequently observed clinical finding of puckering of the skin when stimulated by pinprick, but such a sign should not be interpreted as indicating the presence of an efficient "sphincter." It merely indicates the presence of some sagitally running voluntary muscle.

It is our view that the only effective sphincter capable of providing rectal control is the pubo-rectalis muscle, and the preservation of its integrity is the chief consideration in operative repairs.

Perineum. – No distinctive pattern is followed, and no inference as to the internal anatomy can be made. Most often the natal cleft is obliterated; there is usually a midline raphe, or less commonly a dimple, or a pigmented patch at the expected anal site (Fig. 18).

The perineum may bulge on crying, especially in patients with a pelvic floor paralyzed from sacral agenesis, but there is no meconium coloration visible through the skin.

Investigations.—1. Urine Microscopy.—The meconium patch on the diaper and the "black eye" of the urethra are almost diagnostic of a fistula. Voided urine is more likely to show meconium staining than is urine obtained by catheter, as the meconium is prevented from mixing with urine in the bladder by the protection of the vesical neck sphincters. However, if urine has not been passed and collected, a catheter specimen should be obtained at the time of the preoperative micturition cystourethrogram and the urine examined for the telltale meconium color or epithelial squames and lanugal hairs.

2. Invertography.—The gas shadow remains high near the pubococcygeal line, where the terminal rectum lies cephalic to the levator

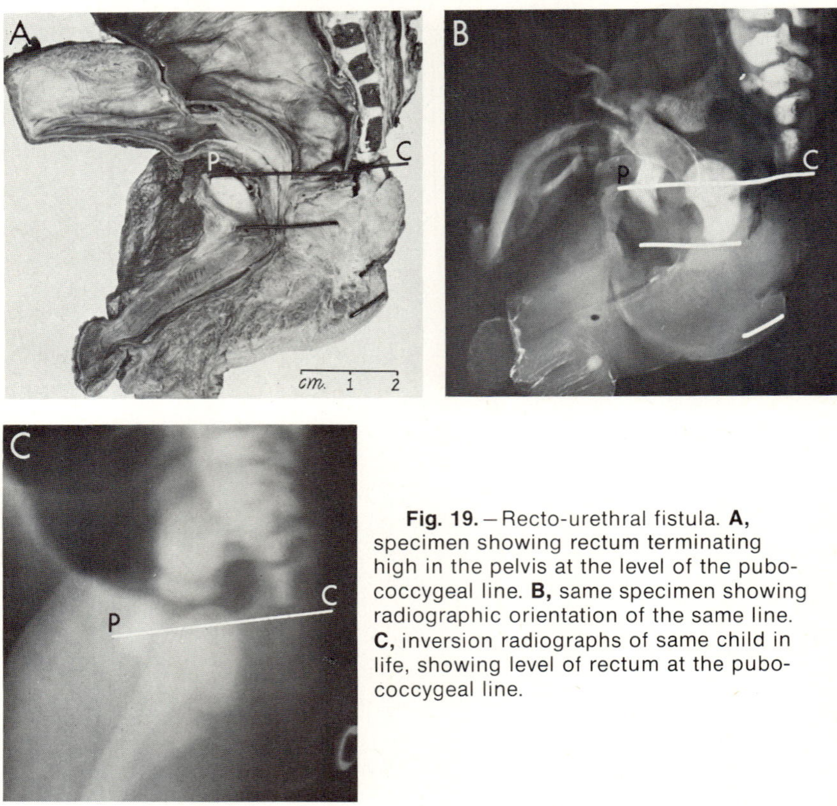

Fig. 19.—Recto-urethral fistula. **A,** specimen showing rectum terminating high in the pelvis at the level of the pubococcygeal line. **B,** same specimen showing radiographic orientation of the same line. **C,** inversion radiographs of same child in life, showing level of rectum at the pubococcygeal line.

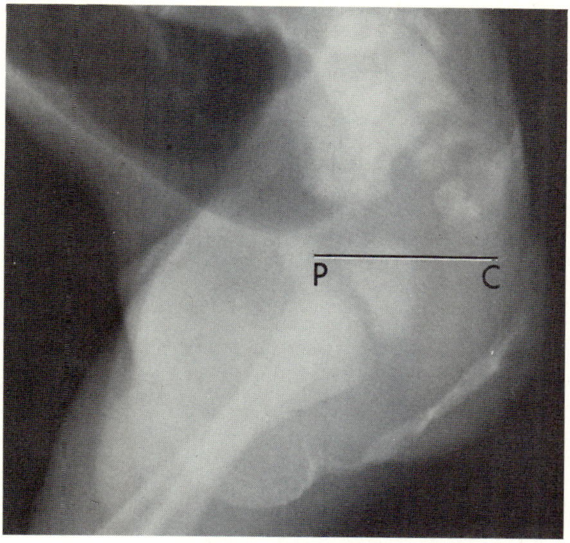

Fig. 20.—Recto-urethral fistula—high level. Rectum terminates cranial to the *P/C* line. Note the projection of the *P/C* line through the upper quarter of the ischial bone in the presence of sacral agenesis.

diaphragm. The usual fistula at the verumontanum is not visible, but the gas content of the terminal patent rectum provides a rounded shadow of the gut at or just below the level of the P/C line (Fig. 19); a fistula near the bladder neck is also invisible, but the shadow of the terminal gut lies cranial to the line (Fig. 20). The gas shadow is always above the "I" point and overlies the upper quarter of the ossified ischium (Fig. 21).

The presence of gas in the bladder is certain evidence of a fistula into the urinary tract, although not necessarily a recto-urethral fistula. Recto-vesical fistulae are, however, very rare (see Fig. 99).

3. Micturition Cystourethrogram.—This investigation may be performed in the pre- or postcolostomy period. If the diagnosis is not clear cut, on the basis of other tests, it should be undertaken preoperatively. The fistula may fill with radiopaque medium, at the P/C line, spilling through into the rectum (Fig. 22 and see Fig. 104), but unless the fistula is clearly seen in its entirety, its level of issue should not be presumed. A recto-bulbar fistula may permit spillage from the urethra to the rectum, and, if accompanied by a strong contraction of the pubo-rectalis muscle, the dye may be milked up to a level which closely approximates the P/C line and may fallaciously suggest a high level lesion (see Fig. 34). Occasionally, if the fistula is

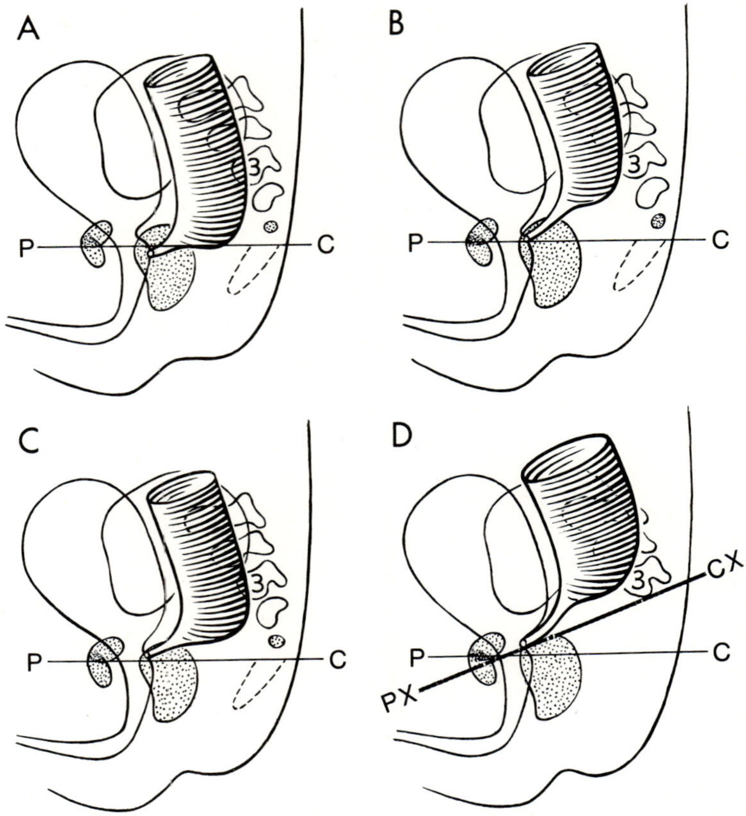

Fig. 21.—Relation of rectum and recto-urethral fistula at various levels to the pubo-coccygeal line. **A,** rectum and fistula on the *P/C* line. **B,** rectum and fistula slightly cranial to *P/C* line. **C,** rectum and fistula well above *P/C* line. **D,** *P/C* is correct projection of this line through the upper quarter of ischium when terminal sacral vertebrae are deficient. *PX/CX* is an incorrect and misleading projection.

very fine or plugged with meconium, it may not actually be seen, but the type of malformation may still be suspected by a characteristic and almost diagnostic posterior angulation of the urethra at the site of the fistula (Fig. 23). Micturition cystourethrography may indicate associated urinary abnormalities, especially defects of the uretero-vesical valves and reflux (see Fig. 137).

4. Assessment of Sphincters and Nerves.—As in all rectal deformities, the clinical tests of the integrity of the sphincters and their innervation are essential. These are described in Chapter 8, Diagnosis and Investigations.

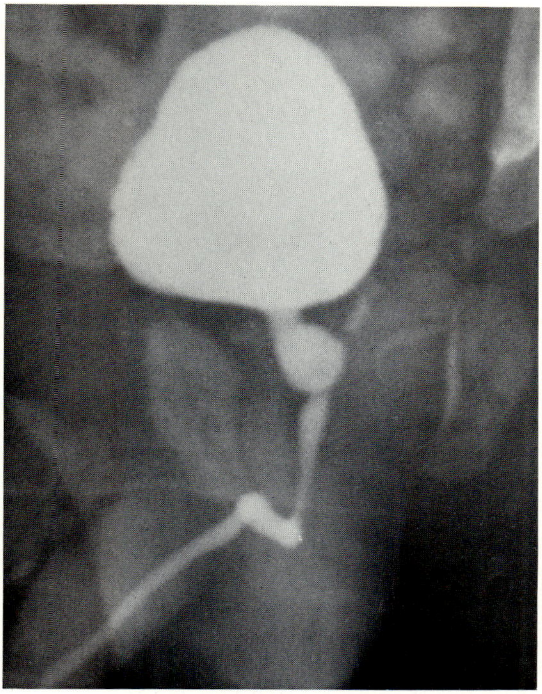

Fig. 22.—Recto-urethral fistula. Micturition cystourethrography showing jet of opaque medium in fistula.

Fig. 23.—Recto-urethral fistula. Micturition cystourethrography showing angulation of the urethra at the site of the fistula.

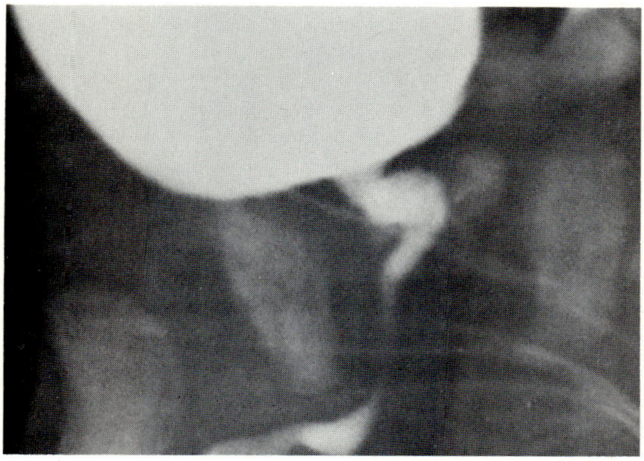

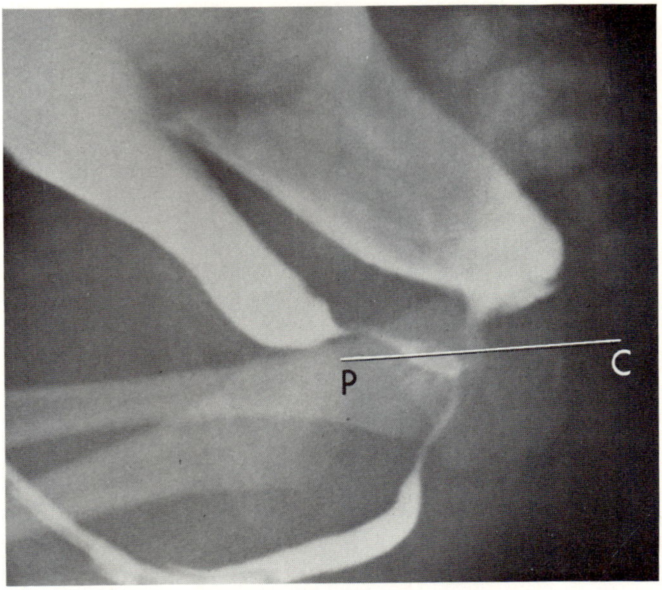

Fig. 24. – Recto-urethral fistula, Injection urethrogram and cologram via a colostomy to show the fistula and the relation of rectum, fistula and angulation of urethra to the *P/C* line.

5. Cologram.—Radiopaque material introduced into the distal limb of the colostomy when the infant is well, combined with a further voiding cystourethrogram, may be indicated if doubts as to the level of the fistula still exist (Fig. 24). Good pictures are also obtained if some dye is aspirated and air introduced. This provides dye-stained shadows which can then be related to the bony landmarks.

6. Documentation of Urinary Tract.—In the weeks following establishment of the colostomy, the state of the urinary tract should be checked by regular urine microscopy and culture and by intravenous pyelography, blood urea nitrogen estimation and, in some patients, by isotope I^{131} Hippuran renograms.

7. Cystourethroscopy.—This investigation is frequently desirable if the site of the fistula is not clear, and to define the size of the fistula. The fistula is often difficult to locate as the ostium is so fine and hidden in the verumontanum or inferior crest. Endoscopy can generally be deferred until the day of the operative procedure of rectoplasty, unless required earlier in the assessment of urinary anomalies.

Management.—The pubo-rectalis sling is the only effective sphincter available for subsequent continence. Its preservation is the prime consideration in choice of operative procedure. We, therefore, find ourselves at variance with many earlier authors who indicate scant reference to the pubo-rectalis, and who stress the importance of the "external sphincter," because our dissections show only a poorly developed external sphincteric mechanism represented by some sagittal strands of muscle beneath the perineal skin. Similarly, we cannot agree with the techniques as described and depicted by Nicolai and Rehbein (1963). (See Fig. 117, *A*, in which the bowel appears to be brought through the levator diaphragm behind the pubo-rectalis.) Rehbein (1967) specifically redesigned his technique for this very eventuality (see Fig. 117, *B*). The pubo-rectalis hugs the urethra intimately at and just below the fistula, and the dissection to define the plane for the mobilized rectum must remain in immediate juxtaposition with the urethra.

Further, any approach solely from the perineum is to be strongly deprecated. Most surgeons have inherited patients operated on "elsewhere" by this technique, by which irreparable damage has been done to the pubo-rectalis by the deep dissection in the small perineum required in finding the lower rectum.

Finally, in order to avoid the problems of urinary infection through the fistula after establishing a colostomy, a laparotomy with division of the fistula, combined with colostomy (but no rectoplasty), has been used on occasions (Partridge and Gough, 1961). However, the scarring resulting from this initial pelvic dissection makes the important step of defining the pubo-rectalis in the subsequent rectoplasty more difficult. The risk of urinary infection can be minimized by other means, but, in certain rare circumstances, it may be appropriate to divide the fistula.

The recommended procedure is as follows:

(i) Transverse colostomy in the newborn period.

(ii) Adequate clearance, by washouts, of the distal limb of the colostomy postoperatively beginning on the operating table to avoid urinary tract infection.

(iii) Completion of investigations as to the exact anatomy of the fistula, of the urinary tract, and of the sphincteric nerve supply, performed over the next 3 months—clinical tests of urinary continence, micturition cystourethrography, colography through the colostomy, regular urine checks, intravenous pyelography and blood urea nitrogen estimation.

(iv) Persistence of urinary infection following the colostomy, despite adequate cleansing and emptying of the distal limb of the colon, antibiotic therapy and possibly neomycin instillations into the distal colon, may necessitate division of the fistula and possibly earlier completion of the rectoplasty than is usually planned.

Precautions in the diagnosis of urinary infections of serious consequence comprise the following:

(a) The obligatory use of bladder specimens obtained by needle aspiration.

(b) A thorough cleansing of the colon and a radiographic check of colon for filling defects of meconium masses (see Fig. 113), which, if found, must be removed by appropriate patient irrigation of the distal colon via the colostomy.

(c) Full investigation of the upper urinary tract to detect additional malformations.

Furthermore, a baby who thrives despite infection discovered in the lower tract may well be cleared of urinary infection by intensive antibiotic therapy, even in the presence of other nonurgent deformities of the urinary tract (see Chapter 12).

(v) A meticulously performed rectoplasty preceded by panendoscopy, preferably at 12–15 months of age. Louw (1965) reports successful rectoplasty procedures undertaken by him at 3–4 months by using the sacro-perineo-abdominal technique, and the program may be so advanced for social or geographical reasons.

(vi) Closure of the colostomy 3 months later, after graduated digital dilatation and patient stretching of the pubo-rectalis sling by the parent.

The decision whether to perform a colostomy at birth and a rectoplasty later or to do a one-stage rectoplasty at birth is discussed in Chapter 9, along with consideration of other high rectal abnormalities.

As to the techniques of rectoplasty, the choices are as follows:

(a) Abdomino-perineal rectoplasty (Rhoads, Piper and Randall, 1948) or its subsequent modifications (see Chapt. 9).

(b) Abdomino-perineal rectoplasty through buttock incision (Sauvage and Bill, 1965) (see Chapt. 9).

(c) Submucous resection and abdomino-perineal or abdomino-sacro-perineal pull-through (Rehbein, 1959, 1965, 1967) (see Chapt. 9).

(d) Sacro-perineal or sacro-abdomino-perineal rectoplasty (Stephens, 1953, 1963) (see Chapt. 9).

(e) Sacro-abdomino-perineal rectoplasty, combined sacro-perineal approach with Rehbein procedure (Kiesewetter, 1966, 1967) (see Chapt. 9).

We prefer the sacro-perineal technique of Stephens, for reasons discussed in Chapter 9. If the fistula and rectum reach comfortably to the pubo-coccygeal line or lower, the whole operation can be performed through the sacro-perineal incision. If the rectum fails to reach the level of the pubo-coccygeal line or if the bowel exhibits a terminal megacolon, abdominal mobilization of extra length of bowel is required. This may be combined, if necessary, with excision of the segment of megacolon. It is recommended, however, that the pubo-rectalis tunnel be defined first via the sacro-perineal route. The additional "mucosal sleeve" technique of Rehbein for the abdominal portion of the operation has considerable merit and can be safely used following definition of the pubo-rectalis sling from the sacral route.

Rare variants of recto-urethral fistula are as follows:

1. In our series, one infant possessed an anomaly which is difficult to explain embryologically. This male infant (Fig. 25) had a normal rectum, anal canal and anus, opening at the normal site, and a long wide fistula arising from the urethra at the level of the verumontanum and which issued into the anterior wall of the rectum at a point approximately 2 mm. cranial to the valves. The urethra distal to the original fistula was of microcaliber and will require dilatation prior to closure of the fistula. There was also present a tracheoesophageal fistula.
2. Brenner (1915), Le Duc (1965), and Santulli (1970) each describe a patient with a normal anus but, in addition, a recto-urethral fistula.
3. Swenson and Grana (1962) describe 2 patients, each with two recto-urinary fistulae, one into the urethra and one into the bladder.
4. Lee (1944) depicts an extraordinary deformity with a colourethral fistula, an imperforate anal membrane and a colo-neurenteric canal communication (Fig. 26).

Fig. 25.—Urethro-anal fistula. Micturition cystourethrography showing wide fistula between midposterior urethra and anal canal. Note microcaliber of the bulbous and penile parts of the urethra. (Hemostat tip lies in anal canal near orifice of fistula.)

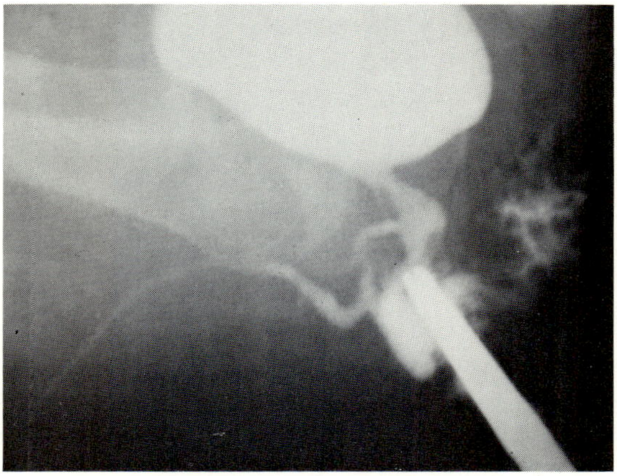

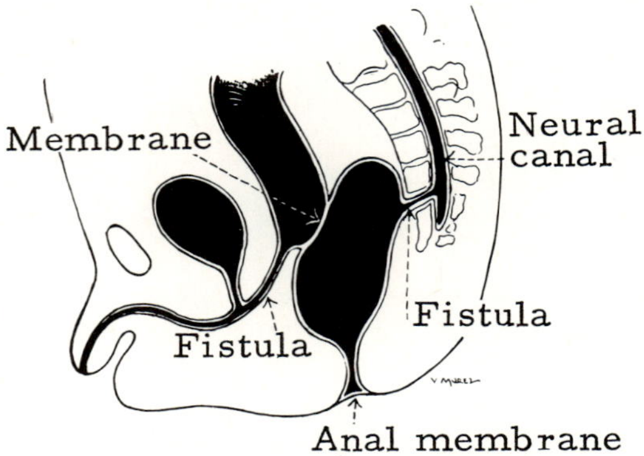

Fig. 26.—Rare rectal anomaly. Recto-urethral fistula, recto-neurenteric canal communication and imperforate anal membrane. (Reproduced with permission from Lee, M. J.: Am. J. Dis. Child. 68:182, 1944.)

2. Rectal Atresia

Anatomy.—In this rare condition, the terminal patent bowel ends blindly at any level, and the rectum beyond exhibits a deficiency which may be short and membranous, or long and stringlike, attaching to the anal canal. The anus and anal canal are normal, in correct relationship to the intrinsic sphincters and to the pubo-rectalis.

These levels of termination do not match those described on the basis of the embryology of the cloaca and are more likely to occur at a later stage, after formation of the rectum, from vascular deficiencies. Nixon (1961) and Partridge and Gough (1961) believe it to be a true atresia of the rectum, arising from a vascular accident to the superior rectal branch of the inferior mesenteric artery in a manner similar to that postulated for jejuno-ileal atresia (Nixon, 1956; Barnard, 1957; and Louw, 1959). A "fibrous cord" from the proximal gut to the sacrum or to the distal bowel which, on section, proves to be atresic bowel, is present in some cases, as reported by Stephens (1953), Nixon (1961) and Magnus (1968). However, as yet, ligation of the superior hemorrhoidal arteries of puppies in utero has not resulted in rectal atresia (Louw, 1965).

Freeman (1966) in a review of congenital atresia and stenosis of the colon, however, classifies the lesion as a colonic rather than rectal atresia, on the basis that associated anomalies are common (45–62%) in other rectal deformities, whereas 3 patients with rectal atresia had no associated anomalies, as encountered in colonic atresia.

Convincing evidence that atresia is an acquired rather than a primary developmental error has been displayed in a dissection by

Magnus (1968) of one of our cases. This infant was a female and is described in Chapter 4.

In rectal atresia, no gas or meconium appears in the urine, and the radiograph shows a "high" gas shadow at or above the pubococcygeal line. The lower pouch may be defined by a probe or by radiopaque dye. After establishment of colostomy, the length of the atresic segment may be determined by studies of dye injected down the distal limb of the colostomy (Fig. 27).

Sphincters.—No opportunity has so far presented to dissect the sphincters in a male with rectal atresia, but, as indicated in the dissection by Magnus of a female child (Chapt. 4), all three sphincter components were present. The surgical problem is thus much simpler than in other rectal deformities.

Perineum.—The appearance of a normal anus may mask the presence of the more proximal atresia, until the presence of intestinal obstruction suggests a rectal examination. Diagnosis in some cases has been revealed only by laparotomy for intestinal obstruction.

Management.—After appropriate investigations, as described for other rectal and anal malformations, it should be assumed that all the sphincter components are present at the usual levels in the pelvic floor. The four procedures are as follows:

Fig. 27.—Rectal atresia. **A,** invertogram displaying gas shadow to P/C line and cranial to the I point. **B,** catheter and barium introduced into well-formed anus; opaque medium in colon and rectum run in through a catheter in the colostomy stoma. This filling defect represents a membrane occluding the lumen of the rectum half-way between P/C line and I point.

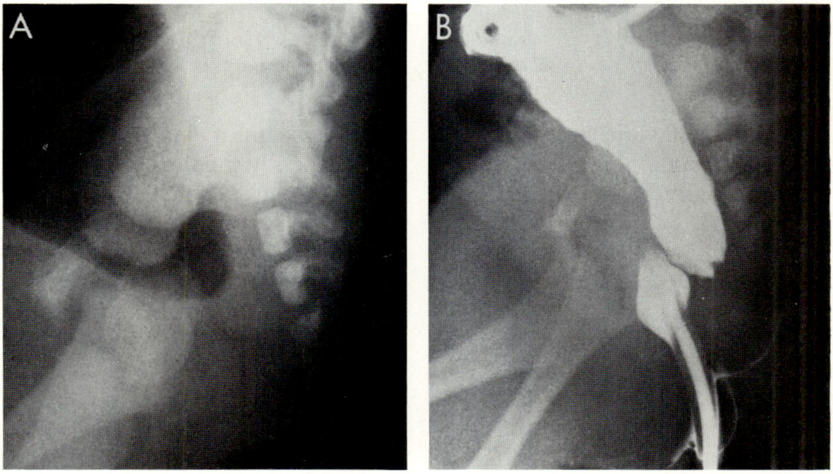

(i) After preliminary colostomy in the newborn period, an abdominal pull-through procedure similar to Swenson's recto-sigmoidectomy for Hirschsprung's disease is performed, i.e., by a sutured anastomosis outside the anus (Santulli *et al.*, 1965). Santulli advised this at 9–12 months of age. Trusler and Wilkinson (1962) and Snyder (1961), however, prefer this reconstruction in the neonatal period, without preliminary colostomy, which they would perform only for sick or premature babies or for those with gross distention as a result of delayed diagnosis.

(ii) Kiesewetter *et al.* (1964) perform a colostomy at birth, followed later by abdomino-perineal pull-through after stripping off the mucous membrane of the lower pouch.

(iii) Brayton and Norris (1958), in 1 case, perforated the atresic segment by a clamp from below, followed by dilatations, and reported a good result. This procedure would seem permissible only when the length of the atresic segment is known to be very short, as demonstrated radiographically by air studies from above and barium from below.

(iv) Nixon (1961) advises an abdominal pull-through procedure by a nonsuture anastomosis, without preliminary colostomy. Louw (1965) performs the same operation but initially defines the puborectalis by the sacro-perineal route of Stephens—with which we agree.

The simplicity of Nixon's operation recommends itself and involves less interference with the sphincters than a Swenson-type recto-sigmoidectomy, which requires some mobilization of the lower pouch in order to turn it out through the anus. The technical details of Nixon's operation are described in Chapter 9. We have not had experience in the management of this deformity. However, on theoretical grounds, we would probably perform preliminary colostomy at birth; at 12 months, Nixon's operation, after first defining the puborectalis by the sacro-perineal route.

B. Intermediate Anomalies

In this group of deformities, the anal canal is agenetic, in whole or in part, and the terminal rectum is either blind or fistulates into a neighboring viscus. The "intermediate" level of these anomalies refers to their complex relationship to the pubo-rectalis muscle—when a fistula is present, it is actually within or through the sling (as in low anomalies), but the termination of the distended bowel is lying on (i.e., above) the sling muscle (as in high anomalies). The intermediate lesions contribute the most controversial issues regarding surgical approach, some surgeons believing that the bowel can be safely approached within the muscular sling from the perineum alone; others, including ourselves, consider that the lesions more closely resemble the high deformities and are treated as such from a supralevator approach. We thus include them in operative descriptions as "rectal deformities."

1. Anal Agenesis

Anal Agenesis (No Fistula).—*Anatomy.*—This developmental defect occurs almost exclusively in male infants. The rectum terminates at the upper border of the bulbo-cavernosus muscle, in close proximity to the urethra, but without a fistula to it (Fig. 28). The rectal pouch may exhibit an anterior fluted protrusion directed towards the bulbous urethra, as if a fistula at one stage existed but closed spontaneously, as shown in one specimen and in x-rays of several patients. A

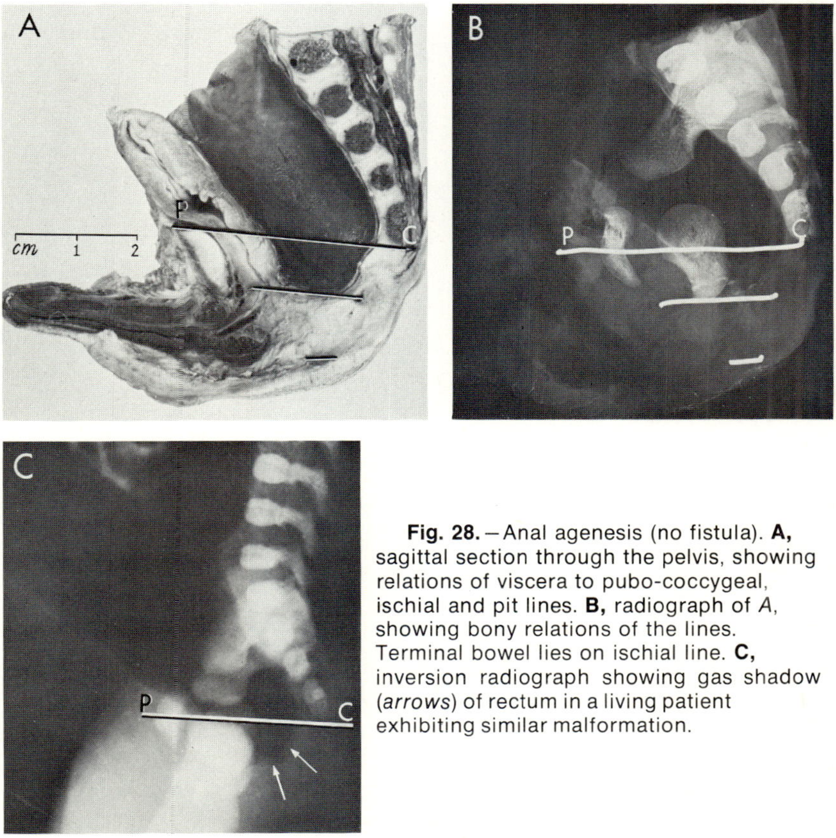

Fig. 28.—Anal agenesis (no fistula). **A,** sagittal section through the pelvis, showing relations of viscera to pubo-coccygeal, ischial and pit lines. **B,** radiograph of *A*, showing bony relations of the lines. Terminal bowel lies on ischial line. **C,** inversion radiograph showing gas shadow (*arrows*) of rectum in a living patient exhibiting similar malformation.

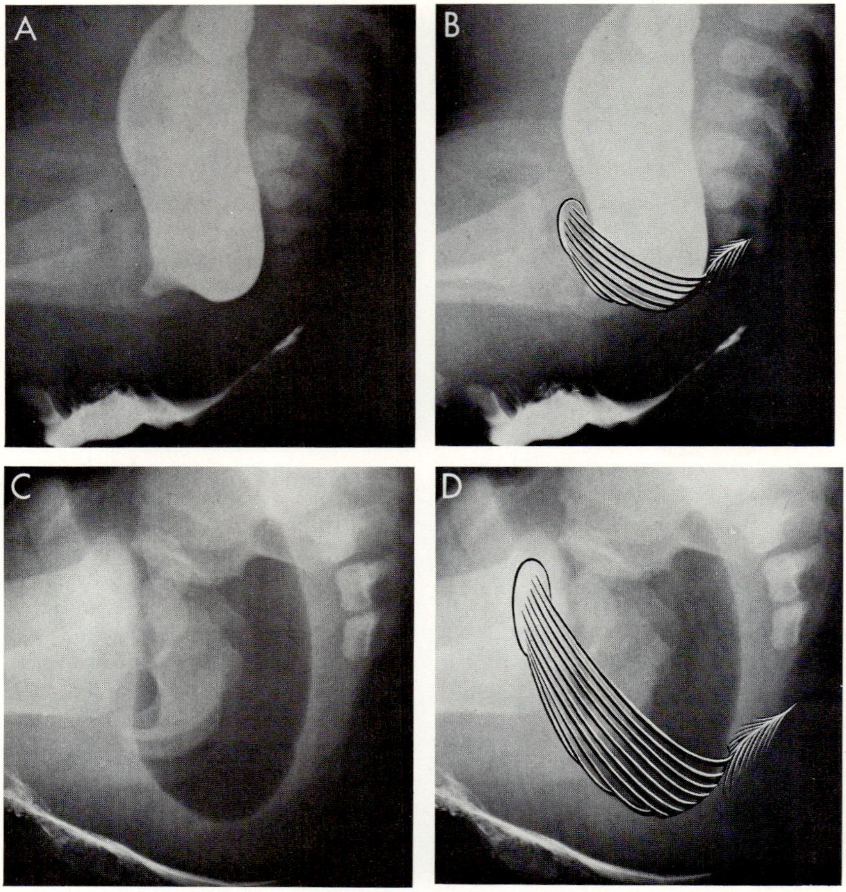

Fig. 29. – Anal agenesis (no fistula). **A,** blind snout at I point is the site of fixation of rectum to the urethra and **B,** pouch of the rectum sits in the pubo-rectalis sling. **C,** same child 1 year later – rectum inflated through catheter in colostomy. Note the distention of the rectal pouch caudally and **D,** the presumed arrangement of pubo-rectalis pressed down by overdistended rectum. N.B.: The snout or beak when present marks the true level for purposes of diagnosis and management in recto-bulbar fistula and anal agenesis (no fistula).

radiologic example is shown in Figure 29. Operative dissections reveal that the anterior wall of the terminal rectum is contiguous with the urethra, and perforation of the urethra is a hazard of surgical mobilization.

Sphincters. – Observations at operation suggest that the sphincter anatomy is similar to that in recto-bulbar fistulae (see below). Kelly's (1968) dissection of anal agenesis demonstrated a lesion very similar in level to recto-bulbar fistula. The levator sling was compressed and

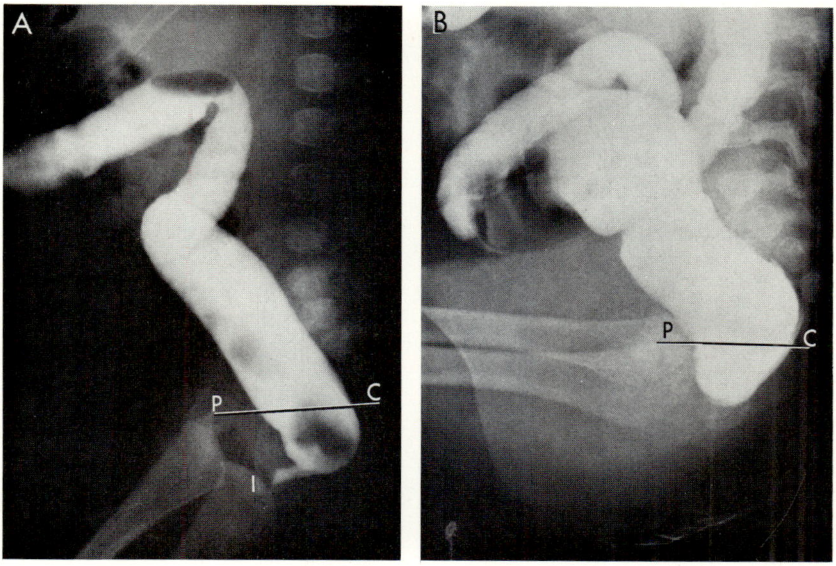

Fig. 30.—Anal agenesis (no fistula). Colograms indicating the level of imperforation at the *I* point below the *P/C* line. **A,** a snout may or may not be present and **B,** at the level of the bulb, but no fistula communicates.

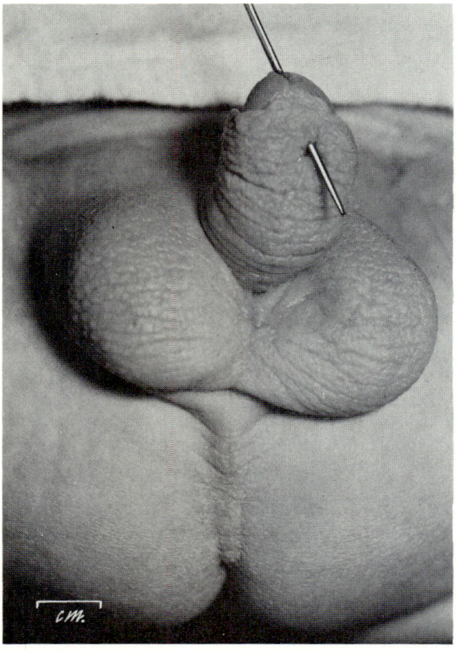

Fig. 31.—Anal agenesis (no fistula). Absence of anal pit, split scrotum and urethral fistula (*probe*) in the floor of the urethra. No connection existed between the rectum and urethra.

foreshortened, and the site of fusion of muscle with the bowel lay well below the P/C line, but above the "I" point. The pubo-visceral sling was disposed around the caudal limit of the gut in a manner identical with that in recto-bulbar fistula (Figs. 29 and 30 and see Fig. 93).

Perineum.—The appearances show no diagnostic features which distinguish the lesion from any other deformity without an external fistula. The anal dimple may be absent or rudimentary, and deformities of the genital folds such as cleft scrotum and urethral fistula occurred in one patient (Fig. 31).

Investigations.—1. Urine Microscopy.—The condition is much less common than a lesion communicating with a urethral fistula. Careful examination of the urine is therefore important in excluding such a fistula, for in anal agenesis the urine should be clear. It should be collected in a pediatric bag, but, if such a specimen is not available, a catheter specimen should be examined prior to operation, and, if negative, then at the time of operation a manual expression specimen may be obtained, still further to exclude a fistula. Voided specimens are more likely to contain meconium than catheter specimens if a urethral fistula is present.

2. Invertography.—This method is essential in this noncommunicating anomaly. Interpretation is easier if a catheter is also passed through the urethra in order to relate the gas bubble to it. The gas shadow lies at or near the lower border of the ossified ischial bone, the "I" point, thus generally distinguishing the lesion from an ano-rectal agenesis higher in the pelvis near the P/C line (see Figs. 28, 29 and 30). However, the anterior protrusion of the terminal rectum varies in length, and rarely the gas shadow may assume a position between the I point and the P/C line, making the distinction between ano-rectal agenesis and anal agenesis difficult. There may or may not be a distinctive anterior "beak" to terminal rectum near the I point.

3. Micturition Cystourethrography.—This method of investigation is advisable to determine the state of the urinary tract and to supplement the evidence for and against the presence of a fistula between urethra and rectum. The urethra is usually normal in appearance, but even this finding may not exclude a fine, one-way or plugged fistula.

4. Further Investigations.—These follow the same pattern as described for recto-bulbar fistula. As a preliminary to operation, in rare circumstances, a telescopic view of the membranous urethra and bulb via the panendoscope may help to solve a point in diagnosis and confirm impressions to date.

Management.—Previously we believed (Stephens, 1963) that provided the surgeon was certain as a result of invertography and needle aspiration that the rectal pouch did not lie above the "ischial line" no colostomy was required, and a one-stage perineal anoplasty could be undertaken in the newborn period. Dissection was kept immediately posterior to the bulbo-cavernosus, using a metal sound in the urethra as a guide; the pubo-rectalis fibers were retracted backwards, and the rectum was anastomosed to a "trapdoor" incision in the perineum. Louw (1965) also advocates newborn perineal anoplasty.

However, further experience has shown that this deep dissection can be very difficult in a small infant, the rectal pouch is firmly attached to the urethra, and the lowermost fibers of pubo-rectalis are vulnerable during mobilization. We believe that the lesion should be considered in the same light as a recto-bulbar fistula (see below). The management and recommendations are therefore colostomy and later sacro-perineal reconstruction, as described for that lesion. Santulli *et al.* (1965) now advise a preliminary colostomy also.

Anal Agenesis with Fistula

Recto-Bulbar Fistula.—*Anatomy.*—Although this is generally described as a very rare condition—only one in Nixon's (1961) hospital series of 323 cases—we have encountered examples in 13 patients, specimens from two of whom became available for dissection. The embryology will be discussed later in this chapter under ano-cutaneous fistula.

The rectum ends at the upper border of the bulbo-cavernosus muscle; from here a fistula may enter the bulb of the urethra below the membranous urethra, or pass distally to the bulb and enter the urethra within the cavernous tissue in its penile part (Fig. 32). In the

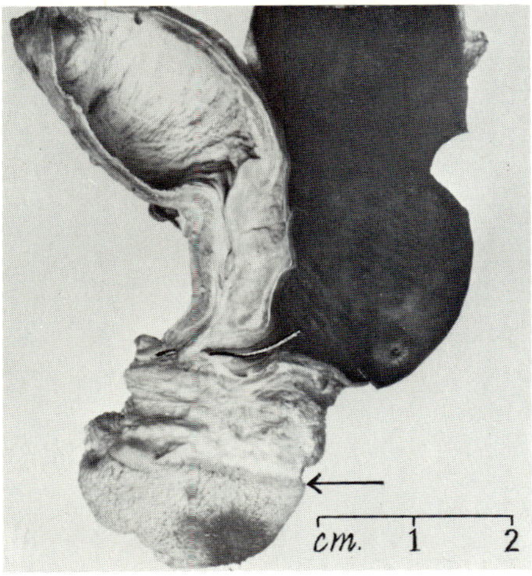

Fig. 32.—Recto-bulbar fistula. Sagittal section of a specimen showing fistulous tract entering the bulbous urethra; bristle indicates the tract; arrow marks the level of the skin of the natal cleft.

recto-bulbar type, the fistula may be quite wide, lying cranial to the pubo-rectalis sling, with the cavernous tissue of the bulb extending posteriorly along the undersurface of the fistula. In the ano-urethral type, the fistula is fine, slips through the open anterior end of the pubo-rectalis sling and the upper fibers of the bulbo-cavernosus muscle and runs forwards in the cavernous tissue.

Sphincters.—(a) Levator Ani.—This muscle is well developed in both its sling and diaphragm portions. In the dissections, the pubo-rectalis was intimately apposed to the caudal end of the rectum down to the fistula, where it fused with the bulbo-cavernosus muscle, although a cleavage plane could be detected between them. The rectum and fistula lay deeply in the bottom of a "basket" made of pubo-rectalis sling and diaphragm (see Fig. 29), but the anatomy differed from that of a recto-urethral fistula, in that the caudal part of the rectum partially penetrated the main bulk of the pubo-rectalis sling and could be compressed by it. The rectum on the bottom of the basket lay at the level of the perineal membrane, by contrast with the recto-urethral fistula, which lies above the sling and the pelvic diaphragm on the pubo-coccygeal line. The recto-bulbar fistula must be regarded as an intermediate group in the high-low classification, al-

Fig. 33.—Various perineal appearances of recto-bulbar fistula. **A,** perineal raphe across the anal pit. **B,** divided raphe (*arrows*) around site of anal dimple; lateral limbs of the raphe converge on cleft scrotum, forming single ridge to midpenis where a blob of erectile tissue overlies a blind sinus, a single raphe continues distally along the penis to the glans. **C,** absence of raphe, umbilicated shallow perineum and thin floor to hypospadiac type of urethra (*arrow*).

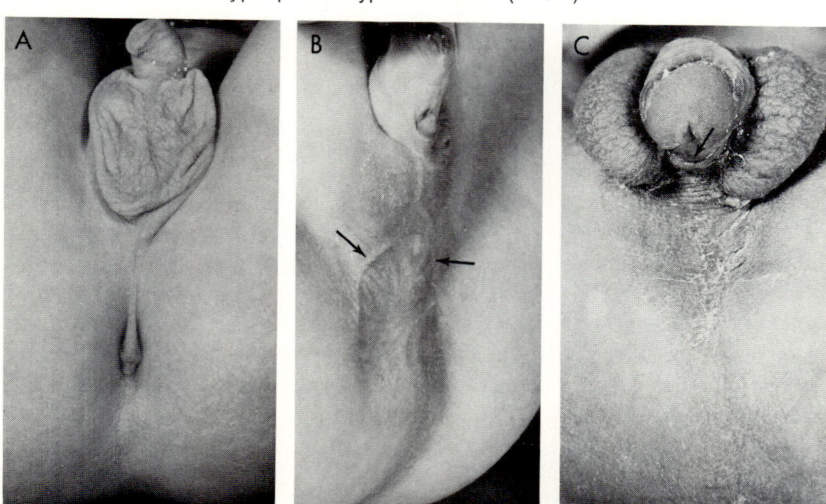

though Swenson and Donnellan (1967) have lowered the high group to include this type. In terms of management, we would agree with this view.

(b) Internal Anal Sphincter.—This sphincter is absent, the rectal muscle coats ending near the cavernous tissue of the bulb.

(c) External Anal Sphincter.—This muscle is identical with that found in ano-cutaneous fistula, i.e., superficial strands of sagittal fibers beneath the skin but not constituting an effective sphincter.

Perineum.—At the normal anal site, there may be no evidence of an anal pit, but sometimes a groove or an absent, weak or double raphe (Figs. 33 and 34). In many patients, there are other deformities of the inner genital folds, such as hypospadias, cleft scrotum, a flimsy floor to the urethra, with an accessory urethral orifice or side hole on the underaspect of the penis. The bulk of tissue palpated between a sound in the bulbous urethra and the finger on the skin of the perineum may be very much reduced in amount.

Gas and meconium can be expressed from the urethra, and a probe passed along the urethra emerges through the back of the bulb and can be palpated in the perineum after its entry into the rectum.

Bourne (1966) described an unusual case of a 25-year-old man who had pneumaturia and fecaluria since birth, and a peno-scrotal hypospadias. The lesion was a recto-bulbar fistula.

Investigations.—The perineal appearances and probe test may present strong clinical evidence of recto-bulbar fistula in some cases, but in others the level of the fistula cannot be judged without further tests.

1. Urine Microscopy.—Voided urine may be obviously meconium stained, confirming the presence of a urinary communication. If urine is not passed spontaneously, a catheter should be passed (at the time of the preoperative micturition cystourethrogram) and the urine examined for color and epithelial squames. Sometimes the catheter preferentially enters the fistula, rather than the posterior urethra, and, although no urine is obtained, the withdrawn catheter is smeared with meconium.

2. Invertography.—Recognizing the errors inherent in inversion radiography when gas escapes freely through the fistula to the exterior, the clinician may still obtain some useful clues from this procedure if gas shadows are found caudal to the pubo-coccygeal line, but he should not be misled by their absence from the expected locations. Gas in the bowel well distal to the P/C line excludes recto-urethral fistula, but because of the possibility of pubo-rectalis contraction, gas at the P/C line does not necessarily mean that the fistula lies at this level. In the typical recto-bulbar fistula, the gas shadow lies well below the P/C line, at or just above the I point overlying the lowest quarter of the ossified ischium (Fig. 34).

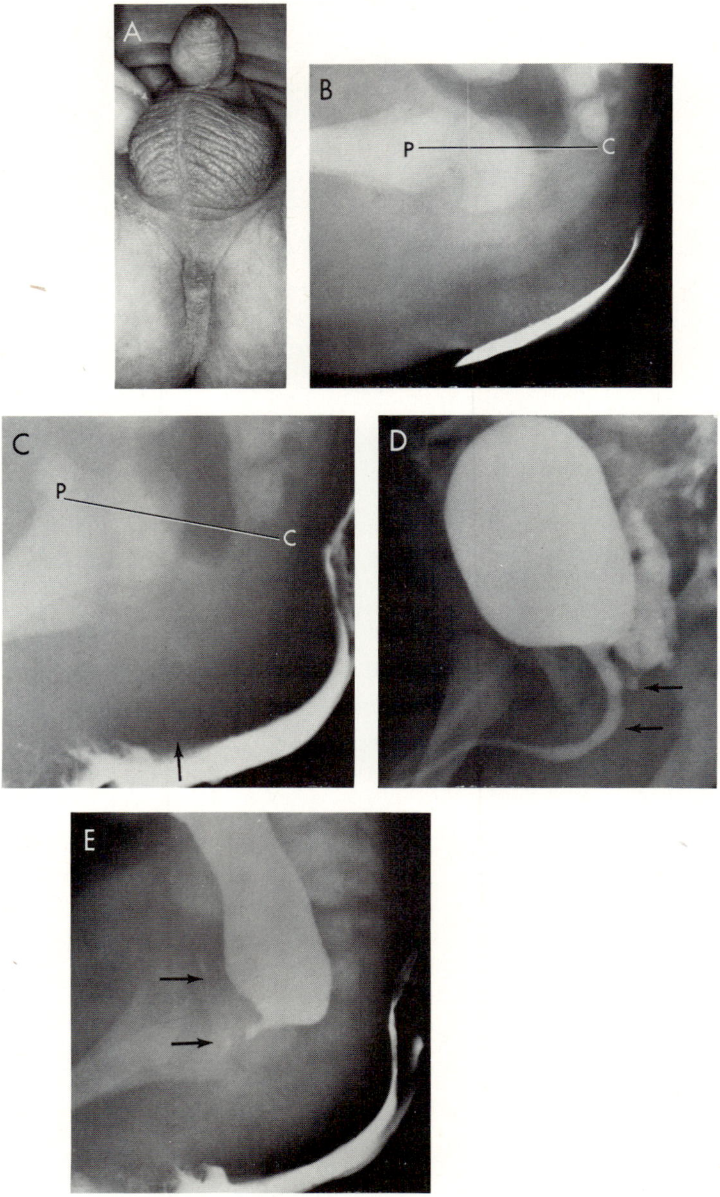

Fig. 34.—Recto-bulbar fistula. Invertography, micturition cystourethrography and colography used to define the site of the fistula. **A,** appearance of perineum—hypertrophic raphe over usual site of anus. **B,** first lateral invertogram shows false

3. Micturition Cystourethrography.—Here again, useful clues may be obtained in the neonatal phase. The procedure may show pooling of contrast material in the rectum or the telltale streak of iodide in the fistula. A radiopaque streak directed posteriorly near the ischial line, on cystourethrography, is positive evidence of the level of the fistula, but a "streak" at a higher level is not always trustworthy (Fig. 34).

4. Assessment of Sphincters and Nerves.—(See Chapt. 8.)

5. Colography.—After establishment of the colostomy, colograms combined with a further micturating cystourethrogram will usually clearly demonstrate the site of the fistula at or just above the "I" point (see Fig. 102).

6. Documentation of the Urinary Tract.—Regular urine microscopy and culture, intravenous pyelography and blood urea nitrogen estimation are obtained over the weeks following colostomy.

7. Cystourethroscopy.—This method confirms the site of the fistula, and the cystoscope may freely enter it in preference to the proximal urethra. This procedure is usually deferred until the reconstruction phase of the proceedings.

Management.—This lesion is intermediate between a "high" and a "low" malformation. Diagnosis can be difficult in the neonatal crisis and the exact site of the fistula confused with that of a recto-urethral fistula. The terminal rectum is intimately related to the pubo-rectalis muscle which blends into the bulbo-cavernosus muscle. Dissection through the small perineum of the newborn babe is liable to damage the pubo-rectalis muscle. For these reasons, we believe the proctoplasty should not be performed under emergency conditions in the newborn, a view supported by Louw (1965).

The recommended procedure is as follows:

(i) Colostomy in the newborn period.

(ii) Clearance, by washouts, of the distal limb of the colostomy in the early postoperative period to avoid urinary infection.

(iii) Completion of investigations as to the exact anatomy of the fistula, of the urinary tract and of the sphincteric nerve supply, performed over the next 3 months, as described above.

(iv) If no urinary infection, sacro-perineal proctoplasty performed

---

level of gas, due to levator contraction. **C,** later invertogram shows gas caudal to *P/C* line, reaching to I point. **D,** micturition cystourethrography shows opaque medium from the urethra lying in the rectum, but the fistula is still not located accurately. Rectum and fistula are squeezed by the pubo-rectalis muscle in the zone between the arrows. **E,** colography via colostomy stoma shows snout of fistula, and opaque medium now showing up course of urethra. Snout leads into the back of the bulbous urethra (*lower arrow*). Upper arrow depicts streak of iodide in prostatic urethra.

at 12–15 months of age is the preferred operation (technique, Chapt. 9).

(v) If urinary infection, proved beyond doubt by needle aspiration of urine from the bladder, persists after appropriate chemotherapy, the proctoplasty program may need to be advanced.

Rare variants of recto-bulbar fistula are as follows: Ramakrishnan (1970) records a patient with an H-type deformity—recto-bulbar fistula plus a normal anus as well; the urethra was also normal. Keith (1908) described a similar situation on autopsy material.

2. Ano-Rectal Stenosis

In the Ladd and Gross classification, type 1 is described as a stenosis at the anus or at a level 1–4 cm. above the anus. We agree with Nixon's (1961) interpretation, that for the majority of male infants who exhibit "stenosis at the anus" the underlying abnormality is one or other form of the common "covered anus."

We have encountered stenosis above the vicinity of the anal valves (Fig. 35 and see Fig. 40), but when stenosis occurs up to 4 cm. within the anus, as described by Gross (1953), it seems more likely that it is an acquired lesion of the terminal rectum and upper anal canal of ischemic origin, such as occurs in stenosis or atresia elsewhere in the bowel. It is this condition to which the term ano-rectal stenosis would seem appropriate.

Nixon (1961) recognizes this intermediate type of stenosis, and

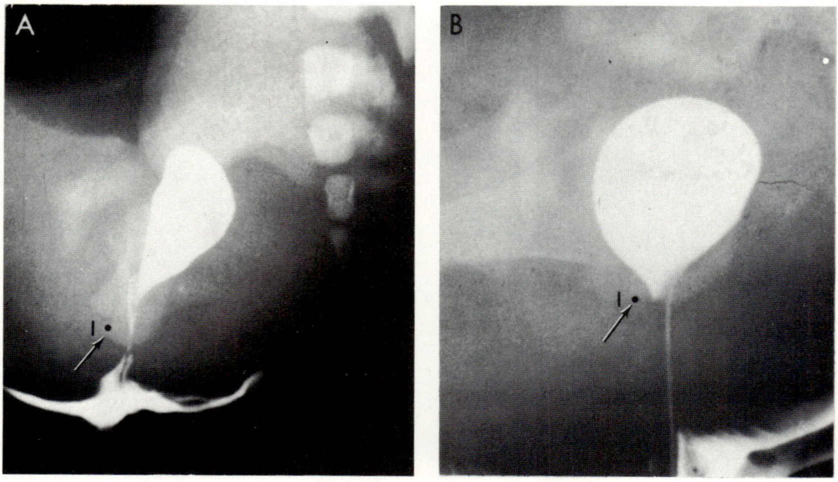

Fig. 35.—Deep ano-rectal stricture (ano-rectal stenosis). **A,** barium instilled into the rectum, anal pit and narrow segment. **B,** upper limit of narrow segment is at the I point.

Santulli *et al.* (1965) list 1 patient (type 4, rectal atresia) in whom the occlusion was incomplete, with a severe stricture just above the levator ani. David (1937) shows illustrations of varying degrees of anal stenosis, in one variety of which the stenosis was 2–3 cm. long. He described the stenosis as being valvular, tubular or membranous.

Management.—In ano-rectal stenosis, internal proctotomy and dilatation are required, the latter for a prolonged period because the degree of associated anal fibrosis creates a rigid, narrow tube.

C. Low Anomalies (Translevator)

Embryologically, these lesions are predominantly "anal deformities."

1. At Normal Anal Site

In the proposed International Classification, two lesions are recognized at the normal anal site. The first is a completely occluded anus. In the discussion determining the classification, it was recognized that two varieties of complete occlusion could occur (1) occlusion by hypertrophy of genital folds ("covered anus—complete") and (2) imperforation of the anal membrane. It was felt that the rarity of the latter lesion, however, should relegate it to the "miscellaneous" group of rare lesions. Consequently, the International Classification lists only the former term.

The second lesion is anal stenosis. Again, it was recognized that the stenosis could be derived from partial covering by the genital folds or from partial perforation of the anal membrane. Again, because of the rarity of the latter, a single term "anal stenosis" was chosen.

For purposes of completeness, however, we now include descriptions of all four lesions.

(i) "Covered Anus—Complete" (International Classification, 1970) (a) Covered anus—complete.—*Anatomy.*—Complete covering of the anal site by genital folds is an uncommon lesion. The anomaly most commonly seen due to the covering process is "anocutaneous fistula," and the major description of that process is described under that lesion below.

In the completely covered anus the perineum has fully developed, the anus has migrated back to the normal site, and the genital folds fuse over the anus by excessive posterior development.

The folds may heap up anteriorly or posteriorly, or fuse as a band in the midline, the latter lesion being described by Bill (1953) is "congenital median band." As pointed out by Bill, however, a day or two after birth a fistulous opening may break down on either side of the band, with the subsequent release of meconium (see Figs. 44 and 45).

Sphincters.—These muscles are identical with those described for ano-cutaneous fistula, an almost identical lesion, to which reference is made below.

Perineum.—The anal pit is obliterated by a midline thick raphe or hypertrophied folds; this is in contrast to an imperforate anal membrane in which, unless the membrane is bulging, the anal pit is present and superficially normal.

Investigations.—A thick median band at the normal anal site is almost diagnostic, but, as there is no visible orifice, the level of bowel occlusion should be confirmed by invertogram films. These show the gas shadow just below the skin marker, well below the I point. Percutaneous needling of the bowel and definition by radiopaque medium, as described by Murugasu (see Chapt. 8), provides the most certain evidence of bowel level.

Management.—Excision of the overlying fold or band, and incision into the anal canal, followed by dilatation, performed in the immediate neonatal period is a simple procedure. A formal "anoplasty" is not required.

(B) IMPERFORATE ANAL MEMBRANE.—*Anatomy.*—The lesion is rare, although referred to frequently in early reports. The perineum is fully developed, and the anus has migrated backwards to the normal site. However, the procto-deal membrane, normally disappearing at an early stage of the embryo may persist. It persists at the site represented in the normal anus by the anal valves and, in the newborn, is not at the anal skin level but up to 1.5 cm. inside the anus (Fig. 36).

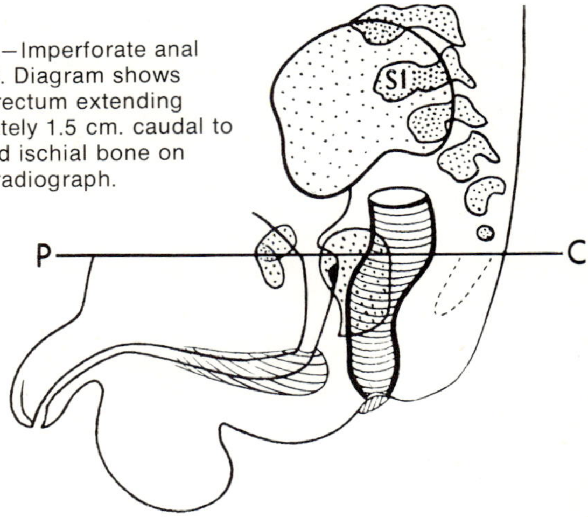

Fig. 36.—Imperforate anal membrane. Diagram shows gas-filled rectum extending approximately 1.5 cm. caudal to the ossified ischial bone on inversion radiograph.

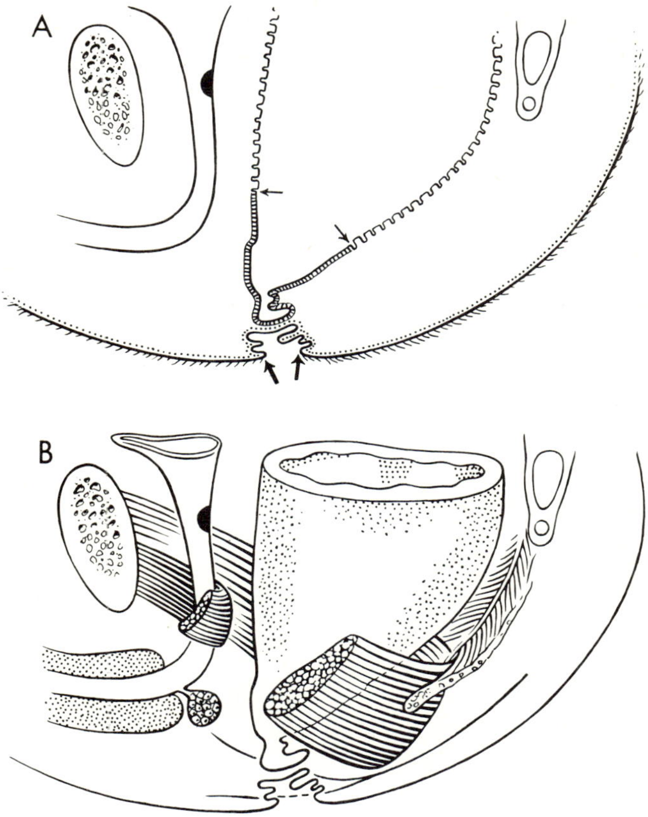

Fig. 37.—Imperforate anal membrane. **A,** composite diagram drawn from serial sections, showing the structures present. Above the light arrows, the lining is columnar epithelium with goblet cells and crypts of Lieberkühn; below the arrows, the epithelium is stratified columnar. **B,** three-dimensional diagram showing the disposition of the voluntary muscle (pubo-rectalis) about the rectum. (Reproduced with permission from Magnus, R.: Australian Paediat. J. 2:165, 1966.)

The epithelial components of the structures are well shown in a serial dissection by Magnus and Stephens (1966) in Figure 37.

Sphincters.—(a) Levator Ani.—This muscle was found to be almost normal in two serial dissections, Stephens (1965) and Magnus and Stephens (1966), the pubo-rectalis surrounding the terminal rectum and forming a normal ano-rectal ring. However, at the caudal extremity, the fibers swept into and around the sides and posterior aspect of the imperforate membrane. The caudal muscle bundles at this site were intersected by the coattails of the longitudinal muscle coat of the rectum (Fig. 37).

(b) Internal Anal Sphincter.—The normal internal sphincter lies predominantly below the anal valves; in imperforate anal membrane, neither the circular nor the longitudinal coat extends beyond the membrane, and no internal sphincter is formed around the skin-lined anal pit, although the distal end of the smooth muscle may be slightly thickened cranial to it. The longitudinal fibers end in a fibromuscular knot below the circular coat or peter out as "coattails" through the circular coat above the membrane.

(c) External Anal Sphincter.—Two layers can be identified. Surrounding the bowel at the level of the membrane is a collar of voluntary muscle intimately blending with the sling of the pubo-rectalis, except anterior to the rectum where fibers converge towards the midline. They probably represent the deep external sphincter. More superficially, a thin band of sagittal fibers passes from coccyx to the bulbo-cavernosus muscle. It is not disposed as a definite superficial sphincter. In the dissection by Magnus and Stephens (1966), the external sphincter was a thin strip of voluntary muscle arranged in the form of a "Y," the stem attached posteriorly to the coccyx and dividing immediately behind the anal pit into two limbs which ran forwards on either side of the pit. These fibers then took a parallel course to end in the fat of the perineum. This arrangement of these superficial fibers would hardly merit the term "sphincter."

Perineum.—Superficially, the appearance may be normal, as the anal pit is formed. The presence of intestinal obstruction may be the first lead to a digital examination of the rectum, which reveals the membrane at about 1 cm. inside the anal verge. When the infant strains, a thin membrane may appear as a bluish bulge (meconium). Denis Browne (1951) has described a variety in which posterior fusion of the genital folds produces a fine central raphe on the membrane, on one or both sides of which there may be some fine dimples which may be patent. The usual membrane is a thin diaphragm of two epithelial layers, about 1 cm. in diameter. Another type is a tough fibro-muscular knot of tissue lying between the rectum with its muscle coats and the apex of the anal pit, without actual membrane formation.

Investigations.—Invertography.—This method shows the gas shadow at the lowest level of all anal anomalies, namely the "pit line," 1–2 cm. caudal to the lower border of the ischium and its I point (Fig. 38 and see Figs. 36 and 97).

Management.—All authors agree that the appropriate procedure is a simple perineal anoplasty, followed by dilatation. Opinions differ slightly as to whether the membrane should be formally excised or

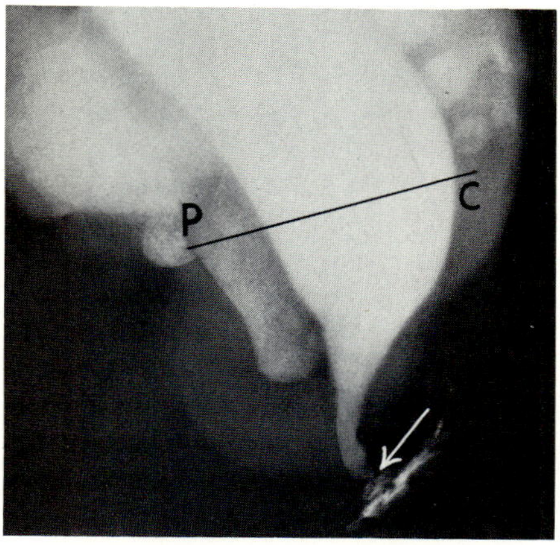

Fig. 38. – Imperforate anal membrane. Contrast medium in anal pit and in rectum displays the diaphanous membrane as a thin-filling defect indicated by arrow. (Reproduced with permission from Magnus, R.: Australian Paediat. J. 2:165, 1966.)

incised by a cruciate incision. In the authors' view no skin should be excised in the first instance.

(II) "ANAL STENOSIS" (PROPOSED INTERNATIONAL CLASSIFICATION, 1970). (A) COVERED ANAL STENOSIS. – This lesion is another variety of the "covered anus" process. The genital fold may partially cover the anus with minimal projection of the "fistula," either anteriorly or posteriorly, the anal orifice itself then presenting as a stenotic one. This form of anal stenosis is the commonest type (Figs. 39 and 40).

Fig. 39. – **A,** Stenosis of the anus: persistence of part of anal membrane and **B,** covered anus. **A,** normal site, but circumferential stenosis at anal membrane. **B¹,** anus covered by sagittal "bucket handle" bar. **B²,** hypertrophic raphe covers and projects anus anteriorly. **B³,** hypertrophic raphe covers in the anterior quadrants of the anus, projecting orifice posteriorly.

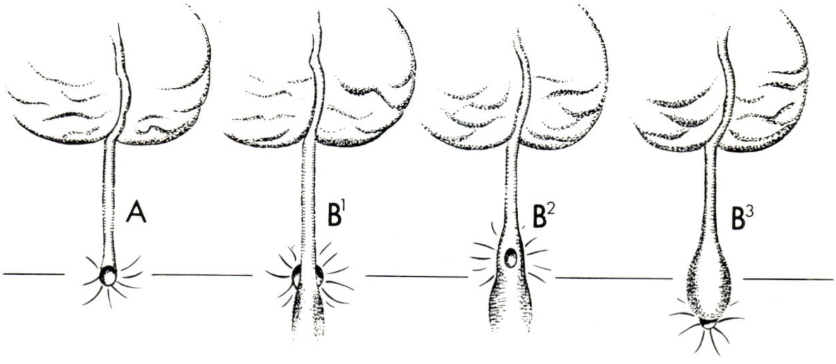

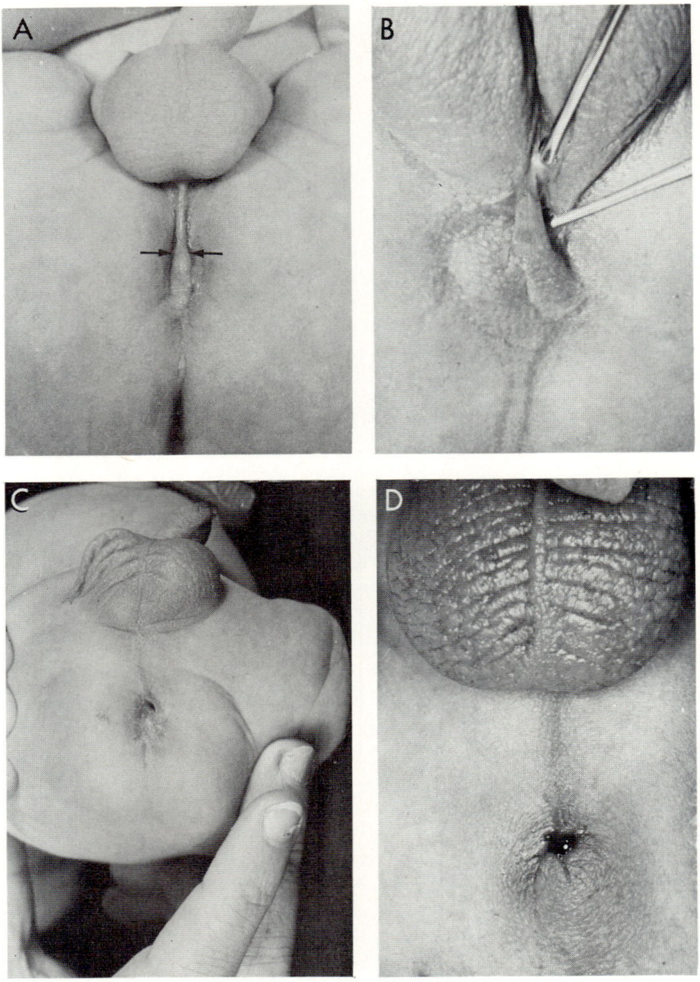

Fig. 40.—Anal stenosis. Perineal variants. **A,** bucket handle—stenotic orifices (*arrows*) on either side—covered anal stenosis. **B,** variant of bucket handle—stenotic orifices on one side and anterior—covered anal stenosis. **C,** ano-rectal stenosis—circumferential stenosis extending into the rectum. (Note also phocomelia.) **D,** anal membrane stenosis. Plug of meconium at the anal membrane.

The "microscopic anus" of Denis Browne is possibly one such variety.

Similarly, if the hypertrophied bar described by Bill (Bill and Johnson, 1953 and Bill *et al.*, 1958) as "congenital median band" covers the anus posteriorly and anteriorly, but not completely, a bucket-handle appearance is produced with two lateral orifices.

Management.—Management should be carried out as follows:

(i) Incision of hypertrophic genital folds and incision and minimal excision of a median band, or rearrangement of perianal skin

(ii) Postoperative dilatation

(iii) Late trimming of tags if a cause of pruritus (see Figs. 115 and 126).

(B) ANAL MEMBRANE STENOSIS.—This defect has features identical with those described for imperforate anal membrane, except that the membrane is partially perforate (Figs. 39 and 40). As discussed in Chapter 7, minor degrees of stenosis may not be seen in large hospital series because they are treated by the family doctor. However, it is not uncommon for this lesion to be overlooked and for the child to present later with chronic distention, ribbon stools, fecal impaction and secondary megacolon, requiring prolonged washouts and re-education (Stephens, 1956). In 2 patients exhibiting large terminal reservoirs in our series, recto-sigmoidectomy of these reservoirs was required, despite adequate dilatation, the restoration of a supple anus and prolonged washout therapy.

Invertography is not necessary, as the condition may be diagnosed from the clinical appearance. In 1 female patient, small metal stitches were inserted into the membrane to identify the level radiographically. The small markers are shown in Figure 58, lying at the pit line.

Management of Anal Membrane Stenosis.—The condition requires dilatation only; any associated skin tags may be excised at a later date.

Further Management of All Stenotic Lesions.—The relatively minor nature of these lesions may tend to undertreatment, with resultant severe degrees of secondary megacolon. Dilatation with sounds used by the surgeon must be undertaken daily in hospital, until the orifice is sufficiently large to admit the parent's little finger and until all accumulated fecal content has been washed away. Further dilatations first with the little finger and then with the larger digits are required daily, then three times per week and at longer intervals, depending on the response. In the dilatation phase, daily enemas and weekly washouts are necessary; after the anus is adequate in size and suppleness, enemas, occasional washouts, and suppositories are needed locally, and petroleum emulsion orally to ensure that stools are kept soft, and accumulations and impactions are prevented. Because of the tendency for the stenosis to recur, digital examinations by the parent are continued about once every 2 weeks and later every 3 or 4 weeks for at least a year, with occasional checks by the surgeon, even after the anus is adequate in size. Neglect and reaccumulations lead to secondary megacolon, which requires prolonged management along the lines indicated.

To avoid these repeated dilatations Bacon and Sherman (1952) prefer an anoplasty in which the anus is enlarged by a posterior sphincterotomy; the edges of the cut mucosa are sutured posteriorly to the sphincter muscles to keep the anus open. We agree that stenosis associated with covered anus is better treated in this way, but we adhere to a policy of dilatation for circumferential membrane type of stenosis.

2. At Perineal Site

At any site forward of the normal anal position two types of external orifice may be found—an anal orifice of normal dimensions and a fistulous orifice.

(I) Anterior Perineal Anus.—*Anatomy.*—The anus has a normal appearance but is situated more anteriorly than usual. The rectum and anal canal are fully formed but lie in close proximity to the posterior or membranous urethra. The anatomy is abnormal, in that the perineum has not developed its full sagittal length, and the anus has not been displaced by it to the normal site.

Sphincters.—All the muscles are presumed to be fully formed and bear a normal relation to the anal canal, as judged by digital examination and the complete continence exercised by the child.

Perineum.—The anus appears to be normal but in a forward position. There are no accompanying defects of the genital folds. The orifice is supple and normal in dimensions. If the anal orifice is stenotic, it must be postulated that it conforms to the variety of anal membrane stenosis in an abnormally placed anus or that the genital folds cover in the back quadrants, in which case it would strictly be classified as a variety of covered anus.

Management.—No treatment is required for the anterior anus, which is otherwise normal.

However, if the orifice is slightly narrowed, dilatations may be required, or a "cutback" procedure may be called for to enlarge the rim of the orifice. No attempt should be made to transplant the anus for "cosmetic reasons," because it is not on view, is clean, the procedure is unnecessary and may damage a perfectly functioning set of sphincters.

(II) ANOCUTANEOUS FISTULA (COVERED ANUS – INCOMPLETE). – *Anatomy.* – This classic lesion is the most common of the anal deformities. Denis Browne (1951) and Stephens (1953), following the explanations of Wood Jones (1904), refer to this malformation as a "covered anus," to suggest the embryological concept of the formed anal canal being "covered" by genital folds which are ectodermal in origin. In the male, the inner genital folds close in the anterior urethra by a process of midline fusion, which begins posteriorly at the anus and extends anteriorly to form the perineal raphe from anus to frenulum. If the perineum has fully developed, with migration of the anus back almost to the normal site, excessive posterior fusion of the folds may cover the anus and project a fistulous tract a short distance anteriorly in the perineum; with partial development of the perineum, the covering process may roll the fistula more anteriorly in the raphe to the scrotum or even to the ventral surface of the penis as far forward as the base of the glans (Stieda, 1903); with agenesis or very rudimentary development of the perineum, the rectum remains close to the urethra, and the fistula then communicates with the bulb of the urethra (recto-bulbar fistula) or with the penile urethra (Fig. 41). The farther the migration of the anus backwards (i.e., the greater the perineal growth) the shorter becomes the perineal fistula. With full migration to the normal site, there may be no fistula, but abnormal posterior fusion of the genital folds in this situation results in the covered anus variety of anal stenosis (see Figs. 39 and 40).

Whereas the medial genital folds have been held responsible in the above description, Tench (1936) believed that the fusion process involved a combination of the lateral genital folds and premature

Fig. 41. – Covered anus in the male. The normal caliber rectum ends at or caudal to the lower border of the ossified ischium. The fistula is directed from this level to the skin or to urethra at or distal to the bulb.

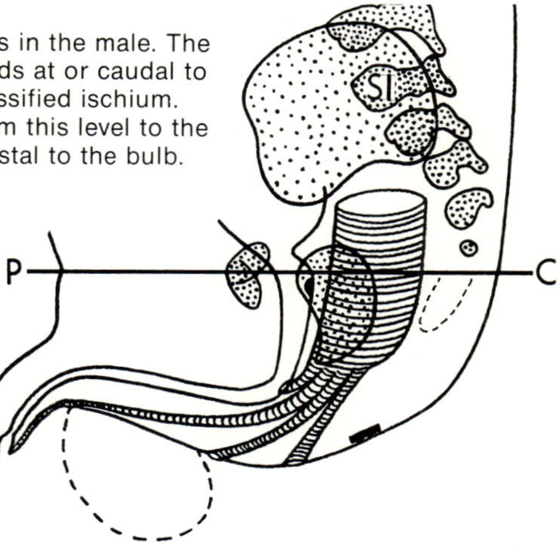

fusion of the anal tubercles. Bill *et al.* (1958) and Bill and Johnston (1958) supported this concept. The anal tubercles are, in our view, only specialized parts of the genital folds arranged around the anal orifice. Possibly both mechanisms are active, and Nixon (1961) suggests that as the medial folds form the urethra their fusion excessively in a posterior direction might be expected to produce a recto-bulbar fistula, whereas the more common ano-cutaneous fistula, regularly associated with a normal urethra, might be due to lateral fold fusion. It is true that a recto-bulbar fistula is often associated with a special form of hypospadias, i.e., the posterior shift and excessive posterior fusion of the medial folds have not "left enough over" to complete the urethra anteriorly.

The special form of "hypospadias" associated with recto-bulbar fistula is one in which the floor of the penile urethra is thin and opens to the skin by a side orifice beyond which the raphe and the urethral lumen continue to their normal destinations. It may, therefore, be caused by a defect of the medial folds rather than the lateral folds which, in this special form of hypospadias, have formed the raphe in the skin to the frenulum.

In the common forms of ano-cutaneous fistula, the anal canal is of normal caliber and correctly located in the pelvis and perineum and is complete to the level of the anal valves. Superficial to this level, the canal is suddenly reduced to a tube of a few millimeters in diameter and is covered by skin and conforms to several patterns.

From the anterior aspect of the terminal normal canal, the squamous-lined fistula usually runs forward a variable distance and opens in the perineal raphe anywhere from adjacent to the anal site to the ventral surface of the penile shaft. Most commonly, the opening of the tract issues behind the scrotum (see Fig. 44, *A*). It is superficial, being covered by thin skin. Meconium or epithelial plugs may be seen in the lumen through this fine translucent skin or at the orifice, not immediately after birth but at 24 hours, when signs of abdominal distention appear.

Sphincters.—(a) Levator Ani.—The levator complex is essentially normal, the pubo-rectalis sling around the lower rectum and the first half centimeter of the fistula (Fig. 42). The most caudal fibers around the neck of the narrow tract are traversed by strands of the outer longitudinal muscle coattails of the rectum. These tails continue for a few millimeters along the tract of the fistula, mingling with a delicate circular sphincteric ring of voluntary muscle surrounding the neck of the fistula. However, Stephens (1953) states that in the serial sections it was not possible to distinguish between the most caudal fibers of the pubo-rectalis muscle and those of the deep part of the external anal sphincter at the neck of the fistula. Fowler

(1957) demonstrated such "coattails" in the normal anal canal, formed from both the longitudinal muscle of the rectum and the levator diaphragm, which penetrate both the internal and external anal sphincters and the pubo-rectalis muscle. As this dysplasia is infrequently associated with sacral agenesis, the muscle is normally innervated.

(b) Internal Anal Sphincter.—No internal sphincter has been found in dissections, the inner circular muscle of the rectum terminating at the junction of the rectum with the fistula.

(c) External Anal Sphincter.—For discussion of the vexed question of the nature of the external sphincter, the reader is again referred to the previous section on recto-urethral fistula.

Nixon (1961) has stated that in the male the external sphincter is fully formed, but Stephens found in his dissections that the only definite fibers were thin, longitudinally running fibers passing on either side of the fistula, from the coccyx to the bulbo-cavernosus. These fibers were quite superficial and ineffective as a sphincter. Bryndorf and Madsen (1959) also stated, "In addition, in the study of several of our patients, we have gained the impression that—as distinct from what is commonly assumed—the anal sphincter does not encircle the normal anal site but extends, in the shape of a 'U,' forward on either side of the ectopic anus." As described above, there may be a deep portion of the external sphincter around the neck of the fistula, but its fibers cannot be distinguished from the lowest fibers of the pubo-rectalis. This concept of the external sphincter is consistent with the postoperative appearance of the anus following a simple "cutback" procedure. When the fistula is laid open and the cut extended into the anus posteriorly, the anal canal gapes, and the

Fig. 42.—Covered anus (ano-cutaneous fistula) in the male. The fistula is a narrow conduit between normal caliber bowel and skin. The pubo-rectalis muscle is related to the bowel, not the fistula, and is the chief muscle of continence.

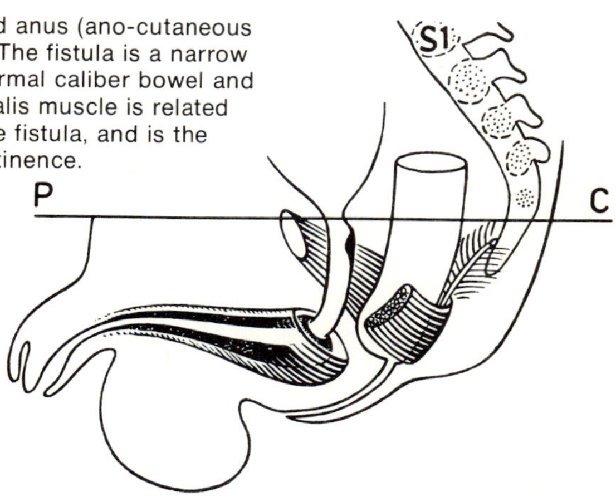

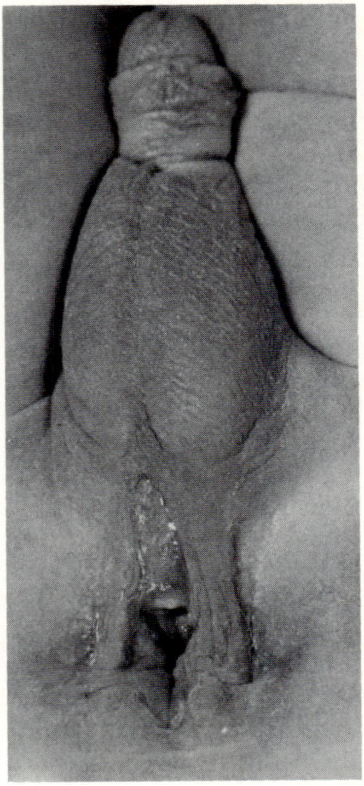

Fig. 43.—Covered anus (ano-cutaneous fistula) in the male. Cutback operation: postoperative view of the anus showing opened-out tract of fistula and the exposed mucosa of the anal canal.

mucosa remains partially exposed (Fig. 43), whereas, if a fully formed sphincter were present, one might expect the superficial fibers to close the anal verge completely, as in a normal person.

Perineum.—Careful inspection of the perineum may be necessary to locate the fine orifice of the fistula. It may be found anywhere from the normal anal site to as far forward as the frenulum of the penis, but the commonest site is behind the scrotum. A "flyspeck" of meconium at the orifice may suggest the site. The fistulous tract may be suggested by a fine bluish line in the perineal raphe or by an obvious bulging with meconium or by white epithelial pearls along its course. The appearance of the normal anal site also varies. If the fistula is well forward, there is usually no anal dimple; in the common fistula behind the scrotum, there may be a rudimentary pit or evidence of the fused genital folds in the form of a hypertrophied raphe or a triangular fold of thickened skin projecting from behind forward (Figs. 44 and 45).

Investigations.—1. Invertography.—Although the usual presentation of an anterior ano-cutaneous fistula is diagnostic of this very low malformation and diagnostic inversion radiography is unnecessary and may be misleading, radiographs are required to establish the state of the sacral vertebrae. The clinical diagnosis of ano-cutaneous fistula transcends the evidence gained from invertography. Inversion x-rays are of confirmatory value when the gas shadows underlie the skin distal to the ischial line. Some confusion may arise from invertography if the pubo-rectalis is in a contracted state at the time of the x-ray or if the gas escapes through the fistula or with packing of meconium in the terminal bowel or if the bowel is collapsed and empty, in which case the appearance may simulate that of a high rectal anomaly (see Figs. 45 and 97).

Indices of suspicion are nonconformity of gas levels to the suspected and regular lines, particularly an overlap of the gas shadow by about one centimeter caudal to the pubo-coccygeal line, this being

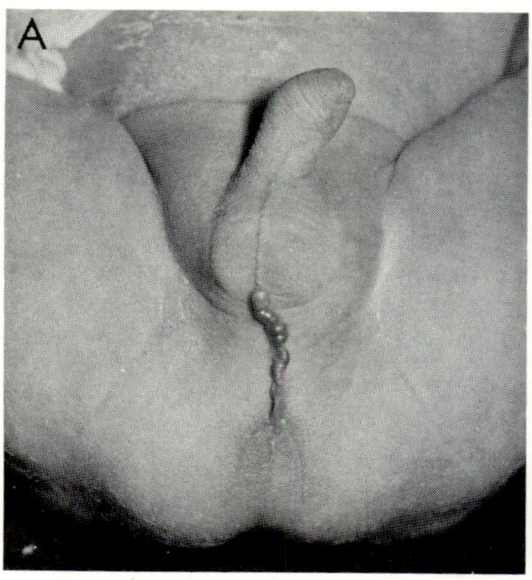

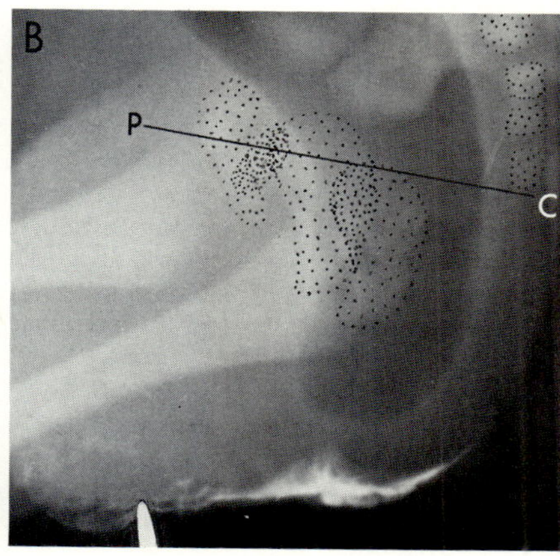

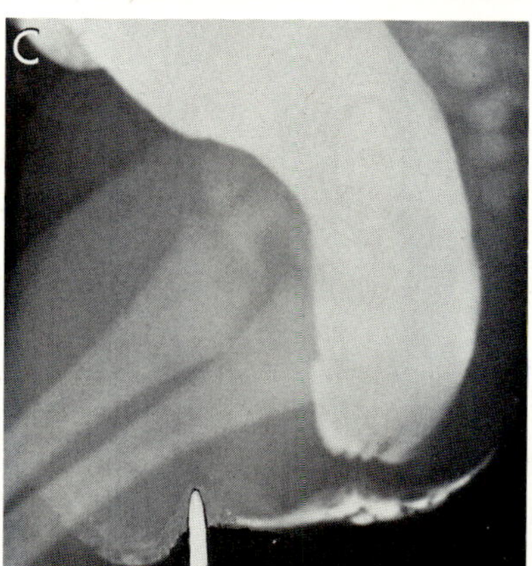

Fig. 44. – Covered anus (ano-cutaneous fistula) in the male. **A,** perineal appearance – meconium tracking anteriorly above the fistula in the raphe, which bifurcates posteriorly around the anal pit. **B,** air introduced via colostomy stoma to show the terminal proximity of the bowel to the skin of the anal pit. Note that this extends well caudal to the ischial ossific centers. **C,** opaque medium more clearly defines the terminal bowel. Marker in **B** and **C** indents orifice of the fistula at the peno-scrotal junction.

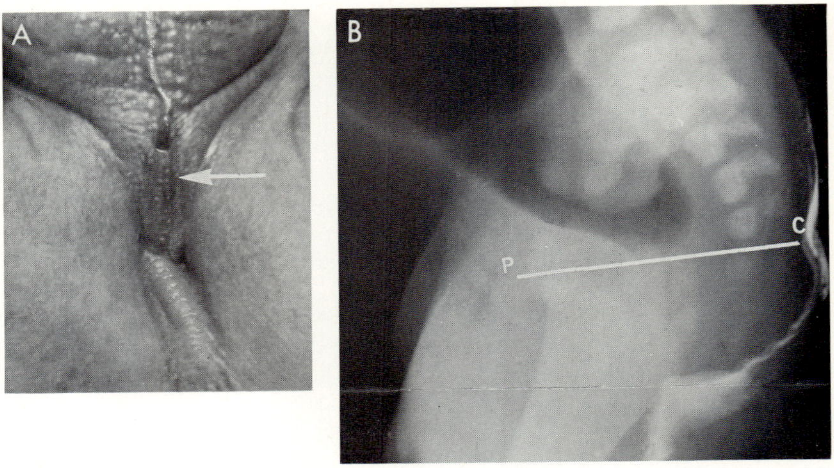

Fig. 45. – Covered anus (ano-cutaneous fistula) in the male. **A,** orifice of fistula issuing on the anterior wall of the anal pit; arrow indicates the ridge caused by the tract of the fistula. **B,** invertogram showing distal limit of gas cranial to *P/C* line; escape of gas from short ano-cutaneous fistula causes unreliable interpretations of an invertogram, as in this patient in whom the gas shadow erroneously suggests a high rectal lesion.

the level of occlusion by the contracted pubo-rectalis muscle. A repeat radiograph may show a different appearance and indicate the true level of obstruction, and, in the presence of an initial high gas shadow, the radiograph should be repeated or ignored, in favor of the more definite clinical identification.

In the usual ano-cutaneous fistula, the gas shadow reaches below the "I" point but may be located more anteriorly than the normal site of the anal canal (compare Fig. 94 with Fig. 90). The segment "I/A" is shortened the farther the fistula lies in the perineum.

2. Fistulograms. – The injection of a visible fistula with radiopaque dye is not strictly necessary, because the anatomy can be predicted in any case; nevertheless, it may be of interest to indicate the depth and lumen size of the covered anal canal, especially in those patients with a very short fistula or with a stenotic anal orifice of the covered type (see Figs. 44 and 101).

3. Other Investigations. – As in all other rectal and anal deformities, the clinical tests for sphincter anatomy and innervation should never be omitted. Over the next 2 or 3 months after operation, the usual check on the urinary tract should be completed – urine microscopy and culture, micturition cystourethrography and intravenous pyelography.

Management.—The pubo-rectalis forms a sling around the terminal rectum, encroaching onto the proximal reach of the fistula. The deep portion of the external sphincter is probably present, although it may not be indistinguishable from the lowest pubo-rectalis fibers; the superficial fibers are ineffectual as a sphincter.

Bearing these facts in mind, the authors do not recommend procedures which attempt to transplant the "anus" backwards through a separate incision within the sphincter muscle. Descriptions of such operations have appeared over many years, generally for "type III deformities with recto-perineal fistula." (Crowell and Dulin (1940), Bacon and Sherman (1952), Gross (1953), Potts *et al.* (1954), Hanley *et al.* (1954), Rhoads and Koop (1955), Santulli (1963) and Sauvage and Bill (1965).

Assuming that these authors' operative descriptions refer to the ano-cutaneous fistula described above, a perineal exploration to mobilize the rectum must involve a dissection within the pubo-rectalis—an unnecessary and possibly damaging step, because the muscle already bears a normal relation to the rectum. The risk of damage is accentuated if the "sphincter muscle" is divided and then reconstituted "to achieve the desired anatomic result." That the dissection in these transplant operations is at least as deep as the pubo-rectalis is suggested by the operative maxim of Santulli (1963), that "it is important to have a urethral catheter in place in order to help identify the urethra and avoid injury to it during the mobilisation of the anterior rectal wall." Potts *et al.* (1954) make the same point.

On the contrary, the concept of the covered anus only requires that the fistula be unroofed by a simple "cutback" to the anal dimple (Denis Browne, 1951, 1955), which is then dilated, no deep dissection being required (see Fig. 121, *B*). This can readily be performed in the neonatal infant under local anesthesia. The technique is described in Chapter 10. This simple operation is supported by Denis Browne (1953), Stephens (1953 and 1963), Bryndorf and Madsen (1959), Louw (1959 and 1965), Nixon (1961), Partridge and Gough (1961), Sommerschild *et al.* (1964), Kiesewetter *et al.* (1964), Bielowicz (1965) and Santulli *et al.* in their recent review (1965). The last authors, however, state that "it may be necessary to divide the anterior commissure of the external sphincter ani muscle."

Other authors, while not advising a transplantation procedure, perform a more formal perineal proctoplasty than a simple cutback: Ravitch (1952), Bradham (1958), Brayton and Norris (1958) and Trusler and Wilkinson (1962).

The recommendations of the authors are as follows:

(i) A simple "cutback" procedure soon after birth.

(ii) Postoperative dilatation.

Rare variants of ano-cutaneous fistula are as follows:

1. Nixon (1970) described a patient with a covered anus, with the fistulous tract *deep* to the scrotum before opening to the skin.

2. Moore and Lawrence (1952) described an infant with both recto-perineal and recto-vesical fistulae.

3. We can find no record of a true "recto-perineal fistula" alone, i.e., a high rectal dysplasia with a long fine fistula to the perineum, although such a deformity may be fallaciously thought to exist on evidence gained from fistulography should the pubo-rectalis be contracted at the time.

CHAPTER 4

Individual Deformities in the Female

(Anatomy, Sphincters, Clinical Appearance, Investigations and Rationale of Management)

AS IN THE PRECEDING CHAPTER on male deformities, the descriptions which follow are based on clinical and operative experience, combined with dissections on postmortem material.

Noncommunicating developmental defects are rare in females, and information regarding the sphincter anatomy is meager, but it is assumed to be similar to that described in males. Diagnosis depends on radiographic techniques. On the other hand, communicating anomalies are very common, and characteristic appearances in the perineum enable diagnosis to be made on clinical grounds alone. Emphasis is laid in this chapter, therefore, on the diagnostic significance of the various orifices, for it is found that the internal anatomy can be predicted with confidence from the external appearances (see Figs. 75 and 76).

As in the preceding chapter on deformities in male infants, discussions on management are confined to the rationale of treatment for each anomaly and the recommended choice of operative procedure. Details of decision between one-stage rectoplasty versus colostomy and delayed rectoplasty for rectal dysplasias, the operative techniques with advantages and disadvantages and the pre- and postoperative care are discussed in Chapters 9 and 10.

The order of description follows that of the "Proposed International Classification 1970," and reference should be made to the introductory paragraphs of the preceding chapter.

A. High Anomalies (Supralevator)

1. ANO-RECTAL AGENESIS

ANO-RECTAL AGENESIS (NO FISTULA).—In all respects, including management, this rare developmental defect in females resembles that in the male and will not be separately described. In females, the terminal blind end may lie at any level, being carried down to a variable extent by the müllerian ducts. Occasionally, there may be a blind strand connecting the rectal pouch to the vagina or perineum.

Rare variants of rectal agenesis are as follows:

1. Vesico-intestinal fissure occurs in female infants and is described in Chapter 13.

2. In reviewing seven unusual forms of imperforate anus in females, Snyder (1966) described two females with blind-ending rectums (see Fig. 51). In 1 patient, the vagina was also atretic in its midportion, and she presented with an abdominal tumor because of hydrometrocolpos. Colostomy and, later, abdomino-perineal rectoplasty were performed, but the baby died at 6 months of age of associated major anomalies. In the second patient, the rectum ended blindly near the fundus of the bladder, and the urethra and double vaginae joined a common cloacal cavity. This infant also had tracheo-esophageal fistula and other malformations.

3. Mahoney and Chamberlain (1940) recorded the very rare event of an "imperforate anus" in association with imperforate vagina, occasioned by a transverse vaginal septum. The infant presented with hydrometrocolpos.

4. In their review of colonic atresia, Trusler *et al.* (1959) included 1 female patient with no rectum, the colon ending blindly (see Chapt. 3).

Fig. 46.—Recto-vesical fistula. The rectal fistula lying cranial to the pubo-coccygeal line separates the two müllerian ducts.

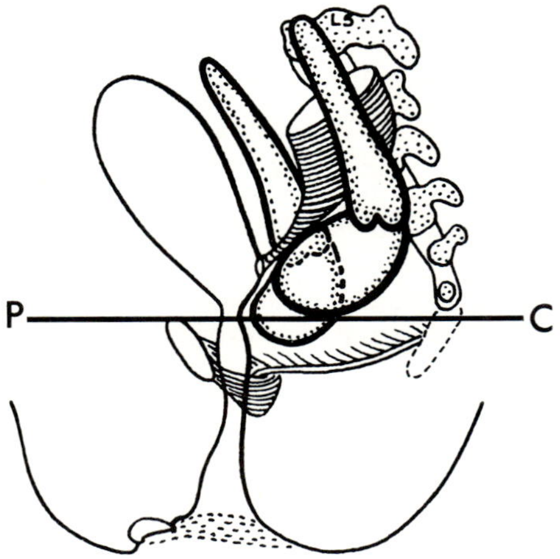

Ano-Rectal Agenesis with Fistula

(i) Recto-Vesical Fistula.—*Anatomy.*—Such a rectal opening is very rare in the female, and we have seen only one living child with this particular abnormality. However, autopsy specimens have been studied, as indicated in Figures 46 and 47. The rectal fistula opened into the base of the bladder between two completely separate müllerian systems. The separate, rudimentary and short vaginae opened also into the bladder, the outlet of which was the common cloaca, and each possessed a cervix, uterus and tube.

Fig. 47.—Recto-vesical fistula—female. **A** and **A**[1], hemisection of pelvis showing rectum (*r*) and rectal fistula entering base of bladder (*b*); part of right vagina (*v*) is seen also entering bladder. **B** and **B**[1], view of "trigone" of bladder (*b*) and internal urethral meatus (*m*). The orifices of the rectal fistula (*r*) and left vagina (*v*) are identified. Other pits are not identified.

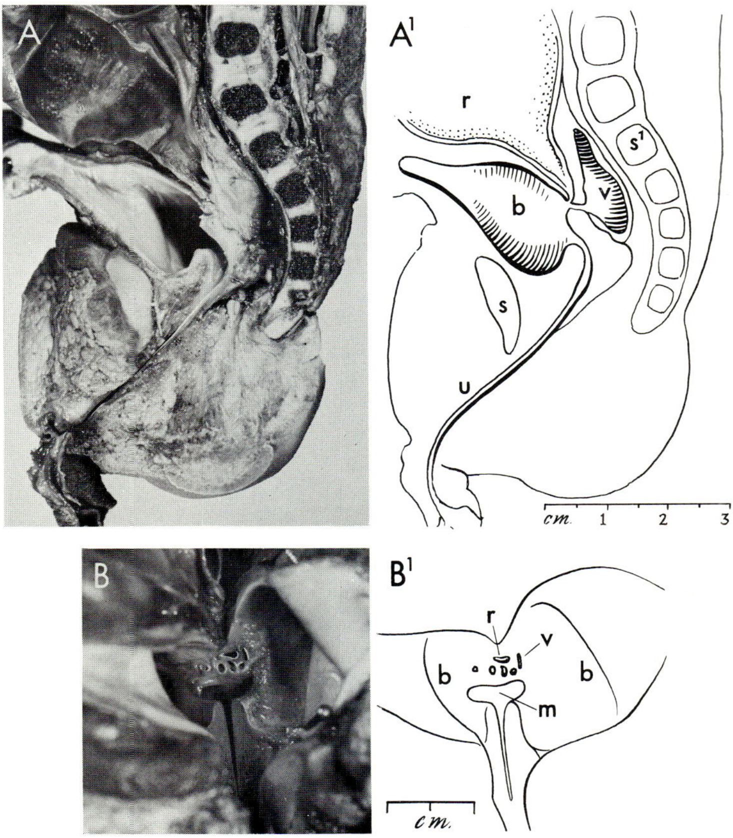

The sphincter anatomy was identical with that found in recto-cloacal fistulae (see next anomaly).

Management.—Investigation, management and recommendations are identical with those described for recto-cloacal fistulae (see next anomaly); in addition, however, persistence of urinary infection may call for division of the fistula, as in the male.

Rare variants of recto-vesical fistula are as follows:

(i) In two of the 3 cases of recto-vesical fistulae in females encountered by Trusler and Wilkinson (1962), there was no vagina, as also in Louw's case (1965), and hence only one orifice is seen in the perineum, that of the urethra.

(ii) A double fistula problem—recto-vesical plus recto-cloacal fistulae (Rehbein, 1970).

(II) RECTO-CLOACAL FISTULA.—*Anatomy.*—The orifice of the cloacal canal at birth is usually about 1 cm. in diameter or less, and the cloacal canal is elongated. The urethra enters obliquely into the anterior wall and is of normal caliber. A short vagina enters the vault of the cloacal canal, and its opening may be partly obscured by a hymenal fold. At the cranial end of the vagina the cervix protrudes into its lumen (Fig. 48). Fusion of the two müllerian systems may not occur or they may remain separate, in which case two vaginae and two cervices may be seen with an anteroposterior or obliquely oriented septum between the two at the apex of the cloaca. Gough (1959) described an unusual variety in which the cloacal canal is globular with no vaginae, and two ill-formed uteri enter directly into the canal. Of

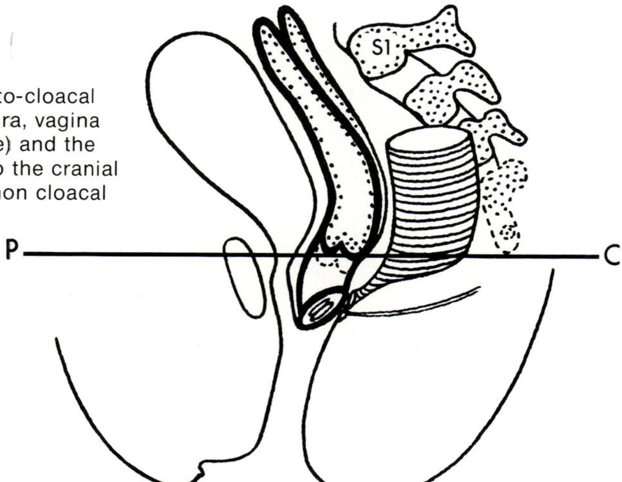

Fig. 48.—Recto-cloacal fistula. The urethra, vagina (single or septate) and the rectum issue into the cranial end of the common cloacal canal.

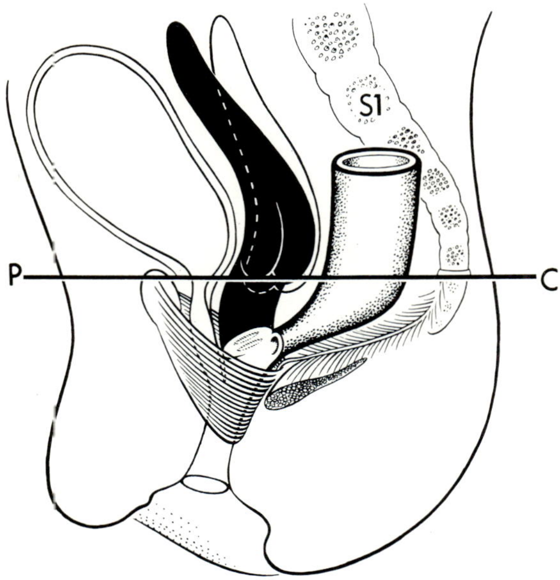

Fig. 49. – Recto-cloacal fistula. The pubo-rectalis muscle and levator diaphragm are disposed around the cloacal canal and caudal to the fistula.

our 8 cases, there was a single vagina in 3, septate vaginae in 2 and double uteri and vaginae in 3.

The urethrae may be long enough for effective sphincter control, or so short that the patient is incontinent. The rectum opens by a moderately stenotic orifice at the cranial end of the cloacal canal in the midline posteriorly, or, if there are two vaginae, immediately distal to the septum between the two.

Sphincters. – (a) Levator Ani. – The arrangement is similar to that described in recto-urethral fistula in the male (see Chapter 3). Surrounding the upper portion of the cloacal canal is a single collar of voluntary muscle, representing both the pubo-vaginalis and pubo-rectalis sections of the levator (Fig. 49). Cranially it lies close up to the caudal surface of the rectal fistula, meeting with the involuntary muscle of the rectum and laterally and posteriorly fuses closely with the cloacal walls; its action as a sphincter is on the cloacal canal rather than on the rectal orifice. The remaining portion of the levator diaphragm is disposed normally from its bony attachments laterally and posteriorly to a midline raphe extending from the pubo-rectalis anteriorly to the coccyx posteriorly. It supports the pelvic floor but has no compression action on the rectum. Sacral agenesis, common in this group, has the same effect on the levator muscle and its nerve supply as that described in recto-urethral fistula in the male (see Chapter 3).

(b) Internal Anal Sphincter.—No trace of this sphincter has been found, the inner muscle coat of the rectal wall terminating at the cloacal wall without forming a thickened ring.

(c) External Anal Sphincter.—Longitudinal anteroposterior bundles are found only beneath the perineal raphe, as in recto-urethral fistula, but they do not constitute a competent sphincter mechanism.

Perineum.—One orifice only is found in the perineum; it lies in the posterior half of the vestibule, which may be short in anteroposterior dimensions, with clitoris anterior and fourchette posterior to it. It is completely surrounded by moist red epithelium. There is usually no sign of an anal dimple, although a raphe may be found. Meconium-stained urine emerges through the common cloacal opening.

Investigations.—1. Invertography and Plain X-rays of the Spine.—Invertography is unnecessary, as the internal anatomy can be predicted from the perineal appearance of a single orifice; in any case, interpretation of the radiographs is misleading because the gas readily escapes through the fistula. Radiographs of the vertebrae, especially the sacrum, are required.

2. Micturition Cystourethrography.—In the first few weeks, this method becomes necessary in the assessment of urinary continence because the cloacal malformations may be associated with incomplete development of the bladder neck and urethral sphincters (see Chapter 12). Because of the angulation of the urethra and the internal location of the orifice, coudé gum elastic catheters should be used to negotiate the passage to the bladder.

3. Assessment of Sphincters, Nerves and Sacrum.—In all rectal anomalies, the assessment of sphincteric integrity and innervation (see Chapt. 8) is essential to management, but especially so in the high lesions in female infants. Recto-cloacal fistulae are frequently associated with severe sacral defects which may result in neurogenic lesions of bladder and levator ani.

4. Colography.—Either in the pre- or postcolostomy period, colography is required to determine the caliber of the terminal gut and the presence of secondary megacolon, especially in patients who have discharged feces through the cloaca for several weeks or more. The fistula lies at or above the P/C line.

5. Documentation of the Urinary Tract.—Because of the frequency of associated urinary anomalies, the state of the urinary tract should be documented by intravenous pyelography, blood urea nitrogen estimation and by renography; these, with the micturition cystourethrogram, can be performed in the first few weeks of life. Apart from that produced from urinary anomalies themselves, however,

urinary infection is not as common as in the male because the female fistulae enter the genital rather than the urinary tract. Nevertheless, urine microscopy and culture should not be omitted.

6. Vaginoscopy.—This method defines the actual site and size of the fistula and also confirms the vaginal anatomy (septate, etc.). The actual rectal fistula may be difficult to locate amongst the confusion of orifices. This can be done in the neonate at the time of the colostomy.

Management.—In this and all communication deformities in the female, the orifice of the fistula is larger than in the male, and immediate obstructive crises are uncommon, and operation is not an urgent concern. The gas and soft feces escape readily at first, and treatment may be unwittingly deferred. Once the bowel content hardens, especially when the baby is switched from breast to cow's milk, fecaliths accumulate, and the rectum becomes large, overdistended, sluggish, necessitating energetic measures to evacuate the content and sometimes radical excision at the time of the rectoplasty operation.

In the neonatal period, although decompression is partly achieved through the fistula, we still prefer a colostomy because of the dangers of secondary megacolon and because of the technical advantages of performing the rectoplasty at a later stage (see Chapt. 9). The rationale of surgical treatment is identical with that discussed under recto-urethral fistula to which the reader is referred. An additional reason for deferring the definitive rectoplasty in some patients is the occasional presence of a large mucocolpos which complicates the pelvic dissection; it also adds to the difficulty in determining the state of urinary continence.

In patients seen beyond infancy, in whom defecation has been allowed to continue through the fistula, we still advocate a temporary period of colostomy defunctioning prior to a rectoplasty, partly to reduce the caliber of the gut and partly to protect the newly channelled pubo-visceral sling after rectoplasty from too-rapid dilatation and stretching.

The recommended procedure is as follows:

(i) Transverse colostomy in the newborn period.

(ii) Postoperative clearance, by washouts, of the distal limb of the colostomy to avoid cloacal contamination and possible urinary infection.

(iii) Completion of investigations as to the exact anatomy of the fistula, of the urinary and genital tracts and of the sphincteric nerve supply, performed over the next 3 months—clinical tests of continence, micturition cystourethrography, colography, urine analysis, intravenous pyelography and blood urea nitrogen estimation.

(iv) Rectoplasty at 12–15 months of age. As in recto-urethral fistulae in the male, the same choice of operative procedure offers, and we favor a combined sacro-abdomino-perineal approach (Chapt. 9).

(v) Closure of the colostomy 3 months later, after graduated digital dilatation and patient stretching of the pubo-rectalis sling.

(vi) The genito-urinary defects may then require correction—vaginoplasty or correction of urinary incontinence (Chapt. 12). Vaginoplasty should not be undertaken until long after rectoplasty has been completed. During childhood and adolescence, spontaneous widening and shortening of the canal may render operations unnecessary, although a large mucocolpos would demand early drainage (Stephens, 1967).

Rare variants of recto-cloacal fistula are as follows:

These have been reviewed by Lowsley (1948), Gough (1959), Stephens (1961, 1966) and Snyder (1966).

1. We possibly have 1 patient with a recto-urethral fistula, or else a rare variety of cloacal fistula, and 1 patient each is reported by Mayo and Rice (1950), Hanley *et al.* (1954) and Brayton and Norris (1958), but no details are provided.

Our female infant (female by sex chromatin and chromosome

Fig. 50.—Recto-cloacal fistula. Rectum and urethra join the cloacal outlet; the vagina is hypotrophic and opens between the urethral and rectal orifices (*crossed arrow*). The uro-genital sinus is covered in almost to the clitoris (*black arrows*).

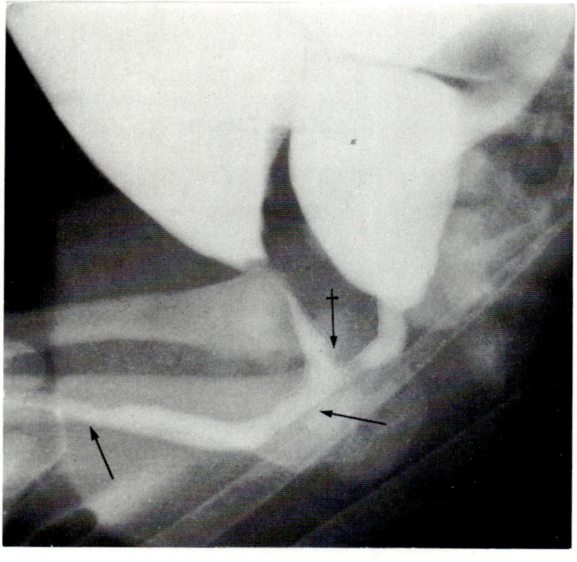

studies) appeared to have a long recto-urethral fistula (Fig. 50). The rectum was voluminous and spiralled into the pelvis to enter the urethra anteriorly. At the operation for rectoplasty, the fistula was found to enter the urethra, but cranial to the fistulous opening was a tiny stenotic orifice opening into a minute vagina and uterus. It is a moot point, therefore, whether the common conduit opening to the exterior should be called a "urethra" or a "cloaca"; if the latter, this child's deformity is a recto-cloacal fistula. However, the conduit appeared radiologically and functionally to be a urethra. This infant also exhibits thin or absent abdominal muscles and megacystis. There is also exomphalos and universal mesentery, and the labia and phallus are large. At present, she survives following exomphalos repair, colostomy, rectoplasty and finally closure of colostomy.

2. Gough (1959) described 18 cases over a 10-year period at the Hospital for Sick Children, London. Apart from the recto-cloacal fistula, the cases included the following:

(a) A wide vesico-cloacal orifice with urinary incontinence and absence of uteri and tubes.

(b) Mucocolpos presenting as an abdominal tumor (1 patient also had a double rectum).

(c) Cloaca with a minute external orifice.

(d) Cloacal fistula between double uteri into the septum between vaginae but accompanied by a cystic duplication of the rectum.

(e) Pseudohermaphroditism.

(f) Cloacal orifice with a tubelike phallus.

In all cases, there were accompanying malformations, such as renal dysplasia, agenesis of urethra, megacystis, congenital heart disease, tracheo-esophageal fistula and sacral and other vertebral anomalies.

3. Recto-cloacal fistula, with nonadrenal female pseudohermaphroditism, 2 cases (Sieber and Klein, 1958). These cases were unusual in that the cloacal opening was at the anal site rather than in the vestibule. In one, a urethra continued through a phallus, but an additional urinary opening communicated with the cloacal canal.

4. We have encountered 1 case of recto-cloacal fistula associated with vesico-intestinal fissure, described under this heading in Chapter 13.

5. Snyder (1966) reported in detail 7 female patients with unusual varieties of cloacal malformation and reviewed the possible embryology. These reports are summarized in Figure 51. Cases 1 and 2 appear to have conditions similar to the usual forms described above, with, however, a cloacal canal of small caliber. One infant had an abdominal mass from hydrometrocolpos. At 1 year after abdomino-perineal rectoplasty, one child is continent, and one incontinent.

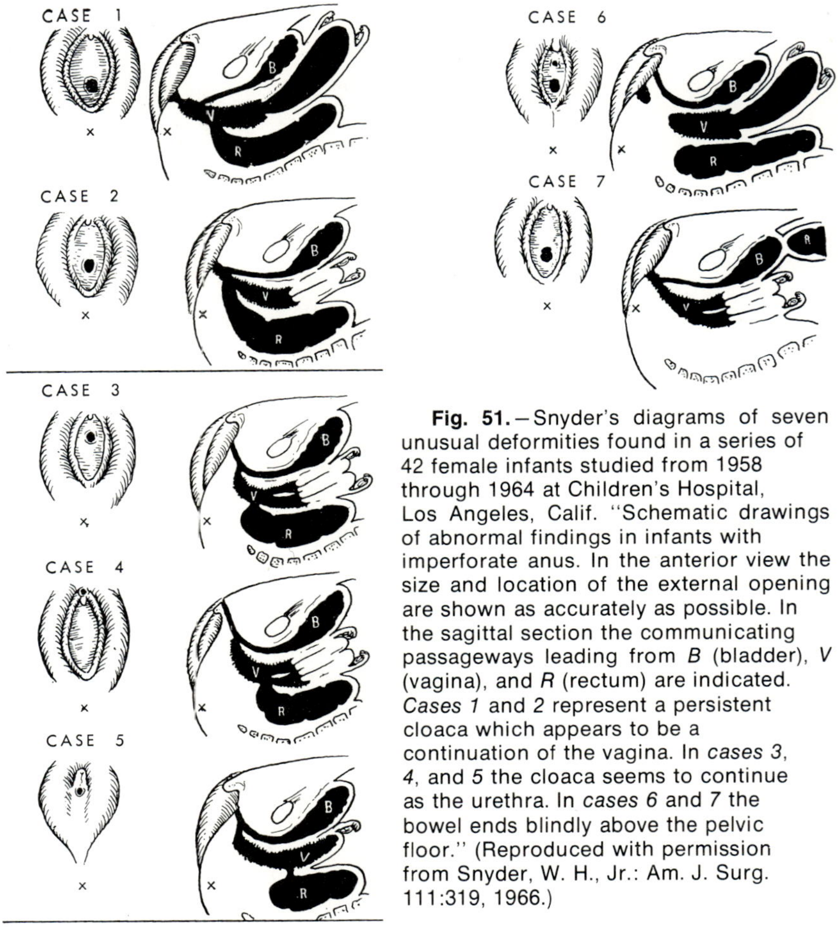

Fig. 51.—Snyder's diagrams of seven unusual deformities found in a series of 42 female infants studied from 1958 through 1964 at Children's Hospital, Los Angeles, Calif. "Schematic drawings of abnormal findings in infants with imperforate anus. In the anterior view the size and location of the external opening are shown as accurately as possible. In the sagittal section the communicating passageways leading from *B* (bladder), *V* (vagina), and *R* (rectum) are indicated. *Cases 1* and *2* represent a persistent cloaca which appears to be a continuation of the vagina. In *cases 3, 4*, and *5* the cloaca seems to continue as the urethra. In *cases 6* and *7* the bowel ends blindly above the pelvic floor." (Reproduced with permission from Snyder, W. H., Jr.: Am. J. Surg. 111:319, 1966.)

In Cases 3, 4 and 5, the cloacae appeared to be continued into a penile or clitoral urethra, and in 1 patient (Case 4) this was epispadic in character, opening on the anterior aspect of the glans clitoris. Two children died of multiple deformities, and the child in Case 5 is alive and continent after abdomino-perineal rectoplasty and vaginoplasty. Cases 4 and 7 are examples of imperforate rectum without fistula, although patients with a condition similar to that in Case 7 would present with one cloacal opening. As in all series, Snyder's patients had many malformations in association.

6. A double fistula problem—recto-cloacal plus recto-vesical fistulae (Rehbein, 1970).

7. Cartledge (1970) depicts a recto-cloacal fistula with a narrow rectal orifice, huge megarectum, and absent appendix (and foreshortened colon).

(III) RECTO-VAGINAL FISTULA.—In the International Classification (1970), only *high* recto-vaginal fistulae are included in the high (supralevator) group of anomalies, whereas low recto-vaginal fistulae are listed in the intermediate group. We agree with this, as the surgical approach to low fistulae is controversial—some surgeons preferring a supralevator approach, others preferring to operate directly from below via the perineum. However, as described below, both lesions are embryologically identical and with essentially the same anatomy, and, for convenience, we describe both levels together in this section.

Anatomy.—The vagina and hymen are usually normal, although occasionally the vagina may be divided into halves by a midline septum above the site of entry of the fistula. The bladder and urethra are normal. The rectal fistula opens in the midline into the posterior wall of the vagina. It may be at any level in the vagina, from the posterior fornix to near the hymen, but most commonly is in the lower one third of the vagina (Fig. 52). In many classifications (see Chapter 6), high vaginal fistulae are considered embryologically as recto-cloacal anomalies in contradistinction to those fistulae in the lower portion of the vagina, which are erroneously considered "low" anomalies of the ectopic type and due to failure of migration. However, embryologically, they are both rectal deformities and, in any case,

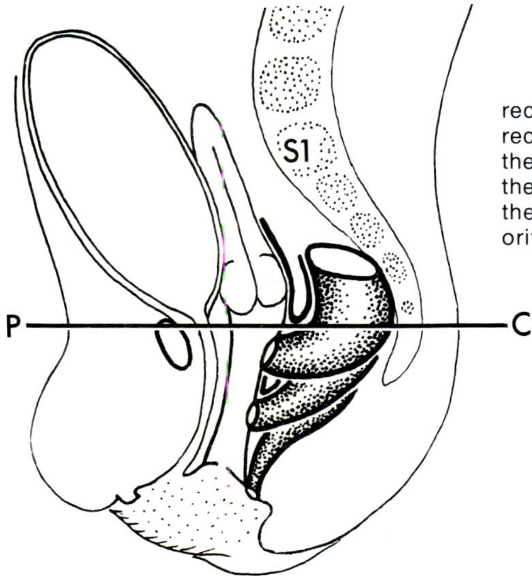

Fig. 52.—Recto-vaginal and recto-vestibular fistulae. The rectum issues into the back of the vagina at any level or into the vestibule contiguous with the posterior wall of the vaginal orifice.

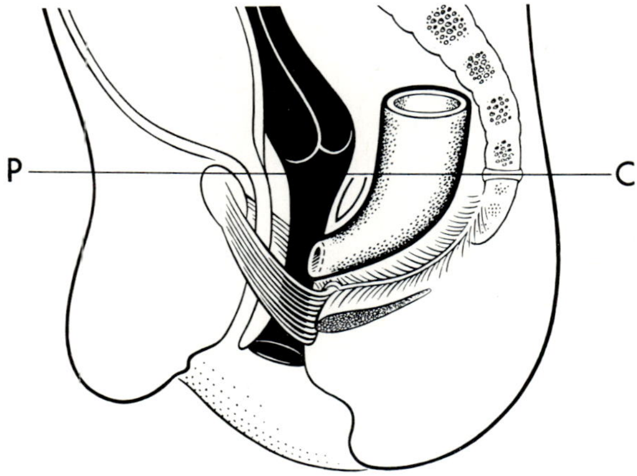

Fig. 53.—Recto-vaginal fistula. The pelvic diaphragm and the pubo-visceral sling lie caudal to the fistula, whether the fistula is high or low.

the bowel and fistula at whatever level lie above the pubo-rectalis sling. We do show these as high and low in the classification, to recognize the "intermediate" nature of the low fistulae, and because we do make a distinction therapeutically.

The orifice of the rectal fistula is usually not difficult to locate as it is moderately large and permits gas and soft feces to emerge freely through it. The baby is, therefore, not immediately obstructed but may present later in infancy because of the unusual exit of feces from the vagina or because of an obstructive episode.

Sphincters.—(a) Levator Ani.—The muscle arrangement is identical with that in recto-cloacal and recto-urethral fistulae (of the male); the pubo-rectalis is continuous with the pubo-vaginalis fibers immediately caudal to the rectal fistula, adjacent to the vaginal wall (Fig. 53). If the rectal fistula is high in the vagina, the sphincter has no action on the rectal opening; in low recto-vaginal fistulae, the bulk of the collar is carried downwards towards the perineum and remains caudal to the fistula, the most caudal muscle fibers partially surrounding the orifice and providing a degree of continence. Some such patients beyond the infancy period exhibit moderately good control of the fecal exit, although soiling of the vagina is inevitable.

(b) and (c) Internal and External Anal Sphincters.—These rudimentary structures are identical with those in recto-cloacal and recto-urethral fistulae.

Perineum.—Apart from the absence of the anus, the vulva and vestibule, together with the orifices of the urethra and vagina, present a normal external appearance. Meconium issues from the vagina. The site of the absent anus follows no special pattern—there may be a dimple or midline raphe. The distinctive diagnostic feature is that two external orifices only are visible in the entire perineum.

Investigations.—The interpretation of radiographs and vaginoscopy is like that described for recto-cloacal fistulae, apart from the normal position of the urethra. Invertography is unreliable and not required in the diagnosis, and direct or endoscopic examination is more appropriate and sure. The other investigations are as described for recto-cloacal fistula.

Management and Recommendations.—Possibly no other ano-rectal defect has provoked such divergence of surgical opinion as the recto-vaginal fistula.

HIGH RECTO-VAGINAL FISTULA.—Little confusion attaches to the high fistulae, which are accepted as "high" anomalies, their management being identical with that of a recto-cloacal fistula, except that there is seldom anxiety about urinary infection. As the orifice of the fistula may decompress the gut, there is seldom urgency, but, if operation is unduly delayed, the colon becomes a reservoir, overflows and impacts proximal to the fistula. The development of such a secondary megacolon complicates management both before and after the deferred rectoplasty. We, therefore, prefer to do a colostomy, clean out the distal bowel and defer the rectoplasty rather than allow the child to defecate through the vagina—with the attendant persistent soiling, vaginitis and skin excoriation. More particularly, however, our choice for a staged procedure is governed by the technical requirements of the rectoplasty, which are discussed in common with the management of all rectal anomalies (see Chapt. 9).

Our *recommendations* are identical with those for recto-cloacal fistula (see above for details), i.e.:

(i) Transverse colostomy in the newborn period.

(ii) Rectoplasty at 12–15 months of age, and the high supralevator nature of the anomaly necessitates abdominal exploration. Our procedure is sacro-perineal-abdominal rectoplasty (Chapt. 9).

(iii) Closure of colostomy 3 months later, after rectal dilatation.

Authors in support of a staged program, who particularly specify high vaginal fistulae, are Palmer (1956)—rectoplasty at 1–4 years; Kiesewetter *et al.* (1964)—rectoplasty late but not stated when; Santulli *et al.* (1965)—rectoplasty at 9–12 months; Louw (1965)—rectoplasty at 3 months.

Those who support one-stage neonatal rectoplasty are Norris *et al.* (1949), Gross (1953), Rhoads and Koop (1955), Brayton and Norris (1958), Trusler and Wilkinson (1962), Gans and Friedman (1963), Rehbein (1967) and Swenson and Donnellan (1967).

Surprisingly, for high recto-vaginal dysplasia, Potts *et al.* (1954)

advocated anal transplantation from the perineum at 6 months of age, and Snyder (1961) commences with a perineal exploration at 6 months, and, if this proves impossible, the operation is extended to an abdomino-perineal procedure. When the site of the fistula is known to be high, we believe a perineal exploration cannot safely expose the rectum without endangering the pubo-rectalis, which hugs the vagina below the rectum.

LOW RECTO-VAGINAL FISTULA.—In the management of low vaginal fistulae, however, three views are held:

(i) No operation need be performed, as the child may have reasonable continence because the most caudal fibers of the pubo-rectalis partly surround the orifice and vagina. Some children are said to have been continent, regular in bowel habit and symptom free in the uncorrected state, but the confusion of terms and the lack of understanding of the differences between recto-vaginal and ano-vestibular fistula, with their utterly different consequences to cleanliness, undermine the validity of these claims. The fact remains that the recto-vaginal fistula projects feces into the vagina, producing soiling, vaginitis and skin excoriation. If a patient is found to be symptom free and normal in bowel habit, there is obviously no need for urgency about operation, but such a rare event should not set the pattern of management for the majority.

(ii) The anus may be transplanted backwards by a perineal approach. Many surgeons favor this approach, the prevailing view being that the rectum can be safely dissected out from the levator ani from a relatively simple exposure below, that, since it is completed in infancy, dilatations are not remembered by the child and that colonic inertia and entero-colitis are less likely if the rectal orifice in the perineum is adequate in dimensions. The anal transplantation is performed at varying times: Stone (1936), at puberty; Potts *et al.* (1954), at 6 months; Hanley *et al.* (1954), in "weeks or months"; Rhoads and Koop (1955), in "a few months"; Donovan and Stanley-Brown (1958), at 4–5 months; Louw (1959 and 1965), at 4 years; Partridge and Gough (1961), in first 9 months; Snyder (1961), unstated; Lynn and Arcari (1962), when 25 lb. weight or more; Gans and Friedman (1963), at 3 months; Kiesewetter *et al.* (1964), at 6–12 months; Sauvage and Bill (1965), "in first few weeks or months"; Swenson and Donnellan (1967), in the neonatal period.

In the interim period from birth to the time of transplantation, if the orifice of the fistula is adequate in size, no treatment is given, apart from that for constipation. If the orifice is stenotic, most authors favor simple dilatations, but Louw (1965) performs a Denis Browne "cutback" to open the orifice definitively backwards into the perineum. The enlarged orifice tends to resume its forward tilt into the posterior vaginal wall and remains within the vestibule, so that later transplantation remains necessary, but the orifice functions well during early childhood.

In the technique of transplantation, many variations have been introduced. In Stone's operation (1936), the levator was divided and sutured in front of the rectum. Subsequent techniques vary only slightly, but almost all surgeons utilize a method similar to that described by Santulli (1969) and discussed in Chapter 10. We seriously disagree with this technique, most importantly because the rectum is mobilized well above the pelvic floor "posteriorly and laterally well up into the hollow of the sacrum," a dissection that must involve dislocation of the levator fibers. Reference to the anatomy detailed above indicates that the pubo-rectalis is intimately related to the posterior vaginal wall at or caudal to the fistula. We do not agree that the integrity of the muscle can be guaranteed by approaching it in this position from below.

Further, as indicated in the discussion of ano-cutaneous fistula in the male, stress is often laid, in these transplant operations, on the *external* sphincter, a structure which we find to be frequently flimsy and rudimentary.

However, in the technique described by Nixon (1961), in Chapter 10, and those described by Louw (1965) and by Swenson and Donnellan (1967), the anatomy is properly considered by keeping the dissection superficial to the pelvic floor, by tunneling anterior to the pubo-rectalis and by considering the external sphincter as only of minor importance.

(iii) Because of the intimate relationship of the pubo-rectalis to the vagina and fistula, *our recommendation* is a sacro-perineal approach for the low vaginal fistula. The operation can be performed through this sacro-perineal exposure, which fully defines and protects the pubo-rectalis, and the abdomen need not be opened, the whole operation being performed from the back. Because of the technical details required to conserve the sling (see Chapt. 9), we prefer to perform this operation at 12–15 months, after a colostomy in the newborn period, as for high vaginal fistulae. Santulli *et al.* (1965), in a recent review, have altered their approach and now suggest colostomy, followed by abdomino-perineal rectoplasty at 9–12 months. It is interesting to note that Carter and Lyall, in 1940, described the repair of a low vaginal fistula via the sacro-coccygeal approach; however, they make no mention of the levator ani during the dissection, except to show an illustration of the muscle being sutured in front of the rectum.

In other respects, our management is identical with that described for recto-cloacal fistula.

Rare variants of recto-vaginal fistula are as follows:

1. Moore and Lawrence (1952) mention 1 patient with a double fistula, i.e., both a recto-vaginal and a recto-perineal fistula.

2. The same authors mention a patient with a recto-vaginal fistula and hydrometrocolpos.

3. Colo-vaginal fistulae (2 patients) were reported, in association with absence of rectum and partial absence of colon, by Trusler *et al.* (1959), and are described with other examples of colonic atresia in Chapter 3.

4. Several authors report an H-shaped configuration of a recto-vaginal fistula, but with the anus continuing patent to the normal site (Loufti, 1970; Nixon, 1970; Ramakrishnan, 1970; Mishalany, 1970). This combination is almost identical with our description of the perineal canal, in which the fistula is into the vestibule (easily confused with a low vaginal fistula). Santulli (1970) also reports a similar anomaly, but the anus is stenotic.

5. Recto-vaginal fistula and ectopia vesicae are described by Santulli (1970).

2. Rectal Atresia

This lesion is a very rare one, and the anatomy, clinical appearance and management are identical with those described for the male (see Chapter 3). Only two examples of this lesion in the female have been seen by us, and only 15 cases are recorded in almost 3,000 cases reviewed in the literature.

Magnus (1968) has dissected the sphincter anatomy of 1 infant, and we describe the findings in full because of the important part they play in suggesting the etiology of this lesion. The infant had multiple atresias of both small and large bowel and died a few days after birth. Serial sections were cut through the whole pubis at intervals of 10μ. The perineum and vulva were normal, and there was a normal anal pit with anal valves and pink mucosa cranially. In the brain, the corpus callosum and gyrus cinguli were absent. There were multiple atresias of the small bowel, and yet the lowest isolated segments contained green meconium. The ascending, transverse and descending colons were absent, but two isolated segments of the sigmoid colon were present. The rectum was a blind, pear-shaped structure 17 mm. long by 8 mm. in diameter (Fig. 54, *A*) and connected to the anal canal by a fibro-muscular band. The epithelium of the rectum was normal columnar with goblet cells and crypts. Similarly, in the anal canal, the epithelium was normal, with stratified squamous below the valves, and there was a 3-mm. strip of stratified columnar epithelium cranial to the valves.

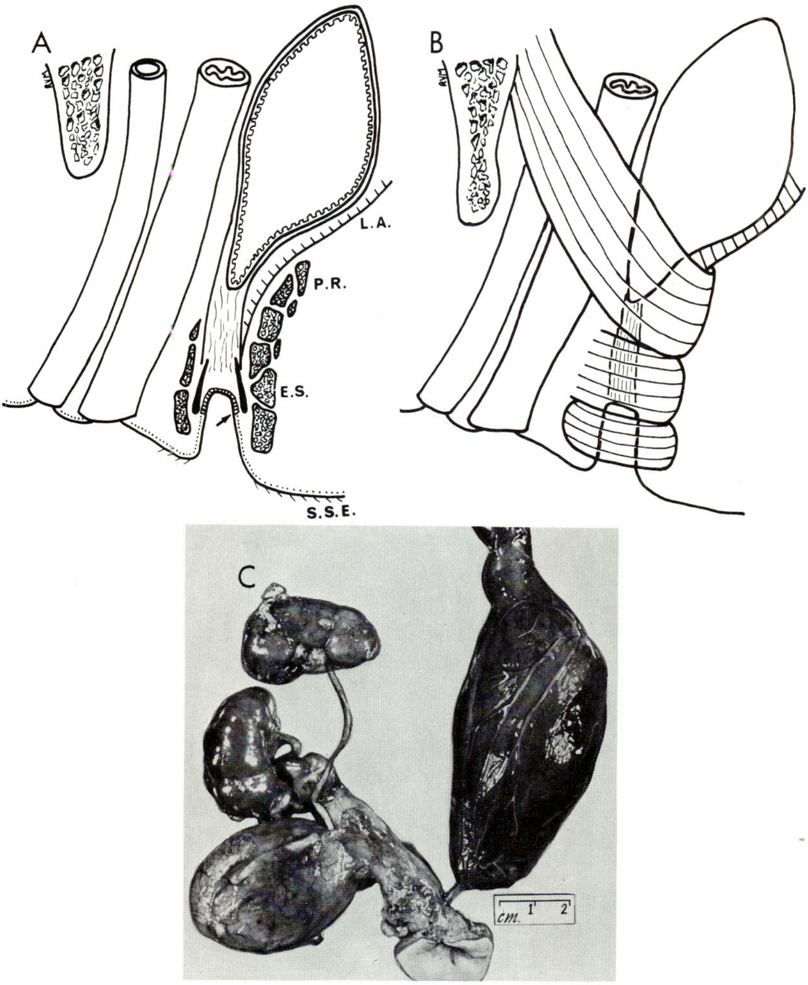

Fig. 54. – Rectal atresia. Pelvic organs of a baby who exhibited multiple atresias of small and large bowel and rectum (see text). **A,** isolated rectal segment showing no attachment to the sigmoid and a long fibro-muscular connection to a well-formed anal pit. Arrow indicates anal valves and a lower margin of internal sphincter muscle. *E.S.* = external sphincter. *P.R.* = pubo-rectalis. *L.A.* = levator ani. *S.S.E.* = stratified squamous epithelium. **B,** voluntary muscle of pubo-rectalis and external sphincter normally disposed around the atresic zone. **C,** another specimen showing atresic rectum and normal appearance of anal pit. The vagina and bladder are anterior and normal in appearances. (*A* and *B* reproduced with permission from Magnus, R.: J. Pediat. Surg. 3:593, 1968.)

The rectal wall was invested in normal, circular and longitudinal muscle coats, and there was smooth muscle in the fibrous band between rectum and anal canal. There was a thick circular smooth muscle terminating caudally at the anal valves, and cranially, with the smooth muscle in the fibrous band, representing the internal sphincter; the levator ani muscle was normal, including a pubo-rectalis disposed around the lower rectum and fibrous cord; the external sphincter was similarly well developed (Fig. 54, *B* and *C*).

The evidence for an atresia rather than agenesis is as follows:

(i) Both the internal and external sphincters were present in the specimen, unlike those in agenesis.

(ii) The fact that there is stratified columnar epithelium above the line of membrane breakdown (anal valves) indicates that the gut lumen from both hindgut and proctodeal pit has developed normally; the site of atresia is thus more proximal than that expected from embryological agenesis of rectum. In an embryological defect, one would expect that either or both components of hindgut and proctodeum would be deficient, and the anal membrane would not break down.

(iii) A fibro-muscular band is commonly seen between blind segments of small intestine, believed now to be of acquired origin. In this baby (Fig. 54, *A*), there was bile in the lower segments, proving that the gut had once had a lumen.

Magnus further suggests the approximate time that the atresias may have developed, between the 65-mm. stage and the 112-mm. stage (13th–14th week), i.e., much later than a developmental defect, because the lumen of the digestive tube is normally complete by the 56-mm. stage. This evidence is based upon the following:

(a) The level of the internal sphincter. Fowler (1957) found that the internal sphincter is above the anal membrane site at the 65-mm. stage and well below the valves at the 125-mm. stage. In this specimen (Fig. 54, *A*), the sphincter lay at the valves, indicating that the rectal wall had developed to beyond the 65-mm. stage.

(b) Bile in the bowel. Bile does not begin to secrete until about the 56-mm. stage.

(c) Absent gyrus cinguli and corpus callosum; this portion of the brain begins to develop about the 112-mm. stage.

Management.—Management is identical with that described for the male (see Chapter 3).

B. Intermediate Anomalies

The concept of the "intermediate" level of anomalies is the same as in the male and the introductory paragraph therein (see Chapter 3) should be read.

1. Anal Agenesis

Anal Agenesis (No Fistula).—An imperforate anus without fistula ending blindly at the radiographic I point of the pelvis is a rare lesion in the female. In all respects, the condition is identical with that of the male and will not be further described (see Chapter 3).

Anal Agenesis with Fistula

(i) Recto-Vaginal Fistula (Low).—For the convenience of the reader, this condition has already been described with the high vaginal fistula.

(ii) Recto-Vestibular Fistula.—The reader is referred to the section on terminology (Chapt. 6), in order to distinguish this fistula from an ano-vestibular fistula and others of the cloacal complex.

Anatomy.—The rectum usually terminates below the pubococcygeal line or, less commonly, at the line, and from its anterior wall arises a narrow fistula to the vestibule, 1–2 cm. in length, immediately adjacent to the posterior wall of the vagina. The "intermediate" nature of the anomaly is because the fistula itself is translevator, opening as it does in the vestibule, but the distended terminal bowel is supralevator. Further, the length of the fistula varies so that

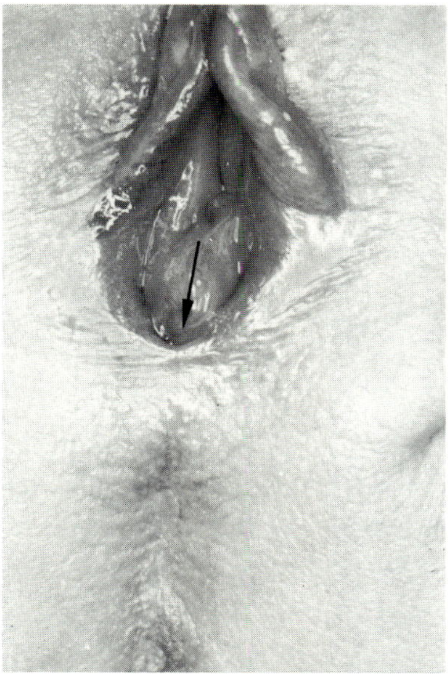

Fig. 55.—Recto-vestibular fistula. The narrow orifice (*arrow*) of the fistula is tucked under and hidden by the posterior border of the vestibule.

in marginal cases it may be difficult to decide whether to place the anomaly in the high recto-vestibular group or the low ano-vestibular group.

The vagina may be double, in which case the fistula is fine and delicate and lies in the most posterior part of the septum, between the two vaginae.

Sphincters.—(a) Levator Ani.—No specimen of this unusual type has been available for dissection, but on clinical grounds the levator sling appears to resemble that pertaining to a moderately low recto-vaginal fistula, i.e., the upper fibers of the pubo-rectalis muscle engage the terminal rectum, the remaining fibers gripping the fistula.

(b) and (c) Internal and External Anal Sphincters.—The state of these sphincters is not known, but presumably they are rudimentary, resembling those of a recto-vaginal fistula.

Perineum.—The perineal appearances are identical with those of an ano-vestibular fistula (see below) (Fig. 55); however, a probe passed into the fistula is naturally directed in a strictly cranial direction in immediate proximity to the vaginal wall and is restrained from turning posteriorly beneath the perineum. There is no posterior mobility in the rectum (Fig. 56, and see Fig. 106, *A*). The vagina is usually double, in which case the fistula lies in the posterior part of the septum, between the two vaginae.

Investigations.—Inspection of the perineum revealing three orifices in the vestibule, combined with probe tests, defines the condition, and invertography in the newborn period is unnecessary. However, a cologram through the colostomy may confirm the lowest level of normal caliber rectum and indicate the length of the fistula.

The investigations are identical with those outlined for recto-cloacal fistula. The length of the fistula may be measured by a Foley catheter marked in centimeters (Fig. 56). By this test, a distinction can be made from the ano-vestibular fistula, which is less than 1 cm. long. We have not confirmed as yet whether retrograde injection of the fistula with radiopaque material will prove of practical help; it may prove useful in distinguishing the length of the narrow fistula, and, as in recto-vestibular, ano-vestibular and ano-vulvar fistulae, this technique is open to error because of the compression effects of the encircling muscle sling (Fig. 57 and see Fig. 107).

Management and Recommendations.—As the terminal bowel is cranial to the main mass of the pubo-rectalis muscle, the management is similar in principle to that for recto-cloacal fistula. Unlike the procedure appropriate to an ano-vestibular fistula, it is not advisable to attempt to dilate or "cutback" the vestibular orifice, as the thin wall and intimate relation of the fistula to the posterior vaginal wall result in rupture of the common septum between fistula and vagina, converting the two orifices into one recto-vaginal orifice.

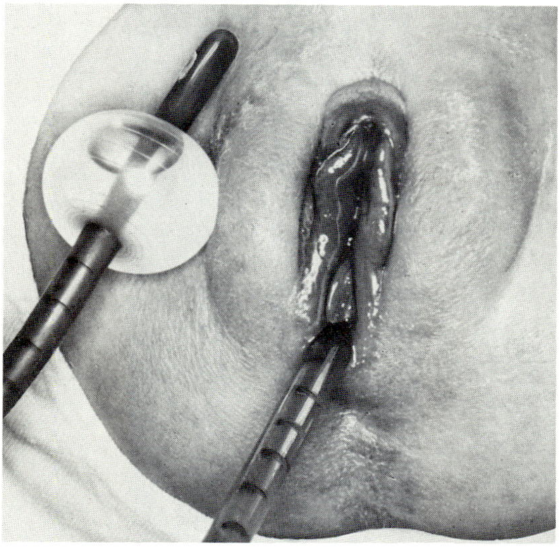

Fig. 56.—Recto-vestibular fistula. The length of the narrow segment of the fistula is measured by the Foley catheter technique: insert the catheter, inflate the balloon, draw back and measure.

Fig. 57.—Recto-vestibular fistula. Retrograde injection of vagina and rectal fistula. The recto-vestibular fistula is 1.0 cm. long (*lower two arrows* in **A**), but, because the pubo-rectalis compresses the distal end of the rectum (**B**), the fistula has the misleading appearance of much greater length (*upper* and *lower arrows* in **A**). Barium clearly shows the contours of the vagina, the filling defect of the cervix and the vestibule.

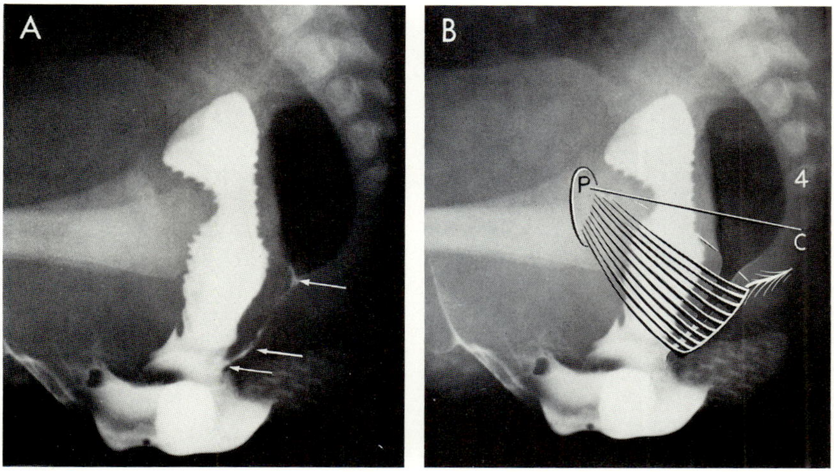

Even though an adequate perineal opening might be achieved, the acquired vaginal fistula then requires treatment. For these reasons we perform a colostomy at birth, and a rectoplasty by the sacro-perineal operation at 12–15 months.

Sometimes the fistula is relatively short and mistaken for an ano-vestibular lesion. A cutback procedure on the orifice may be undertaken in the first instance, but subsequent inability to dilate the fistula, or splitting of the vaginal wall, indicates the true state, and, at this stage, a colostomy should be performed, with subsequent rectoplasty.

2. Ano-Rectal Stenosis

In the female the condition is identical with that in the male (see Chapter 3), and will not be further described.

C. Low Anomalies (Translevator)

As in the male anomalies at this level, all constitute "anal deformities," and the bowel has penetrated the pubo-rectalis sling. In addition to the anomalies at the normal anal site, and further forward in the perineum in the female, there are several additional deformities which open in the vulval area and are separately described.

1. At Normal Anal Site

(i) Covered Anus – Complete (including imperforate anal membrane).

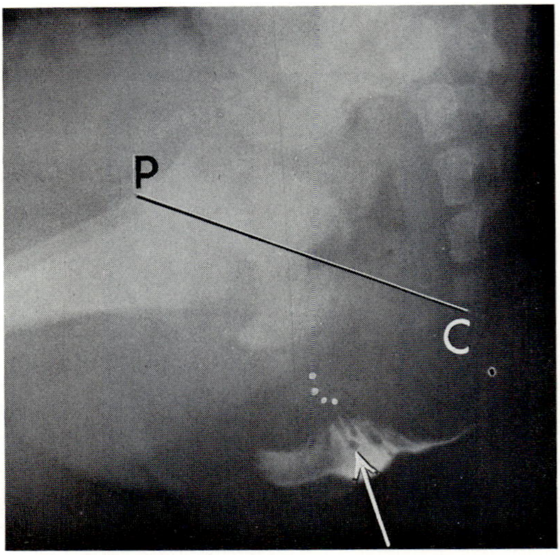

Fig. 58. – Anal membrane stenosis. White dots demarcate the edges of the membrane in relation to the anal pit (*arrow*). Dots overlie small wire sutures inserted into the edges of the membrane.

(ii) ANAL STENOSIS (covered anal stenosis and anal membrane stenosis, Fig. 58).

No special features of these lesions differ from those already described for the male (see Chapter 3) to which the reader is referred. Each group includes the anal membrane deformities. We have not actually seen a completely occluded anus of the covered type in the female.

2. AT PERINEAL SITE

(I) ANTERIOR PERINEAL ANUS.—The anatomy of this lesion and its sphincters is identical with that of the male (see Chapter 3). Taken together with the other variety of anterior anus in females, the vulvar anus, an anterior anus is more commonly encountered in females than in males.

The anterior perineal anus is normal in caliber and function but lies in an anterior cutaneous position in the dry skin of the perineum. The orifice is skin lined and lies near or may be contiguous with the posterior limit of the vulva which is otherwise normal. (Fig. 59, *A*, *B* and *C*).

Management.—Management differs in no way from anterior anus in the male, which functions normally in its abnormal position. Vulval cleanliness in anterior perineal anus is not interfered with, and transplantation backwards is rarely necessary.

(II) ANO-CUTANEOUS FISTULA (COVERED ANUS—INCOMPLETE).—An anal fistula situated at or near the junction of vestibule and perineal skin, with the bowel extending somewhat backwards behind it, has been variously described as a covered anus (Denis Browne, 1951 and 1955; and Stephens, 1955) or as a type of ectopic anus which has failed to complete its migration. (Nixon, 1961; Partridge and Gough, 1961; and Bill, 1964). Nixon points out that the tract to the anus in the female is lined by mucosa instead of squamous epithelium as in the male and that "the anus is not surrounded by a fully formed external sphincter like the male covered anus." He, therefore, is not convinced that the idea of "covering" is always applicable. However, our experience in the male is that the external sphincter is also incomplete, so that the latter criterion is of limited validity. Furthermore, there are several additional points of evidence that the process of covering applies equally to the female, as described below, and we adhere to Stephens' viewpoint. The reader is referred to the male description of ano-cutaneous fistula in Chapter 3 for a more complete discussion of embryology.

As we believe that the ano-vulvar fistula is only another variety of the covering concept, extending the fistula in this case into the vulva, there is necessarily some overlap in the descriptions which follow.

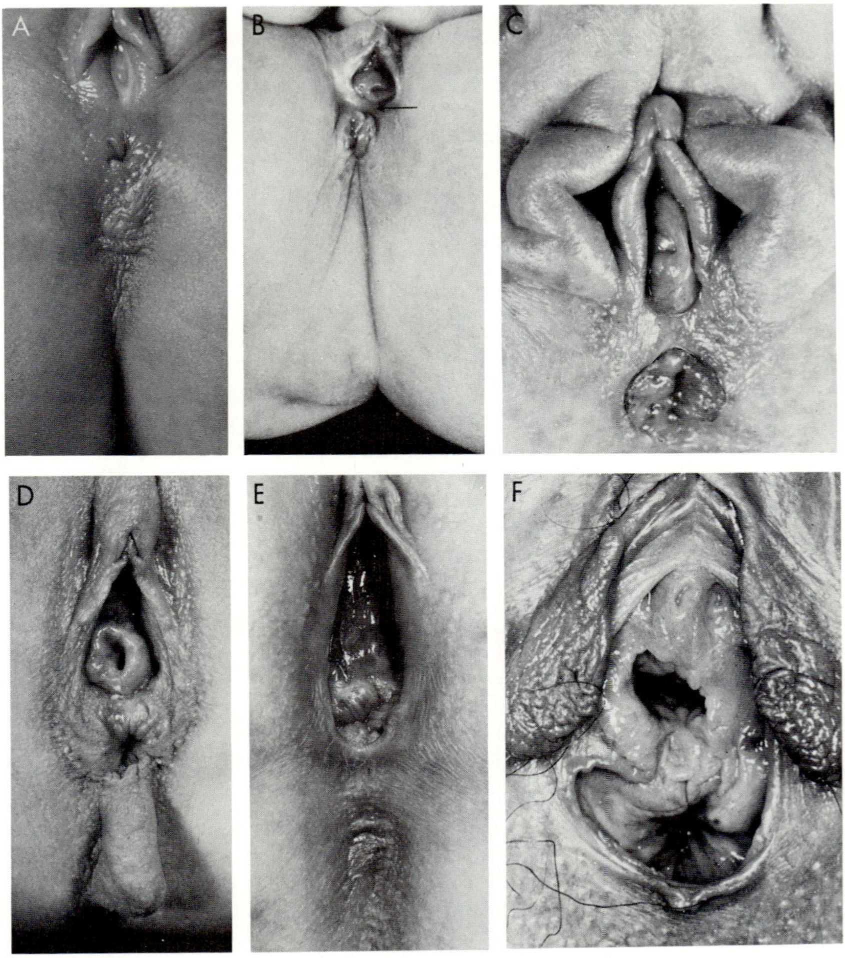

Fig. 59.—Varieties of anterior anus. Perineal (**A**), (**B**) and (**C**), the anus is behind the vestibule; vulvar (**D**) and (**E**); and ano-vestibular fistula (**F**). **A,** normal anus set anterior to the normal site. **B,** untidy anus bunched up behind the vestibule, with narrow perineal skin bridge between (*arrow*). **C,** narrow, deeply set skin bridge between vestibule and anus which lacks its superficial pecten component. **D,** vulvar anus on junction between vestibule and perineum. **E,** vulvar anus of normal dimensions situated in the vestibule. **F,** ano-vestibular fistula after treatment. Married adult with child, with normal bowel control. Anus supple and lying within the vestibule.

Anatomy.—The rectum proceeds through the pelvis normally and arches back away from the vaginal wall in a manner resembling the normal ano-rectal posterior angulation. The rectum is complete to the site close to the perineal skin, a level which is approximately that of the anal valves. From the termination of the rectum, a fistulous tract may extend to any point along the midline of the perineum. Its orifice may lie as far back as immediately adjacent to the normal anal site or as far forward as the vestibule. Any site forward of the normal anal site, but not as far as the vestibule, is referred to as "ano-cutaneous fistula" (the orifice into the vestibular area referred to as "ano-vulvar fistula").

The orifice is stenotic, usually beveled, and projects the ribbon of feces anteriorly. Superficial to the anal site and fistula is a covering of skin which conforms to patterns similar to those seen in the male covered anus.

Sphincters.—The sphincter anatomy is not known to us with certainty, as no specimen has been available for serial sections. However, we may draw the following conclusions, based on operative and clinical experience.

(a) Levator Ani.—Digital examination after operation reveals a strongly contracting collar of muscle surrounding several centimeters of the rectal wall above the outlet. This feeling of compression is deficient anteriorly at a high level, and the suggestion is that the muscle is a normally disposed pubo-rectalis.

(b) and (c) Internal and External Anal Sphincters.—Red mucosa of the rectum is visible after a simple "cutback" operation, in a slightly patulous anal orifice, and it is assumed that as in the male the internal sphincter is absent or rudimentary and that the superficial part of the external sphincter is ineffective as a sphincter to close the anal verge. However, a circumferential squeeze of muscle can be felt at a level below the pubo-rectalis, and this is interpreted as a functional deep external sphincter.

Perineum.—Three orifices are found in the perineum. The appearances provide ample evidence for the "covered anus" concept. At one extremity is a group of lesions in which the anal orifice or fistula exactly resembles the varieties of covered anal stenosis seen in the male, i.e., a stenotic orifice may be found at or near the normal anal site, overhung by a hypertrophied raphe, or bridged over by a midline band. Further sites for the fistulous orifice may be found anywhere in the midline of the perineum, between the normal anal site and the border of the vestibule, and the orifice is narrow and beveled but rarely as fine and tenuous as that of the male. (Fig. 60, *A*). The skin bordering the anterior margin of the anus is usually smooth, dry and

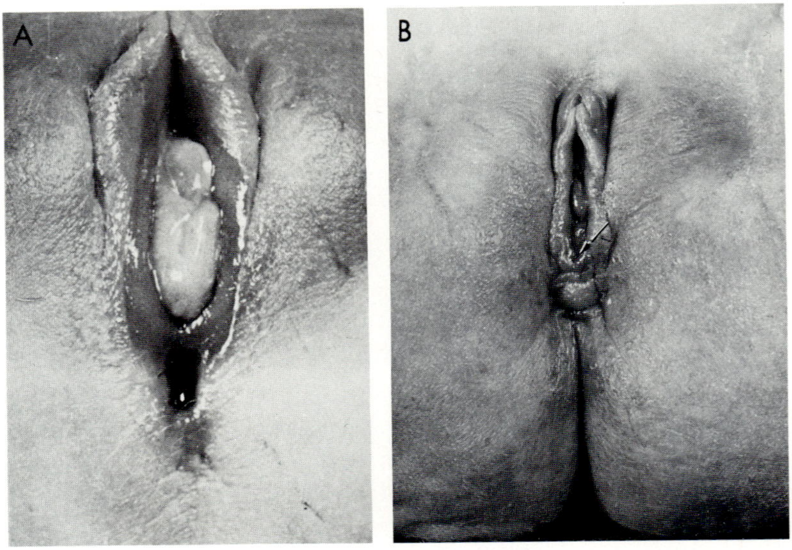

Fig. 60.—Covered anus (female). **A,** ano-cutaneous type. The orifice is stenotic and lies anterior in the perineum, behind the fourchette. **B,** ano-vulvar type. The orifice is stenotic and is projected anteriorly into the posterior margin of the vulva (*arrow*). (See also Fig. 106.)

flat; but, if the orifice is close to the vestibule, its anterior skin margin is formed by a red, wet, narrow and somewhat rudimentary fourchette.

The orifice may be stenotic and set between deep and superficial bifurcations of the minoral tails, the deep forming the fourchette and the superficial partially covering the anus. Ribbon-like stools are laboriously expressed and projected onto the vulva.

Investigations.—No radiographs are necessary in the diagnosis of an ano-cutaneous fistula. The presence of three orifices, combined with the clinical features described above, substantiates the diagnosis. However, the usual investigatory plan of full assessment follows that described for recto-cloacal and recto-vestibular fistulae (see Fig. 107, *B*).

Management.—The reader is referred to the discussions on management of the male ano-cutaneous fistula and an ano-vestibular fistula (Chapter 3), which we believe apply precisely to the female ano-cutaneous fistula. The same controversy exists as to whether to perform a simple "cutback" or to transplant the anus. We favor a simple cutback procedure in the newborn period, which produces a supple and functional anus.

Recently, Pellerin and Nezelhof (1963) and Pellerin and Saied (1969) have reported on the histological findings of the lower rectum and fistulae in this anomaly (and in anterior anus). They were concerned to explain the frequent occurrence of constipation and secondary megacolon, even when the anal orifice was adequate after "cutback." They found that the lower rectum and fistula sometimes contained either no ganglion cells or abnormalities of distribution and number of ganglion cells, with a resulting situation akin to Hirschsprung's disease. It was suggested, therefore, that a very low rectal biopsy should be taken at the time of the cutback; if the wall is normal, cutback operation will be adequate; if abnormal, then these authors recommend an abdomino-perineal rectosigmoidectomy, as performed by Swenson for Hirschsprung's disease. We have not favored this approach.

3. At Vulvar Site

Four deformities may produce an orifice in the vulval area. One, the recto-vestibular fistula, has already been described as an intermediate lesion and is essentially a supralevator anomaly. The remaining three orifices are translevator and are now described.

(I) Vulvar Anus.—The vulvar anus is a variety of anterior anus, but with so little development of perineal tissues that the anal canal opens in the vestibular area. The anal orifice is normal in caliber and function but lies within the vulva, occupying a somewhat expanded region between the vagina and posterior limit of the vulva. The orifice is surrounded by wet, red epithelium of the vulva. The urethra, vagina and other structures of the vulva appear normally oriented.

Occasionally the anus will lie at the junction of vulva and perineum. The posterior margin of the vulva is then interrupted by the lumen of the anus, which is surrounded partly by dry and partly by wet skin. The superficial parts of the minoral tails pass posteriorly behind the anus and may form a ridge or raphe. The deeper parts sweep medially in front of the anus and form a rudimentary fourchette, being formed by the convergence in front of the anus of folds arising from the lateral walls of the vestibule, and the perineum is absent (see Fig. 59, *D* and *E*).

In one specimen of vulvar anus available for histological study, there were the following departures from normal; at the pectinate line, squamous epithelium of the vestibule (without specialized glands) met columnar goblet cell mucosa, and there was no stratified columnar zone; the circular smooth muscle coat was thickened to form the internal sphincter, the lower end of which caused visible pouting of the anus. The external sphincter appeared to be mainly circumcloacal in its distribution, surrounding all structures emerging from the external cloaca. The pubo-rectalis muscle was well represented and appeared to be confluent with the external cloacal sphincter.

This variety may well be termed "anus," since the uro-rectal septum is presumed to be complete and the anal pit formed normally (as evidenced by the presence of the line of the anal valves), function is efficient and its orifice is supple and normal in caliber, although not in its normal location.

Management.—The condition is rare and principles difficult to lay down, but, as the anus is of adequate caliber and possesses normal control, we believe it preferable to leave it in its vulvar site. The situation is exactly comparable to an ano-vestibular fistula after "cut-back," a much more common lesion, and the reader is referred to the management of that lesion (Chapt. 10), for the acceptability of the vulvar site versus the arguments in favor of posterior transplantation of the anus.

(II) ANO-VULVAR FISTULA.—The ano-vulvar fistula is the most forward variety of the covered anus concept in the female, the details of which have already been described in the ano-cutaneous fistula of the female and the male.

Perineum.—The orifice is found at the posterior margin of the vestibule (Fig. 60, *B*), in which location it superficially resembles an ano-vestibular fistula. However, three observations differentiate it from the latter fistula:

(i) Whereas the orifice of the ano-vulvar fistula may have wet vestibular mucosa anterior to it, the margin posteriorly is raised up and formed from dry skin of the perineum and the minoral tails. In the ano-vestibular fistula the orifice is entirely within the wet vestibule.

(ii) The lateral borders of the vestibule may project posteriorly beyond the confines of the vestibule, elongating the fourchette and continuing on posterior to the anal orifice, as a hypertrophied raphe.

(iii) A probe passed into the anal orifice passes preferentially *backwards* beneath the skin of the perineum but also cranially, whereas in an ano-vestibular fistula it slips cranially parallel to the vagina and cannot be induced to pout the skin without undue force and leverage on the probe (see Fig. 106).

On rare occasions, fusion of the genital folds may be so excessive in an anterior direction that the whole of the vestibule and vaginal orifice may be covered completely, and only one small orifice is then visible anteriorly, near the clitoris. No assessment of the various orifices of urethra, vagina or rectum can be made until these folds are separated or divided and the vestibule "uncovered."

Management.—In many papers ano-vestibular fistula, a "vulval anus," and a "recto-perineal fistula in the female" are synonymous terms, implying similar treatment, but this is not so in our classification. Most authors transplant the anus to a more posterior site.

It is our belief that, as in ano-vestibular fistula, even the most anteriorly placed covered anus, as far forwards as the posterior limit of the vulva, functions normally and hygienically after simple cutback of the fistula. On rare occasions, perhaps because of vulvar soiling, a secondary anal transplantation may be necessary.

Rare variant of ano-vulvar fistula. We have encountered 1 patient with ano-vulvar fistula and ectopia vesicae.

(III) ANO-VESTIBULAR FISTULA.—In our experience, this is the commonest anal deformity in the female child. The embryological explanation of this lesion and the empirical distinction made between it and recto-vestibular fistula are described under Classification in Chapter 6 and Embryology in Chapter 5. The description which follows applies to the common anal malformation in the female child, the ano-vestibular fistula. Suffice it to say here that this malformation differs from recto-vestibular fistula only in the length of the narrow segment, being very short in the ano-vestibular type.

Anatomy.—The rectum lies adjacent to the posterior vaginal septum and extends with a well-formed lumen to the vestibule (Fig. 61). It is surrounded by the pubo-rectalis sling, as in the normal, and this may appear to reduce the lumen size by compression; the fistula to the vestibule is very short, however, and constitutes little more than a stenotic orifice for the terminal rectum. Although in the common variety of ano-vestibular fistula, the vagina is usually single, it is occasionally septate, in which case the anal opening is situated posterior to the intervaginal septum.

Sphincters.—(a) Levator Ani.—The pubo-rectalis fibers bear a normal relation to the terminal rectum, wrapping round the back and side walls intimately (Fig. 62). The lowest fibers lie very close to the site of the orifice, directly continuous with the external anal sphincter fibers. The remaining diaphragm part of the muscle is normally disposed. The pubo-rectalis is an effective sphincter, acting upon the lumen of the bowel distally as far as the rim of the orifice.

(b) Internal Anal Sphincter.—In a dissection by one of us (F. D. S.) the muscle coats of the rectum expanded slightly into a rudimentary internal sphincter just above the orifice.

Scott (1966) has dissected four specimens of ano-vestibular fistulae (patients dying from other anomalies). He found a well-developed internal sphincter and an epithelial zone of stratified squamous cells in the terminal bowel; above this, however, he found a zone of stratified cuboidal epithelium, absent in our dissections.

(c) External Anal Sphincter.—Immediately caudal to the lowest fibers of the pubo-rectalis sling, the serial sections showed a narrow collar of voluntary muscle embracing the three orifices of the ure-

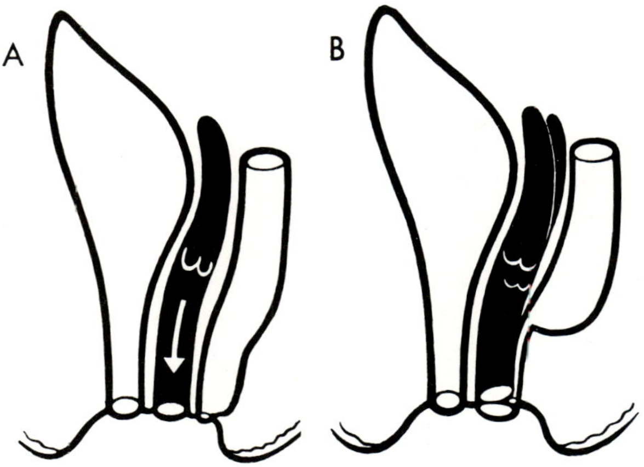

Fig. 61.—Ano-vestibular and recto-vestibular fistulae. **A,** narrow orifice with adjacent normal lumen—ano-vestibular fistula. **B,** narrow orifice with adjoining narrow lumen of long fistula—recto-vestibular fistula. The fistula is close to the vagina (single or double).

Fig. 62.—Ano-vestibular fistula. The pubo-rectalis sling is arranged around the terminal bowel as a sphincter.

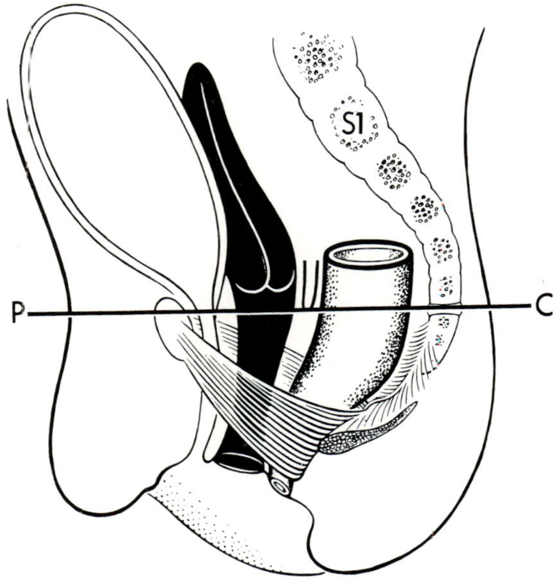

thra, vagina and rectum. It is a cloacal sphincter. Farther back, and immediately beneath the perineal raphe, were longitudinally running voluntary muscle fibers, as are found so characteristically in many other anal deformities.

Perineum.—Three orifices are located in the vulval area (Figs. 63 and 64). The urethral and vaginal orifices appear normal, and the labia and borders of the vestibule show no signs of genital fold hypertrophy. Inspection of the vestibule reveals a third small orifice behind the vaginal orifice, tucked up in the fossa navicularis. It lies completely within the borders of the vestibule, i.e., it is surrounded by red, wet epithelium all around, including posteriorly between the orifice and the margins of the fourchette. It does not extend onto the dry skin of the perineum. Occasionally the opening may encroach a little onto the posterior rim of the vaginal orifice, there producing a small V-defect at this site.

A probe passed into the orifice passes preferentially *upwards* in a cranial direction parallel to the vagina (see Fig 106, *A*), but it also has some limited mobility backwards, but not as directly as in a covered anus.

Fig. 63.—External appearances of ano-vestibular fistula. The vestibule is small. The urethral and vaginal orifices occupy the exposed area, and the narrow orifice of the bowel fistula is tucked up and hidden by the overhanging posterior margin of the vestibule. It is in the vestibule, separate from and posterior to the vaginal orifice. Three patients—**A,** orifice hidden from view. **B,** meconium overflowing from orifice. **C,** associated deformity of perineum, possibly hypertrophic anal tubercles.

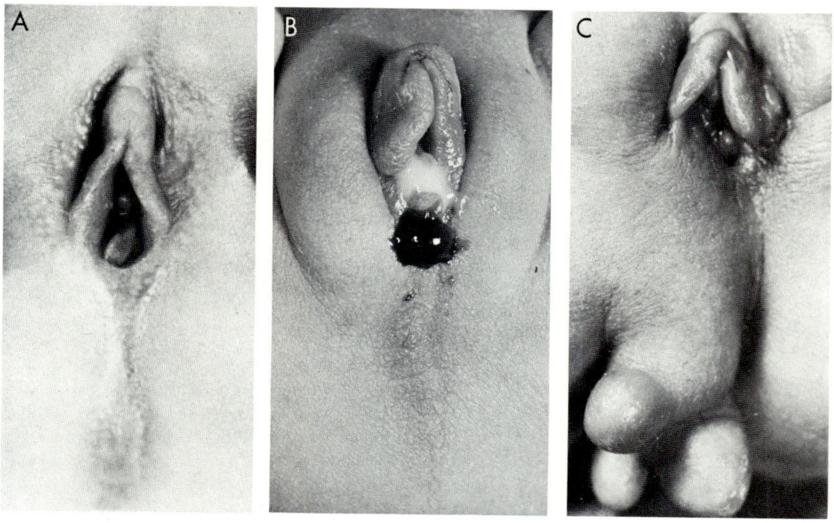

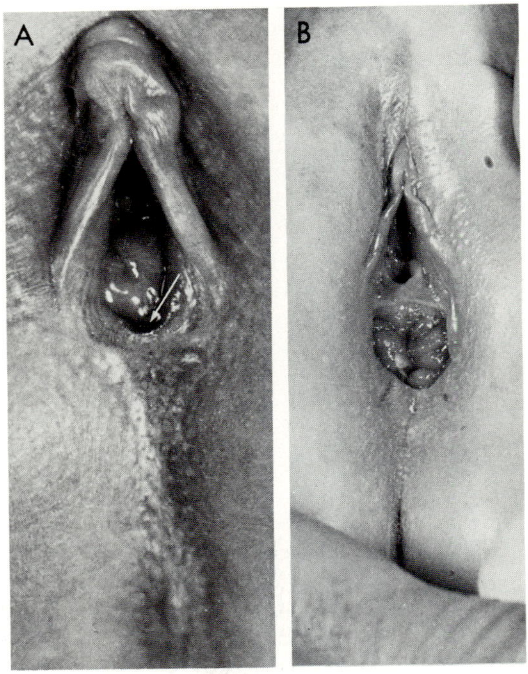

Fig. 64.—Ano-vestibular fistula. **A,** orifice of fistula concealed in vestibule (*arrow*) before cutback procedure. **B,** patulous continent orifice after liberal cutback procedure in another patient.

The fourchette usually overhangs the vestibule, and unless this is retracted backwards, or even divided, the rectal orifice may be overlooked. More rarely, the genital folds may "cover in" the whole vestibule and vagina completely, and no inspection of the vestibule is possible until the genital folds are divided radically (see Fig. 105).

Investigations.—No radiological investigations are essential for diagnosis as the appearance of the three vulvar orifices, combined with the probe test, indicates the type of internal anatomy present (see Chapt. 8 for details). However, other deformities of the spine and urinary tract should be anticipated and investigated radiologically, and the general assessment, as outlined in recto-cloacal and recto-vestibular fistulae should be followed (see Figs. 56 and 57).

Management.—A similar controversy centers on this malformation as on low vaginal fistula, i.e., whether to transplant the orifice out of the vulval area or not. All surgeons agree that treatment is not urgent and that a satisfactory temporary orifice can be achieved by dilatation alone, or supplementary to a simple "cutback" of the orifice of the fistula. Bryndorf and Madsen (1959) in a study of 29 vestibular anuses found that most of them functioned better after dilatation and/or cutback than after perineal transplantation. Four of 6 patients of David (1937) required no treatment, and Brayton and Norris (1958) found that most required no treatment or only dilatation. Brenner (1915) quotes Morgagni's description of a woman living 100 years, bearing several children and never knowing of her abnormality! It is certainly our experience that transplantation is seldom required, and 12 of our 16 examples, observed personally, functioned normally in their vulval positions – no soiling and complete control of feces and flatus (see Figs. 59, *F*, and 127, *B*).

The presence of a fully formed pubo-rectalis around the terminal rectum and its orifice and of a rudimentary cloacal sphincter ensures perfect rectal cleanliness and is responsible for the high degree of continence exhibited by these patients. The firm posterior rim of the stenotic orifice of the fistula requires to be cutback for a short distance and dilatations instituted in the newborn period. Dilatations alone may rupture the weaker anterior rim and the thin septum between the anterior rectal wall and vagina creating a recto-vaginal orifice.

The first few dilatations must be tenderly performed with dilators until it is certain that there is a sufficiently strong septum between vagina and anterior rectal wall and until the caliber accommodates the parent's little finger. Dilatations are continued by the parent until the orifice is adequate in size and supple.

With a strong septum between the vaginal and anal orifices, the feces do not contaminate the vagina; four of our patients are now over 14 years old, without transplantation, and find no inconvenience.

Although we have been satisfied with the cosmetic and hygienic results of simple cutback, it is true that many other surgical groups feel that the vulvar-sited anus is esthetically displeasing and that the vulvar area may be difficult to keep clean. Should feces actually enter the vagina because of an inadequate septum between it and the rectum, there are risks of infection (vaginitis, tubo-ovarian abscess), and, in these circumstances, cleanliness is not possible. We then agree with Nixon (1961), transplantation is necessary. Nixon reserves transplantation for such secondary complications and performs it at about 4 years of age. His technique of perineal anoplasty is described in Chapter 10.

An alternative technique for transplantation favored by us is the sacro-perineal approach. Direct access to the fistula, freer mobilization of the rectum and protection of the pubo-rectalis muscle are afforded by this method.

A list of surgeons who perform transplantation for low recto-vaginal fistulae, and the times at which they do so, is detailed in Chapter 9. For ano-vestibular fistulae, these same recommendations obtain; however, Crowell and Dulin (1940), Harkin (1942), Bradham (1958), Katzen (1962), Sommerschild *et al.* (1964) and Lloyd (1964), all perform anal transplantation routinely (at unstated times); David (1937), at 6 years; Trusler and Wilkinson (1962), at 3–5 years; and Santulli (1963), either between 3–9 months or after 4 years, when the operation is technically easier. Hanley (1965) in a recent paper has delayed his time of intervention to 18–24 months.

We believe anal transplantation is unnecessary, except for secondary complications mentioned above and, further, carries the following risks:

(i) The pubo-rectalis may be damaged in the rectal mobilization via the perineum, with subsequent loss of control, and this contention is supported by the results as reported (see Chapt. 14).

(ii) Transplantation performed in early infancy is unreliable and as Nixon (1961) states, "the submucous layer of the bowel is not strong enough to hold stitches against the forces of straining and defecation, and a proportion of breakdowns with fistula or stenosis occur."

(iii) After transplantation, there is a disconcerting tendency for the anal orifice to move back to the vulvar area, and, in fact, in the attempt to prevent this complication, the technique has been modified many times since Dieffenbach's first description of the operation in 1826 in Vienna.

(iv) The new orifice may permit some degree of mucous wetting, because by transposition the anus is shifted to a site well below the lowest muscle fibers of the pubo-rectalis sling. Hence, the unguarded distal segment of mucus-secreting rectum leaks mucus through the patulous orifice.

A further variant on the theme of treatment of ano-vestibular fistula is reported by Santulli *et al.* (1965), in which "colostomy in the newborn period, followed by definitive perineal repair at 9–12 months" is now advised. However, if the anal orifice can be made to function where it lies, colostomy and transposition are not required.

(iv) and (v) Perineal Groove and Perineal Canal.—In the International Classification (1970), these two lesions do not appear in the basic list but are relegated to the "miscellaneous" rare group. For completeness we include their description here.

(iv) Perineal Groove.—The features common to this group are, firstly, normal formation of the vestibule, including urethra and vagina in its anterior two thirds; secondly, hypertrophic minoral tails which skirt the perineum and course posteriorly to join at the anus or surround it; thirdly, a wet groove in the perineum between the fourchette and the anus (Figs. 65 and 66).

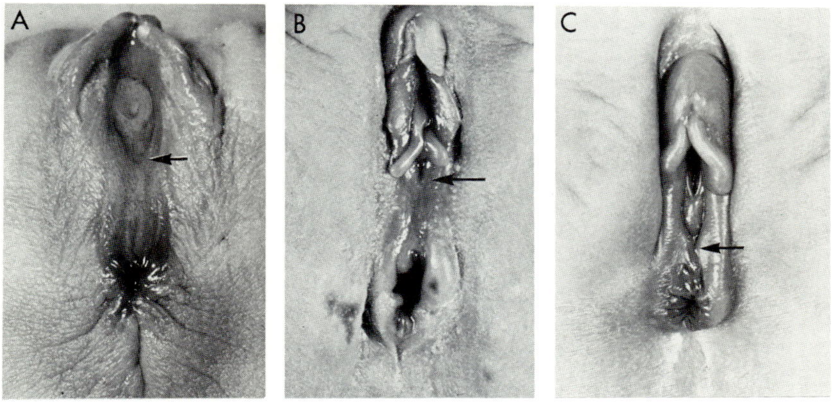

Fig. 65.—Perineal groove. **A,** showing anus enclosed by genital folds and a short sulcus between the vestibule and anus. **B,** a similar deformity, but with a long, shallow sulcus. **C,** a deep sulcus. The fourchette in each case is indicated by an arrow.

Fig. 66.—Perineal groove. Minoral tails border the groove and anus. Deep fourchette formed by perineal mound and a contribution from the minoral tails. **A,** superficial external sphincter ring is open anteriorly. **B** and **C,** on straining, the rectal mucosa prolapses.

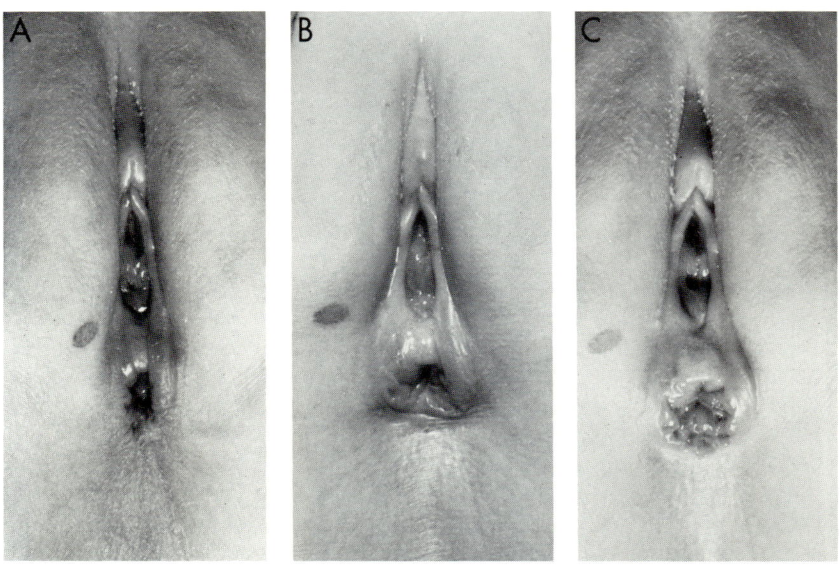

The fourchette lies deeply set at the anterior end of the groove between the inner genital folds.

The sulcus is of variable length and may be deep or shallow; it leads from vestibule to anus and is red and moist.

The labia majora are abnormally long, flanking not only the vestibule but the perineal zone and anus.

The anus is supple, not stenotic, and exhibits ectropion anteriorly, with resulting exposure of the muco-cutaneous junction. The mucosa of the anterior quadrant of the anal canal is in continuity with the wet lining of the central perineal sulcus. On straining, the anterior wall of the anus is inclined to prolapse (see Fig. 66).

The levator ani muscle is normally disposed, the deep external sphincter is present but the superficial sphincter is U-shaped, bifurcating along the sides of the groove.

Management.—No treatment is required for this anomaly. The wet perineal sulcus gradually becomes epithelialized into normal skin.

(v) Perineal Canal.—An apparently normal perineum separates the vestibule from the anus, both of which are normally sited, but deep in the perineum a fistulous communication exists between vestibule and anus (Fig. 67). Its anterior orifice is sited close to the fossa navicularis deep in the fourchette, and its posterior orifice is on the anterior wall of the anal canal, at or superficial to the site of the anal valves. The anus may or may not exhibit some degree of stenosis of its anterior quadrant.

There are other reports of patients, each with a normal anus, and, in addition, a fistula into the fourchette. In Sitkovskii's case (1963), the vestibular fistula joined the normal anus 2 cm. inside the anal verge; Pegum *et al.* (1964) describe a 25-year-old woman with the same anomaly; and Bryndorf and Madsen (1959) illustrate their similar case with a photograph showing a probe between the two orifices.

Chatterjee and Talukder (1969) report from Calcutta 7 children with this anomaly in a total ano-rectal series of 56 patients. Six of the 7 had a normal anus; in the seventh the anus was ectopically placed forward of the normal site. This paper also quotes two additional patients from Swenson (when in Boston) and four from Nixon in London. The paper should be read for clinical detail.

Ninh and Bohn (1970) have encountered no less than 25 patients with this anomaly in 1 year in Saigon. These have presented with an inflammatory abscess in the vulva, which bursts and then discharges feces. The anus was normal, except that some patients developed slight narrowing from inflammatory scarring. The anal end of the fistula lay above the sphincters and valves. They believe the fistula is of congenital origin, often blind at birth, and infection enters from the anal end. The close approximation of rectal wall to fourchette in

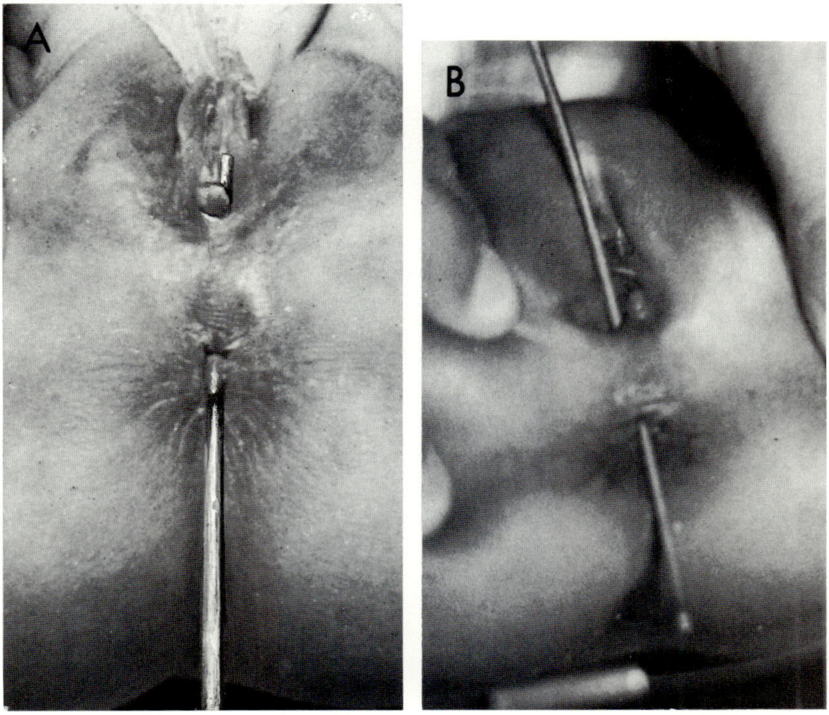

Fig. 67.—Perinea canal. **A** and **B,** sites of entry and exit of probe introduced through the anus along the canal, into the vestibule. (B courtesy of Mr. S. K. Chatterjee, Calcutta, personal communication.)

some patients suggests a congenital aberration rather than a perianal abscess which simply ruptures into the vestibule. In a section through the fistula in one of Chatterjee and Talukder's patients, there were no inflammatory changes.

Management.—The only management required is excision of the tract of the fistula, with oversewing of both the vestibular and anal terminations. Chatterjee and Talukder (1969), however, report on the prevalence of fistula recurrence and advise a "vestibulo-anal pull-through repair" in which, after dissecting out the vestibular fistulous opening, the fistula is drawn back into the lumen of the anal canal and excised. The gut, vagina and vestibule are then reconstituted. Ninh and Bohn (1970) have generally performed a colostomy initially in the presence of gross infection, the repair being delayed.

CHAPTER 5

Embryology

Normal Embryology

Embryology of Cloaca

The internal and external cloacae of the human embryo undergo a continuous but distinct series of changes, with transformation from an embryological rendezvous of the urinary genital and rectal systems to the more familiar anatomical arrangement in which the urethra and genital ducts are entirely separate from the rectum and anus. These changes are effected in an orderly chronological manner, rarely failing to achieve the miraculous perfection of the separate systems (Fig. 68).

A coronal septum is formed to divide the cloaca into urinary and rectal passages. It is made up of at least four different components. It starts cranially and ends caudally, each component being built sequentially upon the other. Two of the processes divide the internal cloaca and at least two the external cloaca.

Defects, however, in the partitioning of the cloaca cause not only errors of the visceral tracts but also of the pelvic muscles and perineal muscles and sphincters, and the resulting deformities follow fairly stereotyped patterns.

Partitioning of the Cloaca.—While the cloacal membrane separates the internal from the external cloaca in the transverse plane, and undergoes a gradual process of atrophy, the uro-rectal and uro-anal septa cleave the cloacae in the coronal plane. At the 16-mm. crown rump phase of development, the uro-rectal septum has come, the cloacal membrane has gone, the internal cloaca is divided and the external cloaca is a deep pit about to be partitioned by the uro-anal septum.

The Internal Cloaca.—At the 4-mm. stage (4-week embryo), the hindgut expands to form a reservoir or internal cloaca, into which issue the large intestine, the postanal gut, the allantois, and the wolffian or mesonephric ducts. This reservoir contacts the surface ectoderm in the midline between the allantoic stalk anteriorly and the tail fold posteriorly. This is the area of the cloacal membrane,

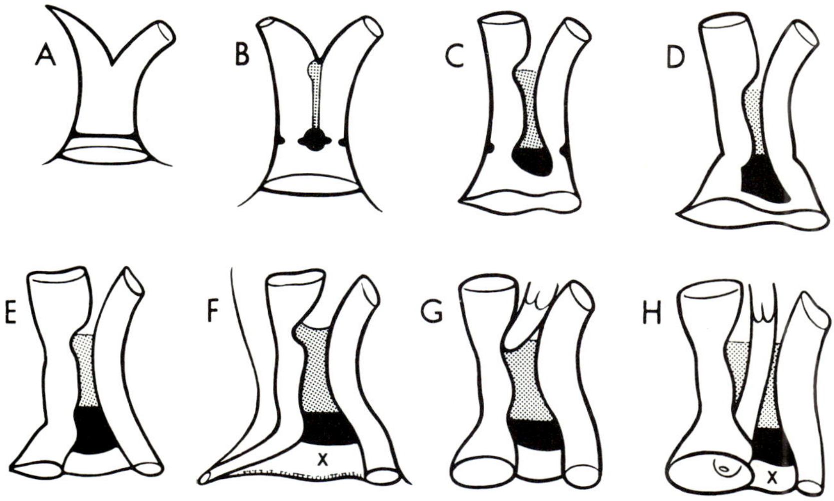

Fig. 68.—Partition of the internal and external cloacae. **A,** undivided internal cloaca at 4-mm. stage. **B,** uro-rectal septum (*hatched area*) complete at 16-mm. stage. **C,** perineal mound (*black area*) forms the deep part of the uro-anal septum which divides the external cloaca. **D** and **E,** inner genital folds now surge medially over the mound to form the anus. **F,** inner genital folds (x) in the male are further supplemented by overlay of outer genital folds which form the midline perineal raphe. **G,** in the female, müllerian ducts penetrate posterior wall of the urethra at 36-mm. stage. **H,** müllerian ducts descend to gain an internal opening in the uro-genital sinus or vestibule.

which is at first ventrally oriented. It recedes caudally from the allantoic stalk, by the interposition of the abdominal wall and the genital tubercle and the unfolding and disappearance of the tail on the dorsal aspect.

The Uro-Rectal Septum.—The partitioning of the internal cloaca, begins in the 4-mm. embryo and is completed in the 16-mm. stage. This septum is developed in two parts (Keibel and Mall, 1910; Stephens, 1963; and Duhamel, 1966) (Fig. 69).

The cranial part of the septum is a crescentic fold which settles deeply into the saddle between the allantois and the hindgut, on the cranial aspect of the cloaca. This crescentic spur was claimed by Tourneux to progress caudally until it met the cloacal membrane. Rathke and Retterer (quoted by Duhamel, 1966) considered that the septum was formed by the coming together and fusion in the midline of two lateral mesodermal folds.

There is no controversy amongst embryologists (Hamilton, Boyd and Mossman, 1962; and Patten, 1953) concerning the progressive craniocaudal march of the septum (Fig.70). Emphasis, however, is

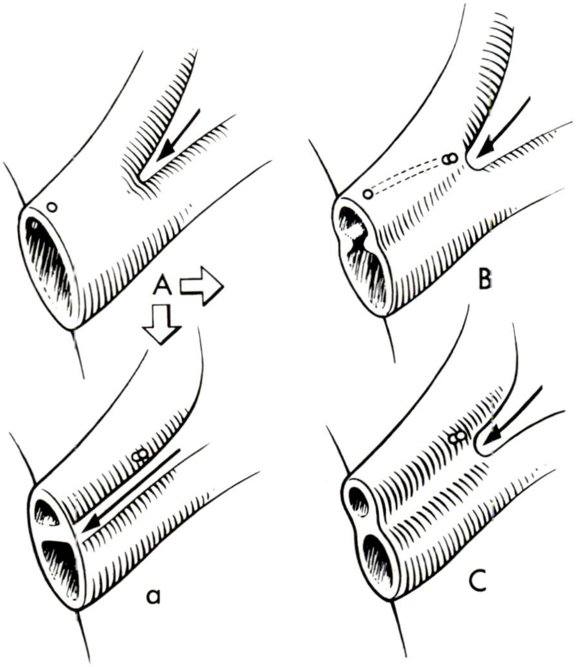

Fig. 69.—Methods of subdivision of the cloaca. **A–a,** subdivision by downgrowth of the ano-rectal septum to meet the cloacal membrane. **A, B** and **C,** subdivision by downgrowth of uro-rectal septum as far as Müller's hillock (verumontanum) and by lateral ingrowths of mesenchyme caudal to this level. (The dotted lines in **B** represent the line of retraction of the orifices of the wolffian ducts from sites near the cloacal membrane at the earliest stage to the later attained level at the verumontanum.)

placed more on Tourneux's method, although Keibel and Mall (1912) and Patten (1953) imply that the craniocaudal spur is supplemented by the lateral indentations nearer the cloacal membrane. This combined method of formation of the uro-rectal septum offers ready explanation of many of the congenital abnormalities of the area.

Once the septum is complete, the wolffian ducts proceed to become organized in situ into the vasa deferentia and the vesicles of the male; in the female, they are the guides for the migrating müllerian ducts to the uro-genital sinus, and then they proceed to atrophy. The müllerian ducts penetrate the uro-genital sinus by about the 36-mm. stage and then proceed farther to issue in the vestibule. These changes take place concurrently with the differentiation of the external cloaca.

The External Cloaca.—During the formation period of the uro-

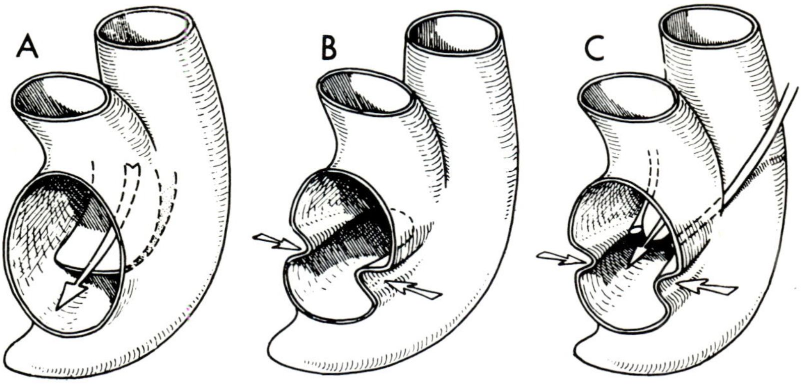

Fig. 70.—Eponymous terms denoting the means of subdivision of the cloaca. **A,** craniocaudal descent of Tourneux fold. **B,** lateral plicae of Rathke dividing the lumen from side to side. **C,** combination of the folds of Tourneux and Rathke. (Reproduced with permission from Duhamel, B.: *Morphogenese Pathologique "Des Monstruosities aux Malformations* [Paris: Masson & Cie, 1966].)

Fig. 71.—Derivations of the component parts of the rectum and anal canal. **A,** male. Internal cloacal rectum (*pale shading*). The uro-rectal septum grows caudally into the external cloaca to form the perineal mound (*P*) and advances the internal cloacal rectum with it into the perineum (*dark shading*). The anal canal below the valves is formed from the inner genital folds (*stippled*) and from the outer genital folds (*crosshatched*) which form the perineal raphe. **B,** female. Similar developments of rectum, except that outer genital folds do not contribute to the formation of the anus. (Dotted horizontal lines in *A* and *B* represent the original level of the cloacal membrane.)

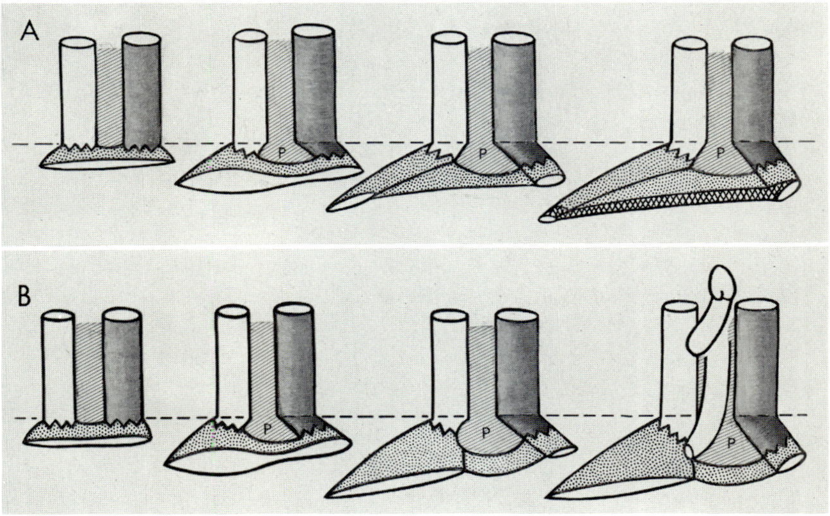

rectal septum, between the 4- and 16-mm. phases, the cloacal membrane becomes deeply set in the perineum as the result of the surface build-up of mesoderm around it. The genital folds form on either side and the genital tubercle on the ventral aspect. The depression so formed is the external cloaca.

When the uro-rectal septum reaches the level of the membrane, the membrane atrophies, and both systems then issue into the common external cloaca.

The Uro-anal Septum.—The process of partitioning now extends caudally into the external cloaca (Fig. 71, *A* and *B*).

The uro-anal septum, or dividing wall of the external cloaca, is again a composite structure. Its deep part is a caudal extension of the uro-rectal septum, and more superficially it is added to by the inward migration and overlap of the genital folds. These sex folds develop differentially in males and females. Caudal to the level of the cloacal membrane, a central mound forms in continuity with, and as an extension of, the uro-rectal septum, separating the orifice of the uro-genital sinus from the anus. This is the primitive perineum of Keibel and Mall (1912). It begins to develop at the 16–50-mm. crown rump length, and as it grows caudally the rectum elongates with it (Fig. 71). The adjoining genital folds proliferate to form projecting lateral borders of the external cloaca.

In the male, the inner medial folds spread medially over the primitive perineum at approximately the 50-mm. stage and tent over the uro-genital sinus to form the bulbous urethra. This is the stage of sex distinction from external appearances. The outer lateral folds also migrate medially, blend into the inner folds and meet in the midline to form the raised-up perineal raphe characteristic of the male. They enlarge locally to form the scrotum.

The deep part of the uro-anal septum in the male is largely responsible for the anteroposterior length of the perineum, while the superficial component formed by the genital folds adds depth.

In the female, the inner genital folds bordering the external cloaca surge onto the mound, as in the male, and together they form the perineum. In the vicinity of the uro-genital sinus, the inner genital folds remain separate and form the labia minora along the anterior third of the sinus, and the minoral tails along the posterior two thirds. These tails converge and overrun the perineal mound to form the fourchette.

Some recent observations on female premature babies (Stephens, 1967) indicate that the fourchette and the central perineum and anterior wall of the anus may sometimes be formed almost entirely from the perineal mound. This structure then protrudes caudally so far that it interposes itself between the minoral tails.

The outer genital folds remain widely separate as the labia majora and do not take part in the formation of the fourchette, although in the perineum the folds may approach each other but rarely meet. In consequence, the female perineum in contrast to that of the male very rarely exhibits a raphe.

The Cloacal Septum.—The cloacal septum of the internal and external cloacae, when complete, is thus a complex structure and consists of Tourneux's spur, Rathke's folds, the perineal mound and the inner and outer genital folds.

The Anus.—The ectodermal part of the anal canal comprises the anal pit and orifice caudal to the site of the anal membrane. This membrane atrophies shortly after the uro-rectal septum has reached the level of the cloacal membrane and is demarcated by the anal valves or pectinate line. The line of the valves is carried caudal to its original site by elongation of the rectum brought about by the formation of the perineal mound between the urethra and the anus. The ectodermal anus then elongates by additional ringlets from the genital folds around the sides and posterior part of the anal circumference. This is the embryological anal canal which should be clearly distinguished from the surgical anal canal which incorporates part of the rectum cranial to the pectinate line as far as the upper border of the pubo-rectalis muscle.

The pectinate line represents the meeting of endodermal and ectodermal components of the anal canal. It originally lies contiguous with the urethral orifice but subsequently migrates in a posterior and caudal direction away from the urethra. The shift takes place by caudal elongation of the rectum supplemented by the growth of the perineal mound in front. It assumes a deeper location when the inner genital folds wrap around the orifice on the superficial aspect creating the pecten, that zone of smooth skin between the pectinate line above and the orifice below.

In the male, the outer genital folds overlie the inner folds on the anterior quadrant of the anus and perineum. The perineal raphe extends in a posterior direction onto the anal orifice where it may appear as a skin tag. In the female, no such raphe occurs because the outer genital folds do not enroach upon the anus or the sagittal line of the perineum.

Components of the Rectum and Anal Canal.—The rectum extends from the 3d sacral vertebra to the anal orifice. The pectinate line signifies the junction of endodermal rectum with the ectodermal anal pit.

The posterior and lateral walls of the rectum are intrinsic to the original internal cloaca; those of the anal pit are intrinsic to the genital folds of the external cloaca.

The anterior walls of the rectum and anus, however, are highly complex structures being formed from no less than five components in the female and six in the male.

From above down, the anterior wall consists of the hindgut, Tourneux's spur and Rathke's folds; then the perineal mound occupies the deep part of the anterior quadrant, supplemented in the male by the inner and outer genital folds. In the female, the perineal mound may form the whole of its anterior quadrant or it may be the deep component overlapped superficially by the inner genital folds only.

THEORETICAL LEVELS AT WHICH DEFECTS OF DEVELOPMENT OCCUR.—Although the components that form the anterior segment of the rectum and anal canal are distinct, they depend upon appropriate timing for their continuous and complete construction one upon the other. Defects induce a chain reaction in the steps of the ladder of events.

Males

Defect of Tourneux spur	Recto-vesical fistula
Defect of Rathke's folds	Recto-urethral fistula
Defect of perineal mound	Recto-bulbar fistula
Defect of inner genital fold	Ano-urethral fistula
Defect of outer genital fold	Ano-cutaneous fistula

Females

Defect of Tourneux spur	Recto-vesical fistula Separate müllerian ducts
Defect of Rathke's folds	Recto-cloacal fistula Septate vagina or recto-vestibular fistula or recto-vaginal fistula
Defect of perineal mound	Perineal canal
Defect of inner genital fold	Perineal groove
Defect of outer genital fold	Ano-cutaneous fistula
Defect of perineal mound and defect of inner genital folds	Anterior anus—vulvar or perineal
Defect of anal membrane	Imperforate anal membrane or anal membrane stenosis
Defect of anal pit	Anal agenesis

Abnormal Embryology

An understanding of the deviations from the normal course of embryological events and their ultimate effect on the structure and relations of the pelvic viscera is essential to the proper appreciation of the distinction between rectal and anal deformities drawn as long ago as 1904 by Wood Jones.

SUBDIVISION OF THE RECTUM AND ANAL CANAL.—The *rectal group* of malformations consists of those abnormalities intrinsic in the partitioning of the internal cloaca. The termination of the hindgut is found at the level of the verumontanum or higher in the male and, in the female, lies at almost any level in the pelvis, perhaps opening into the cloacal canal or the posterior wall of the vagina or into the fossa navicularis of the vestibule.

The *anal group* of malformations is referable to developmental aberrations affecting the proctodeal pit and membrane, the perineum and genital folds. The deformities comprising this group are the more common, the more easily treated and provide the greater number of satisfactory surgical cures.

(The schemata in Figs. 74, 75 and 76 [see Chap. 6] correlate the usual malformations, with their underlying defects in development, and the stages at which such lapses occur in males and females, respectively.)

Rectal Defects

Males.—Because of the more frequent occurrence of *rectourethral fistulae* in males at the level of the verumontanum than at the bulb and the rarity of fistulae in the membranous urethra between these two levels, some explanation is sought from the manner in which the internal cloaca is subdivided by the uro-rectal septum.

If downgrowth of the uro-rectal septum were the only mechanism involved in cloacal division, it would be expected that the commonest form of fistula in the male would be located at the level of the triangular ligament, the site of the cloacal duct, a structure which represents the last part of the cloaca to be sealed off from the uro-genital sinus. The rarity of such a fistula at this level, however, and the frequency of a fistula at the verumontanum suggest that the subdivision of the cloaca below the verumontanum is effected by a different process from that which separates the gut from the urinary tract cranial to this point. We maintain that Tourneux's uro-rectal septum effects the cleavage of the cloaca only as far as Müller's hillock. In the interval between this level and the cloacal membrane, the second mechanism, in the form of an inward surge of mesenchyme from the sides of the embryo towards the midline (Rathke's folds), operates to complete the cleavage of the urinary tract from the gut. The frequency with which a recto-urethral fistula occurs at the level of the verumontanum, and the rarity of fistulae below this level are explained by the complete failure of the second mechanism. The cloaca remains undivided below the level of lowest point of descent of Tourneux's fold (see Figs. 68, 69 and 70).

The resulting recto-urethral fistula may undergo atrophy; the rectum then ends blindly, remaining attached to the cloaca by fibrous tissue in close proximity to the prostate (see Fig. 74). The term *ano-*

rectal agenesis has been applied to this particular anatomical defect. Communication with the urinary system may persist as a fine fistula opening in immediate proximity to the normal orifices of the ejaculatory ducts and the utriculus masculinus – the so-called recto-urethral fistula. More rarely, Tourneux's fold may be more rudimentary, the rectal fistula, wolffian ducts and prostatic tissue together open into the urinary system at a higher level, with the production of *rectovesical fistulae* and the rarer high type of recto-urethral fistulae (see Fig. 74).

If the lateral ingrowths are partly formed and all but meet to complete the subdivision, a long opening between the verumontanum and the bulb may persist as the cloacal canal, the orifice occupying the posterior wall of the membranous urethra. This is an uncommon recto-urethral fistula, less common than the recto-bulbar fistula, which is a more caudal communication between rectum and bulbous urethra.

In our opinion, the *recto-bulbar fistula* is a perineal deformity involving maldevelopment of the anus and urethra subsequent to partition of the internal cloaca by the uro-rectal septum. In this deformity, the urethra and rectum initially have separate openings which subsequently become enclosed by the genital folds to issue to the exterior through and along a bulbo-urethral conduit (see Fig. 74).

FEMALES. – The cloacal abnormality, caused by failure of subdivision of the cloaca into uro-genital and rectal compartments, is at first similar in males and females. The hindgut and urinary systems remain in direct communication, and their contents are conducted to the exterior through a common cloacal canal (see Fig. 75). The müllerian ducts arriving at the site of the verumontanum at the 35 mm. stage impose female modifications upon this deformity, which is called *recto-cloacal fistula*.

The final definitive anatomical arrangements of the organs which take part in this deformity depend largely on the further migratory capacity of the müllerian bulbs. If migration is arrested, the recto-cloacal deformity persists; the urethra, vagina and rectum issue independently, one behind the other, into the cranial end of the cloacal canal. The urethra is short, the vagina is short and often septate and the rectum issues into the cloaca through a narrow orifice. If migration progresses, the hindgut communication may be incorporated in the actively proliferating and wandering bulbs to form a *recto-vaginal fistula* (see Fig. 75), or it may be advanced with the bulbs to the vestibule, forming the *recto- or ano-vestibular fistula* (Fig. 72).

Sometimes the rectal fistula is occluded in the process, the deformity being then called *ano-rectal agenesis* (see Fig. 76).

Rectal atresia, on the other hand, is more likely to be an acquired

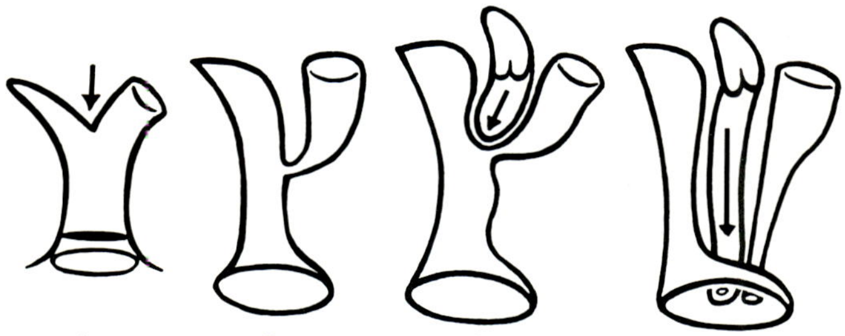

Fig. 72.—Stages in the formation of a recto-vestibular fistula. **A,** internal and external cloaca separated by cloacal membrane. **B,** Tourneux's fold (arrow in *A*) forms a saddle-shaped cleavage of the cloaca as far distally as Müller's hillock. Rathke's folds fail to appear. **C,** müllerian ducts descend upon the undivided cloaca. **D,** müllerian ducts migrate down the posterior wall of the undivided cloaca, carrying the attenuated rectal fistula and orifice with them (short and long arrows in *C* and *D*).

vascular lesion imposed on an already formed rectal canal, similar to the formation of an ileal atresia.

Perineal and Anal Deformities of the Male

Imperforate Anal Membrane and Anal Stenosis.—Imperforate anal membrane and anal membrane stenosis are due to persistence of the proctodeal membrane, wholly or in part. The membrane at fault is situated at the level of the anal valves. The membrane may be diaphanous or up to several millimeters thick. Sometimes it is perforated centrally and the periphery persists as a stenotic ring. In the male, another form of anal stenosis may occur if the genital folds almost cover over the anus and produce a narrowed orifice in the raphe, as in a variety of "covered anus." Finally, these malformations are different in their development from ano-rectal stenosis, which is probably a fault in the tract similar in origin to rectal atresia, i.e., a secondary vascular phenomenon applied to an already formed canal (Stephens, 1968).

Anal Agenesis.—When the cloaca is completely divided at the 16-mm. stage, the anal membrane lies closely approximated to the uro-genital membrane. If the anal pit is absent or rudimentary, the rectum remains imperforate, lying in its original location adjacent to the uro-genital sinus at the level of the upper border of the bulbo-cavernosus muscle; the rudimentary pit may be absent or represented only by a shallow blind dimple on the perineum (see Fig. 74).

Covered Anus—Recto-Bulbar and Ano-Cutaneous Fistu-

LAE.—Covered anus is the term applied to a malformation in which the anus is covered completely or partially as the result of abnormal posterior fusion of the outer genital folds (Wood Jones, 1915).

At the 16-mm. stage of the embryo, when the subdivision of the cloaca is complete, the uro-genital and anal pits normally lie closely approximated, but, in the mature fetus, the anal pit lies considerably posterior to its original site. This posterior migration takes place concurrently with the appearance and interposition of the primitive perineum between the uro-genital orifice and the anus and with the ingrowth of the genital folds over the perineum and uro-genital sinus.

Errors of formation of the anus develop as the summation of defects of combined and concurrent development of the perineum and genital folds, either or both of which may be defective. If the primitive perineum is defective or if the genital folds are set posteriorly or are hypertrophic, the folds may enclose the anal pit. In any case, the lumen of the anus remains patent but is projected anteriorly as a fine fistula to the raphe or to the urethra. The term "covered anus" has been applied to this group of abnormalities. Wood Jones (1915) furnished the embryological explanation for this deformity. In the case of absence or minimal formation of the primitive perineum, the anal fistula is projected into the bulb or floor of the urethra—the recto-bulbar or ano-urethral fistula. In a partially developed perineum, the fistula is rolled anteriorly into some part of the perineal raphe, even as far anteriorly as the frenulum.

That part of the rectum which is derived from the partitioning of the cloaca is normal in dimensions in the covered anus group of anomalies, but the anal contribution is attenuated. The rectum is jammed against the urethra and issues into the back of the bulb directly or into the floor of the urethra by a slender track in the recto-bulbar or ano-urethral fistula, respectively. The rectum is nearer its normal location in the ano-cutaneous type of covered anus, and the nearer the rectum to the normal site the shorter the anal fistula (see Fig. 74).

The genital folds at the posterior site of fusion may be hypertrophic and represented by a sagittal cord of skin across the anal pit, the bucket handle deformity, or by a lump encroaching on the pit from in front or behind or by a mass consisting of a combination of all three (see Fig. 40).

ANTERIOR ANUS.—In this classification the term is restricted to that type of anus which is outwardly and functionally a normal anus but which issues to the skin of the perineum at a point anterior to the normal location.

This anomaly results from defective migration of the anus, consequent upon a relative shortness of the perineum. This anomaly is uncommon, although minor degrees of positioning may pass unrecognized.

Perineal and Anal Deformities of the Female

Perineal Groove, Perineal Canal, Covered Anus, Anterior Anus.—The perineum, being a composite structure formed of the primitive perineal mound and genital folds, may have maximal mound and minimal fold components or vice versa or any combination of both. However, when the major contribution is formed from the mound, the perineum is convex. Perineal deformities in this type are rare. When the mound contribution is minimum, the genital folds assume a major role in the composition and completion of the perineum; if, however, they fail to migrate medially, the perineum remains cleft as a *perineal groove*, the floor being the septum and the sides the genital folds; if the cleft is bridged over by the genital folds, it becomes a canal—the *perineal canal*; if the medial migration of the folds affects a greater extent of the external cloaca, the anus may be covered over in the manner of the covered anus of the male, and its lumen projected anteriorly onto the perineum or vestibule to form the *anocutaneous* or *anovulvar* types of female covered anus (see Fig. 75) (Stephens, 1968).

An anterior anus in the female may be either perineal or vulvar in situation.

The *anterior perineal anus* results from inadequate sagittal length of the otherwise normal uro-anal septum and the perineum and fourchette are slender. The *vulvar anus* is due to agenesis of this same septum, and the perineum is absent and the fourchette rudimentary (see Fig. 75).

The anterior vulvar anus as described in this book is an anus by right, supple and normal in caliber, gaining by normal development and partitioning of the internal cloaca its rightful entry into the external cloaca but remaining in its abnormal situation because of failure of subdivision of the external cloaca by the uro-anal septum. The müllerian ducts descend normally upon the anterior chamber of the already partitioned internal cloaca and descend further caudally in the uro-rectal septum to issue into the vestibule, wedged between but quite separate from the urethra and anus in the unpartitioned external cloaca. The orifice of the rectum is embryologically not a fistula but an anus, albeit abnormal in respect to site and sphincters and epithelium. In past writings, Stephens has not recognized this deformity as an entity separate from recto-vestibular fistula, but here it is included on the grounds of the presumed pathological embryology, its normal caliber and function and its differences from the recto-vestibular and ano-vestibular fistulae.

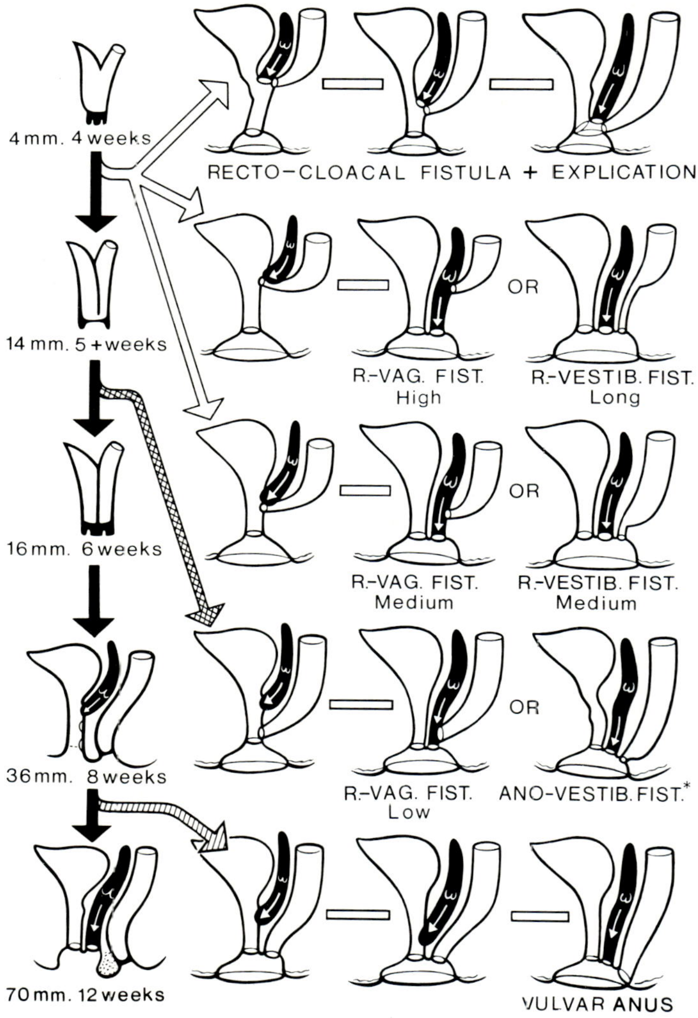

Fig. 73. – Recto-vestibular complex. Concepts of the normal (*black arrows*) and abnormal embryological pathways. White arrows indicate those malformations which derive from the failure of partition of the internal cloaca and which exhibit similar but not identical external appearances. Cross-hatched arrow indicates the possible final deformities which result from persistence of the cloacal canal modified by the intrusion of the müllerian ducts. Hatched arrow indicates the explanation of the anterior vulvar anus. The uro-rectal septum is complete, the uroanal septum is absent. Note that the diagrams in the right-hand column have very similar but not identical features, which usually distinguish them. *Although this deformity is embryologically a recto-vestibular fistula, it is herein called ano-vestibular because of its treatment by perineal anoplasty.

Embryological Differences Between Anterior Anus and Recto-Vestibular Fistula. – The recto-vestibular and recto-vaginal fistulae, by contrast with the anterior anuses, are not merely arrests along a pathway of normal development but examples of the summation of two abnormal processes, one superimposed upon another (Fig. 73). The primary error is a failure of partition of the internal cloaca by the uro-rectal septum, a state common to males and females in the sexless phase of the 16-mm. embryo. Such a deformity would show itself in the male as a recto-urethral fistula. However, in the female, the müllerian ducts descend not upon the anterior chamber of the normally partitioned internal cloaca but on the unpartitioned cloaca, which lacks some or all of the uro-rectal septum. The end result of the intrusion of the müllerian ducts depends upon the intrinsic activity of these structures, which go their own way. Some stop and enlarge at this point to form the recto-cloacal fistula but most descend caudally in tandem with the urethra to open externally in the normal place behind the urethra. In doing so, the müllerian ducts may (1) obliterate the rectal fistula, which remains attached to the vagina as a fibrous cord, (2) incorporate the rectal fistula in the back wall as a recto-vaginal fistula or (3) transport the fistula to the exterior as a recto-vestibular fistula, creating pari passu a useful but abnormal kind of septum consisting of the separate adjacent walls of vagina and rectal fistula. This vicarious and unconventional transposition of the rectum to the external cloaca is entirely dependent upon the vagaries of Müller's tubes. The recto-vestibular fistula becomes endowed with some of the properties of an anus, although its orifice is always stenotic. Its background of development, however, is not that of a true anus arrested in its normal embryonic pathway but that of a rectal fistula hitched by chance for a short ride from one abnormal site to another on the back of the sex ducts in their relentless migration to the exterior. The rectal orifice is moved from one point of arrest to another, on the normal pathway of migration by an unorthodox müllerian mechanism, which operates in the absence of the conventional uro-rectal septum and creates a late, imperfect, and alternative type of separation of the urethra, vagina and rectum (see Fig. 72).

Recto-cloacal fistula is a well-recognized and clear-cut entity (Stephens, 1963), but when the cloacal canal is short this entity may closely simulate the recto-vestibular fistula. Four patients exhibited this deformity. The orifices of urethra, vagina and rectum converge on and issue into an internal cloaca, which is so short that it is a common orifice and canal run into one. This channel then issues on the undivided external cloaca. The rectal orifice is stenotic and has a characteristic ventral slant, the urethral orifice is slanted dorsally, and both lie caudal to the vaginal orifice. These subtle features distinguish this deformity.

The small and large rectal and anal orifices in and around the fossa navicularis of the vulva fall into groups which may be distinguished by subtle, fine clinical features. These abnormal orifices arrive at their sites by different embryological pathways, and an attempt is made to illustrate these presumed paths in Figure 73.

CHAPTER 6

Classification

THE APPEARANCE of a perineum devoid of an anal orifice has traditionally suggested the name "imperforate anus and rectum," a term which has been made to embrace a complex of anomalies in this region. Yet it is often inappropriate, for by far the greater number of malformations of anus and rectum are not imperforate but communicate with either the urinary or genital tracts or actually open to the skin of the perineum. To a greater or less degree, the malformations consist of maldevelopment of the anus, or rectum, or both of these structures, for which the term "ano-rectal defect" or "dysgenesis" would be more appropriate.

Acceptable Criteria

1. The terms used should be simple, and themselves indicate the essential anatomy.
2. They should be accurate and explicit in terms of anatomy, especially in relation to the controlling sphincters, for upon these depend treatment and prognosis.
3. As far as possible, they should conform to the known facts of embryological development of both anus and rectum and associated structures.
4. They should conduce to precision in diagnosis and, therefore, must distinguish between the sexes and between communicating and noncommunicating anomalies.

Suggested Classification

As illustrative of the discrepancies in the nomenclature used by individual writers, we (1963) compiled a compendium of terms in use by contemporary writers during the 1950–1960 decade. The degree of disparity revealed was such as to call urgently for examination and revision of the whole subject of nomenclature.

In April, 1963, we introduced the subject of classification of ano-rectal deformities at a meeting of the Australian Paediatric Association, attended by 20 pediatric surgeons, and advanced proposals for a schedule of terms based upon clinical observations and embryological associations. Most views were expressed in favor of an embryological terminology, and several suggestions were incorporated. This classification, based upon the various embryological processes affecting the hindgut, cloaca, perineum and proctodeal pit, has been the basis of our previous writings (Stephens and Smith, 1963) and is reproduced in slightly modified form in Table 1 (a), and in Figures 74, 75, and 76.

TABLE 1 (A).—CLASSIFICATION BASED UPON EMBRYOLOGICAL CONCEPTS

MALE	FEMALE
Ano-Rectal Deformities	*Ano-Rectal Deformities*
A. Defects of partition of internal cloaca Ano-rectal agenesis	A. Defects of partition of internal cloaca Ano-rectal agenesis
1. Ano-rectal agenesis (no fistula)	1. Ano-rectal agenesis (no fistula)
2. Recto-vesical fistula	2. Recto-vesical fistula
3. Recto-urethral fistula	3. Recto-cloacal fistula
	4. Recto-vaginal fistula
	5. Recto-vestibular fistula
B. Secondary defect after partition	B. Secondary defect after partition
1. Rectal atresia	1. Rectal atresia
Anal Deformities	*Anal Deformities*
A. Defects of the perineum	A. Defects of the perineum
1. Anterior perineal anus	1. Anterior anus— (i) Perineal (ii) Vulvar (vestibular)
	2. Ano-vestibular fistula (syn. anal type of recto-vestibular fistula)
	3. Perineal groove
	4. Perineal canal
B. Defects of the genital folds (covered anus)	B. Defects of the genital folds (covered anus)
1. Covered anus—complete	1. Covered anus—complete
2. Ano-cutaneous fistula	2. Ano-cutaneous fistula
3. Ano-bulbar (recto-bulbar) fistula	3. Ano-vulvar fistula
C. Defects of the proctodeal pit	C. Defects of the proctodeal pit
1. Anal agenesis (no fistula)	1. Anal agenesis (no fistula)
2. Imperforate anal membrane	2. Imperforate anal membrane
3. Anal stenosis—	3. Anal stenosis—
(i) Covered anal stenosis	(i) Covered anal stenosis
(ii) Anal membrane stenosis	(ii) Anal membrane stenosis
(iii) Ano-rectal stenosis	(iii) Ano-rectal stenosis

Unclassified 1. Vesico-intestinal fissure
2. Duplication of rectum and anus
3. Combinations of the usual deformities

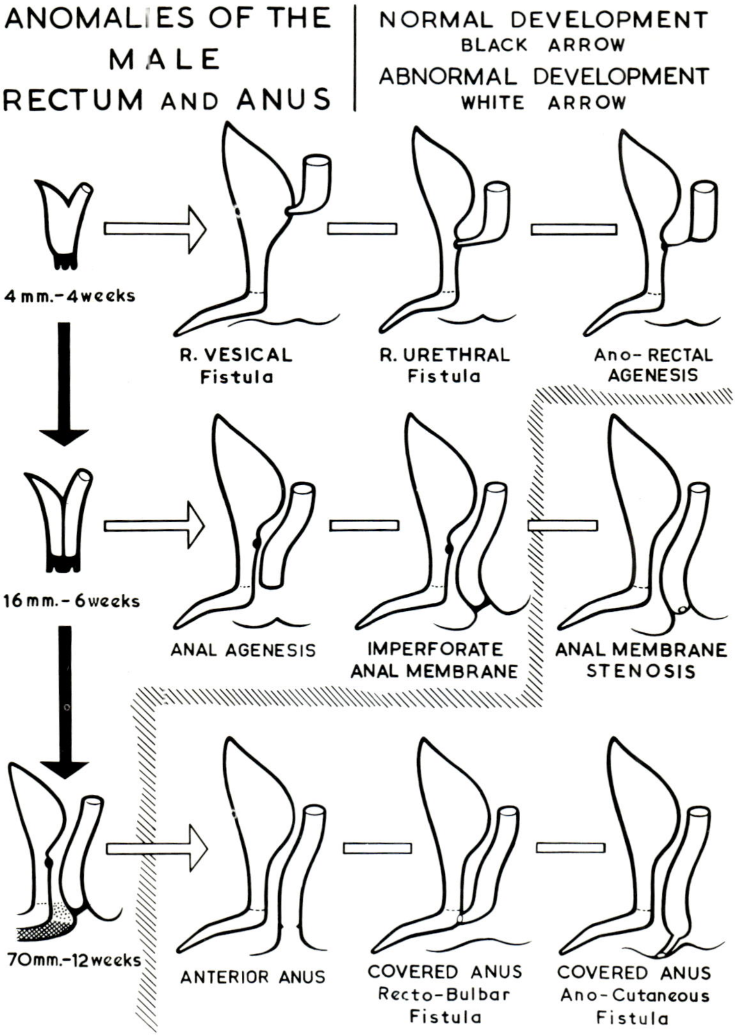

Fig. 74. – Embryological classification in the male. **Upper row,** rectal deformities arising from failure of subdivision of cloaca. **Middle row,** defects in the formation of the anal pit. **Lower row,** malformations derived from concurrent faulty development of the perineal mound (*dotted area*) causing irregular migration of the anus and of genital folds (*cross hatching*) causing anterior projection of anal fistula. Hatched line, diagnostic inversion radiographs are required to define groups shown above the line. Diagnosis of deformities shown below the line is made by local inspection.

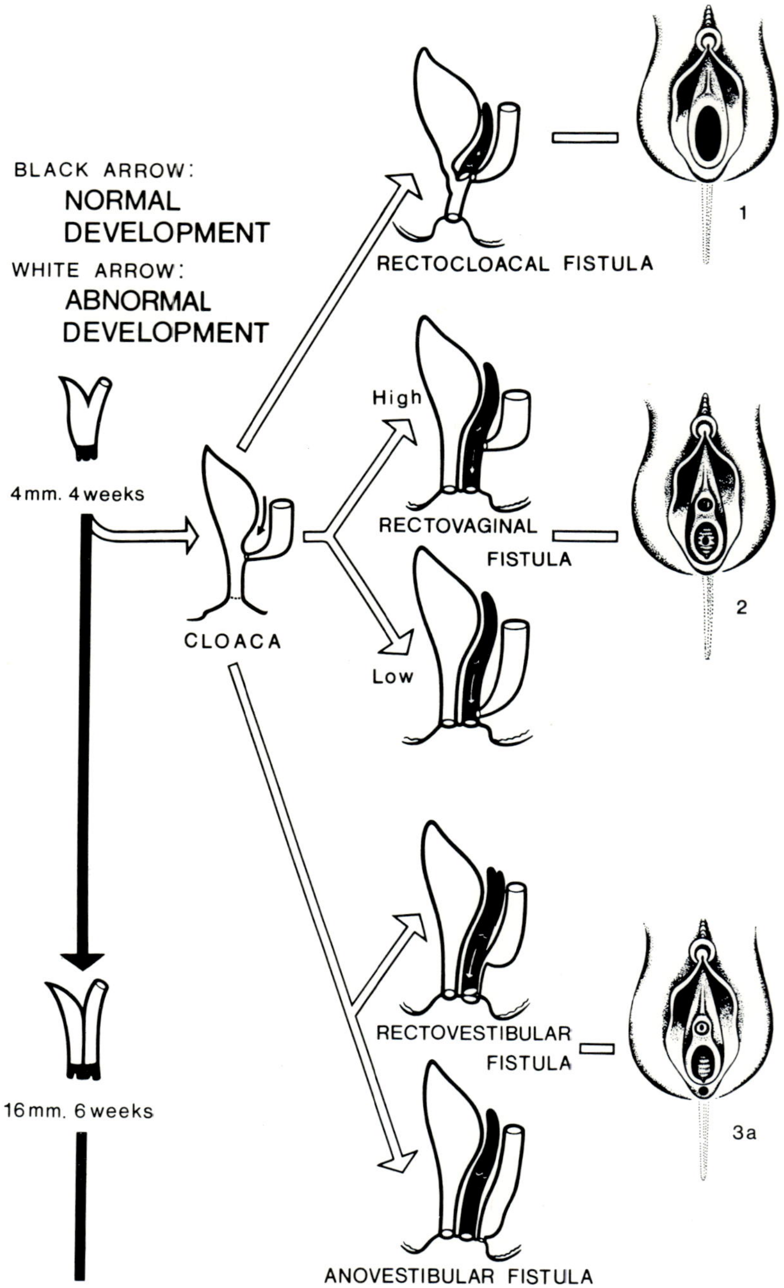

Fig. 75.—Legend on facing page.

An opportunity for a more internationally agreed upon classification at last developed during 1970. In our Hospital in Melbourne, during March 1970, was held a Paediatric Surgical Congress, a principal subject in which was ano-rectal deformities. Over 200 pediatric surgeons from 27 countries attended the symposium on terminology. Preliminary brochures and questionnaires, with diagrams of all the anomalies, had previously been circulated, so that views on terms were received from surgeons in many parts of the world, even in addition to those present at the Congress. A smaller group continued the discussions beyond the main symposium, and an agreed upon classification for international consideration was formulated. This "Proposed International Classification (1970)" is shown in Table 1 (b). In addition to the 200 surgeons who contributed to the main symposium, the smaller group of discussants included Doctors T. V. Santulli; W. B. Kiesewetter; A. H. Bill and S. Gans (United States); Professor J. Louw and Dr. S. Cywes (South Africa); Mr. H. H. Nixon (United Kingdom); Professor F. Rehbein (Germany); Dr. D. Vervat (Netherlands); Dr. G. Grotte (Sweden); Miss R. Magnus and ourselves (Australia).

The basis of the new classification is the anatomical configuration of the visceral deformities in relation to the principal muscle of continence, the pubo-rectalis part of the levator ani muscle. It is basically descriptive of the anatomical orifices and avoids controversies of embryology, especially in low anomalies. The primary divisions are those of the high rectal lesions clearly above the levator muscle (supralevator) and those of the low anal lesions clearly through the levator muscle (translevator), because from almost every point of view (anatomy, embryology, surgical approach, associated anomalies and prognosis), the two levels are fundamentally different. It was recognized, however, that a strictly high-low classification is an oversimplification since there are some anomalies in which the relation of the bowel and fistula to the levator muscle is more complex and "intermediate" in type and where therapeutic considerations are at present more controversial.

This new classification is used as the basis for this book, as outlined in the individual deformities of Chapters 3 and 4, although in some of the sections which follow we have tried to relate these

---

Fig. 75.—Schema of communicating anomalies of the female rectum and anus. **Left column,** stages in development of the normal female pelvic organs (*black arrows*). **Middle column,** congenital abnormalities derived from aberrations of development of the cloaca and perineum (*white arrows*). **Right column,** perineal patterns corresponding with the internal anatomy shown in **middle column**. **1,** recto-cloacal fistula—one external orifice. **2,** recto-vaginal fistula—two external orifices. **3a,** recto-vestibular and ano-vestibular fistulae—three external orifices, the fistulae being stenotic and all within the vestibule. (*Continued.*)

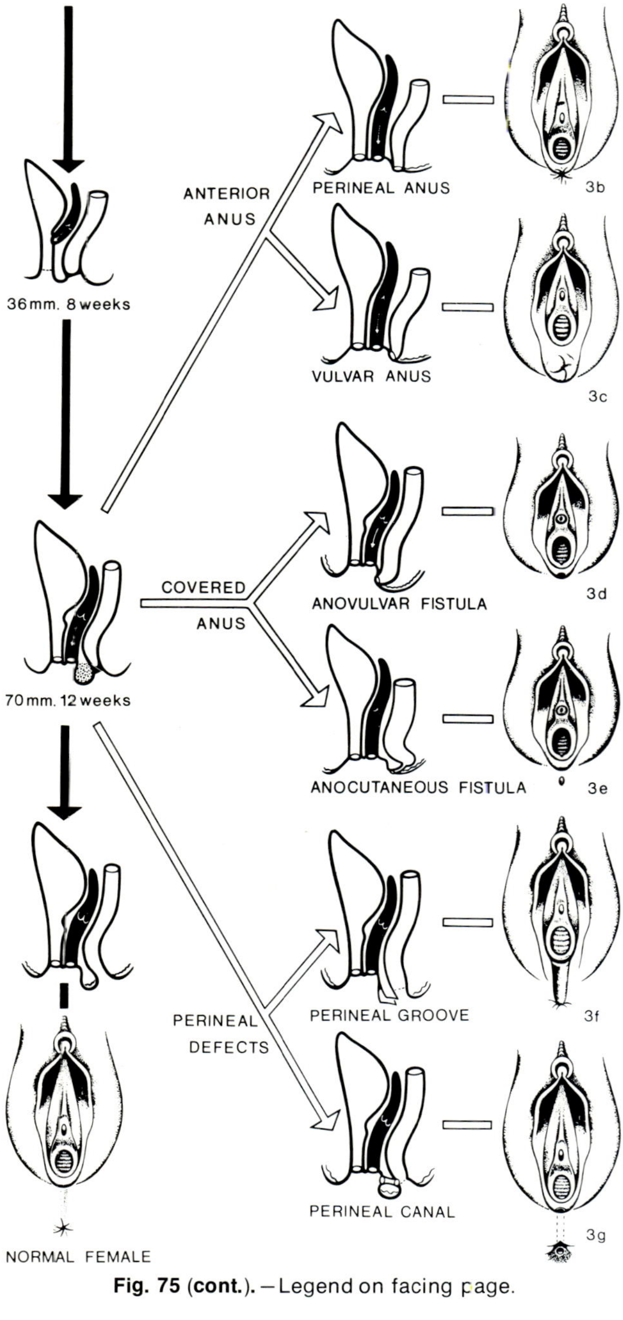

Fig. 75 (cont.). – Legend on facing page.

TABLE 1 (B).—PROPOSED INTERNATIONAL CLASSIFICATION OF ANO-RECTAL ANOMALIES (1970)
(see also Appendix C, inside back cover)

HIGH ANOMALIES (SUPRALEVATOR)

1. Ano-rectal agenesis

Male	*Female*
(a) Without fistula	(a) Without fistula
Ano-rectal agenesis (no fistula)	Ano-rectal agenesis (no fistula)
(b) With fistula	(b) With fistula
(i) Recto-vesical	(i) Recto-vesical
(ii) Recto-urethral	(ii) Recto-cloacal
	(iii) Recto-vaginal—high

2. Rectal atresia
   Male and Female

INTERMEDIATE ANOMALIES

1. Anal agenesis

Male	*Female*
(a) Without fistula	(a) Without fistula
Anal agenesis (no fistula)	Anal agenesis (no fistula)
(b) With fistula	(b) With fistula
Recto-bulbar	(i) Recto-vaginal—low
	(ii) Recto-vestibular

2. Ano-rectal stenosis
   Male and Female

LOW ANOMALIES (TRANSLEVATOR)

1. At normal anal site
   Male and Female
   (i) Covered anus—complete*
   (ii) Anal stenosis†
2. At perineal site

Male	*Female*
(i) Anterior perineal anus	(i) Anterior perineal anus
(ii) Ano-cutaneous fistula (Covered anus—incomplete)	(ii) Ano-cutaneous fistula (Covered anus—incomplete)

3. At vulvar site

Female
(i) Vulvar anus
(ii) Ano-vulvar fistula
(iii) Ano-vestibular fistula

*Includes imperforate anal membrane.
†Includes anal membrane stenosis.

Fig. 75 (cont.).—**3b,** anterior perineal and, **3c,** anterior vulvar anus—both exhibit three external orifices, the anuses being normal in dimensions. **3d,** ano-vulvar fistula and, **3e,** ano-cutaneous fistula—both being examples of covered anus, and both exhibit three orifices, the anal orifice being stenotic and issuing into the fourchette (**3d**) or perineum close to the fourchette (**3e**). **3f,** perineal groove—three external orifices, the anus being nonstenotic and in continuity with the vestibule by a wet perineal groove. **3g,** perineal canal—four external orifices, the anus being normal in appearance and a fine fistulous tract leading from the anterior wall of anal canal to vestibule.

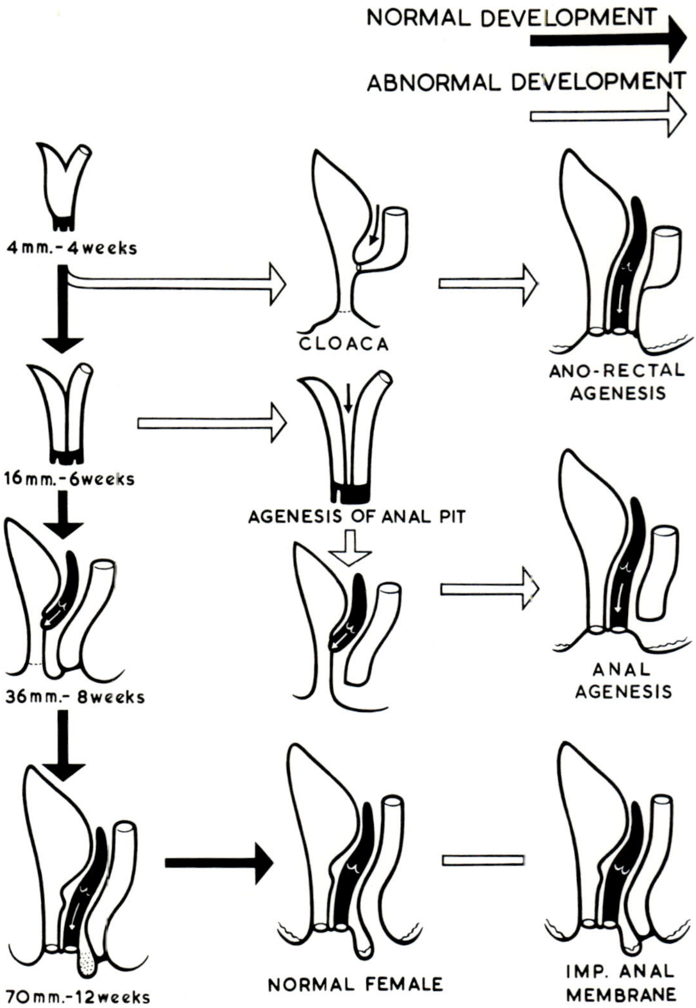

Fig. 76.—Noncommunicating anomalies of the female rectum and anus. **Left column,** stages in normal development. **Middle column,** presumed aberrations of stages of development. **Right column,** the deformities.

terms to the embryological concepts. The classification is shown in Table 1 (b) and is illustrated in Appendix C, Ano-Rectal Anomalies (Proposed International Classification, 1970) in the pouch on the inside back cover.

It was agreed that the less common and rare anomalies be listed in a miscellaneous group. It is noted that the membrane deformities (imperforate anal membrane and anal membrane stenosis) and perineal groove and canal have, in the International Classification, been put in the miscellaneous group because of their rarity, although we have included them in the analysis of figures of incidence and in our descriptive text. These rare patients have been compiled into a list from the literature and our own cases in Table 1 (c).

In *ano-rectal deformities,* the embryological basis is a failure of development of the terminal bowel, both anus and rectum "agenesis," combined with a failure of the partition process which separates the primitive internal cloaca into uro-genital sinus and rectum. Incomplete partition results in fistulous communications between rectum and the urinary or genital tracts. In the male, such fistulae are at the level of the verumontanum or higher. Anatomically, these deformities all lie at or above the level of the levator ani muscle and require a major rectal reconstruction through the pubo-rectalis sling of this vital muscle if continence is to be preserved. In the International Classification they are all supralevator lesions.

The formation of *"rectal atresia"* is believed, however, to be an acquired lesion, perhaps secondary to some vascular accident to the gut after its formation, akin to the formation of atresias in other parts of the gut. The evidence for this hypothesis and the special features of the lesion are discussed in Chapter 4.

TABLE 1 (c).—List of Miscellaneous Rare Anomalies

Both Sexes

1. Imperforate anal membrane
2. Anal membrane stenosis
3. Vesico-intestinal fissure (Chapter 13)
4. Duplications of anus, rectum and genitourinary tracts (Chapter 13)

Variants and Combinations of the Usual Malformations

Male

1. Ano-rectal agenesis (no fistula)
   - (i) Varying lengths of absent colon and rectum
     (Spriggs, 1912; Zaidi, 1959; Trusler *et al.*, 1959; Dickinson, 1967)
     (Also see Duplications, Chapter 13)
2. Recto-vesical fistula
   - (i) Recto-vesical and recto-urethral fistulae (Swenson and Grana, 1965)
   - (ii) Recto-vesical fistula into ectopia vesicae (Moore and Lawrence, 1952)
   - (iii) Recto-vesical and "recto-perineal" fistula (Moore and Lawrence, 1952)
   - (iv) Recto-vesical fistula and vesico-intestinal fissure (Santulli, 1970)
   - (v) Colo-vesical fistula (Trusler *et al.*, 1959)
   - (vi) Recto-vesical fistula and a patent stenotic anus (Prasad, 1970)
3. Recto-urethral fistula
   - (i) Recto-urethral fistula and normal anus (micro-urethra)
     (Our own case, Fig. 25, p. 51)
   - (ii) Recto-urethral fistula and normal anus
     (Brenner, 1915; Le Duc, 1965; Santulli, 1970)
   - (iii) Recto-urethral and recto-vesical fistulae

TABLE 1 (c).—(*cont.*)

TABLE 1 (c).–(*cont.*)

(Swenson and Grana, 1965)

(iv) Colo-urethral fistula and imperforate anal membrane and colo-neurenteric canal fistula

4. Recto-bulbar fistula

(i) Recto-bulbar fistula and normal anus
(Keith, 1908; Ramakrishnan, 1970)

5. Ano-cutaneous fistula

(i) "Recto-perineal" and recto-vesical fistulae
(Moore and Lawrence, 1952)

(ii) Covered anus with the fistulous tract deep to the scrotum
(Nixon, 1970)

Female

1. Ano-rectal agenesis (no fistula)

(i) Ano-rectal agenesis and atretic vagina and hydrometrocolpos
(Snyder, 1966; Mahoney and Chamberlain, 1940)

(ii) Ano-rectal agenesis and common urethro-vaginal cloaca
(Snyder, 1966)

2. Recto-vesical fistula

(i) Recto-vesical fistula and absent vagina
(Trusler and Wilkinson, 1962; Louw, 1965)

(ii) Rectovesical and rectocloacal fistulae (Rehbein, 1970)

3. Recto-cloacal fistula

(i) Recto-cloacal fistula (?recto-urethral) and hypoplastic vagina
(Our case, p. 89; Mayo and Rice, 1950; Hanley *et al.*, 1954; Brayton and Norris, 1958; Snyder, 1966)

(ii) Complicated combinations reviewed by Lowsley (1948); Gough (1959); Stephens (1961, 1966); and Snyder (1966)

e.g., Gough (1959) – wide vesico-cloacal orifice
– double rectum and mucocolpos
– cloaca with minute external orifice
– with pseudohermaphrodism
– with tubelike phallus

e.g., Snyder (1966) – cloacal canal of small caliber and hydrometrocolpos
– cloaca continued into penile or clitoral urethra (and epispadias)
– cloaca with ano-rectal agenesis

e.g., Our own p. 334 – with exstrophy of the cloaca

(iii) Recto-cloacal fistula at *normal* anal site and female pseudohermaphrodism and normal urethra as well
(Sieber and Klein, 1958)

(iv) Recto-cloacal and recto-vesical fistulae (Rehbein, 1970)

(v) Recto-cloacal fistula and megarectum (and absent appendix)
(Cartledge, 1970)

4. Recto-vaginal fistula

(i) Recto-vaginal and "recto-perineal" fistulae
(Moore and Lawrence, 1952)

(ii) Recto-vaginal fistula and hydrometrocolpos
(Moore and Lawrence, 1952)

(iii) Colo-vaginal fistula and absent rectum
(Trusler *et al.*, 1959)

(iv) Recto-vaginal fistula and a normal anus
(Nixon, 1970; Loufti, 1970; Ramakrishnan, 1970; Mishalany, 1970)

(v) Recto-vaginal fistula and anal stenosis
(Santulli, 1970)

(vi) Recto-vaginal fistula and exstrophy of bladder
(Santulli, 1970)
5. Ano-vulvar fistula
(i) Ano-vulvar fistula and ectopia vesicae
(Our case, p. 109 and Fig. 107, *B*)
6. Perineal groove
(Stephens 1968)
7. Perineal canal
(i) Ano-vestibular fistula and normal anus
(Our cases, p. 116; Bryndorf and Madsen, 1959; Sitkovskii, 1963; Pegum *et al.*, 1964; Chatterjee and Talukder, 1969; Ninh and Bohn, 1970)
(ii) Ano-vestibular fistula and anterior perineal anus
(Chatterjee and Talukder, 1969)

In the embryological *anal deformities*, there are developmental faults caudal to a normally subdivided cloaca. These faults affect the formation of the primitive perineum, the genital folds and the proctodeal pit and membrane; in addition, there may be a variable degree of anal agenesis, affecting a portion of the anal canal—an area variously described as originating from the postallantoic gut segment of the rectum (Wood Jones 1904 and 1915) or from the cloaca itself (Keith, 1908). Anomalies may arise from an aberration of any one of these embryological processes, although usually they act in combination. In formulating the basis of an embryological classification, the primary aberration is used to denote a group, even though another process may be added secondarily.

The three primary aberrations of the anus are as follows:

1. The perineal structures between bowel and uro-genital sinus may fail to develop fully, resulting in close approximation of gut to urethra or vagina. The same phenomenon may be considered as a failure of "migration" of the anus backwards from its primitive forward position (Bill and Johnson, 1958; Bill, 1964). In its "pure" manifestation, the aberration results in an *"anterior perineal anus"* in either sex. In females, a *vulvar anus* and an *"ano-vestibular fistula"* are partly referable to the same process, but in addition in the latter, the proctodeal pit has not fully formed. These anomalies are translevator, i.e., low.

2. The proctodeal pit may become secondarily "covered" by abnormal fusion of the genital folds or anal tubercles (Browne, 1955; Stephens, 1953a). The classic examples are *"covered anus—complete," "covered anal stenosis"* and *"ano-cutaneous fistula"* in either sex, and the *"ano-vulvar fistula"* in females; in a *"recto-bulbar fistula"* in the male, in addition to the covering process, there is a lack of development of perineal structures and anal canal, so that the rectum remains anteriorly approximated to the urethra. The embryological details of the covering process are discussed fully in Chapter 5.

3. The proctodeal pit may be incomplete in its development. Absence of the entire pit and terminal anal canal results in *"anal agenesis—no fistula"*; incomplete perforation of the proctodeal membrane may result only in *"imperforate anal membrane"* or *"anal membrane stenosis"* and incomplete development of the pit and/or part of the anal canal may result in *"ano-rectal stenosis."*

Anatomically, the embryological anal deformities, such as anterior anus, vulvar anus and the covered anus group, all perforate the pubo-visceral sling of the levator ani muscle and are thus translevator low anomalies. The three exceptions are recto-bulbar fistula (embryologically, "ano"-bulbar fistula), anal agenesis (no fistula) and ano-rectal stenosis. Embryologically, we believe these deformities are primarily anal in origin, but anatomically the termination of the bowel is seated on the sling in intimate relationship to the muscle and they thus correctly appear in the International Classification as "Intermediate."

Further, the very low occluded anus at the normal anal site, listed in the International Classification as "covered anus—complete," was accepted as the more common cause of complete occlusion at this site; "imperforate anal membrane" also causes complete occlusion at the normal anal site but was considered so rare that it should be listed in the miscellaneous rare group and not in the basic list.

The details of the various embryological processes are discussed in Chapter 5, also by Stephens (1963 and 1967) and, in relation to classification, are shown diagrammatically in Figures 74, 75 and 76.

Modifications in the Female

The subdivision of the internal cloaca in females is complicated by the arrival of the müllerian ducts between the junction of the bowel and the uro-genital passages. The interposition of the descending müllerian ducts joining with the sino-vaginal bulbs thenceforth affects the transfer of the rectal attachment to the cloaca. Persistence of the opening of the rectum into the cloaca without caudal migration of the müllerian ducts results in a *"recto-cloacal fistula."* With further caudal migration of the müllerian ducts, one of two events may occur: The rectal orifice may be incorporated in the posterior wall of the fused müllerian ducts as they migrate caudally, thus creating a separate urethra and vagina while the rectal orifice presents in the posterior wall of the vagina—the *"recto-vaginal fistula"*—or the müllerian ducts may carry the rectal orifice before them to the exterior as a *"recto-vestibular fistula."* Although these deformities are embryologically "rectal" in origin and thus supralevator, in the case of *low* recto-vaginal fistula and recto-vestibular fistula, the bowel is "intermediate" in position with respect to the pubo-visceral sling.

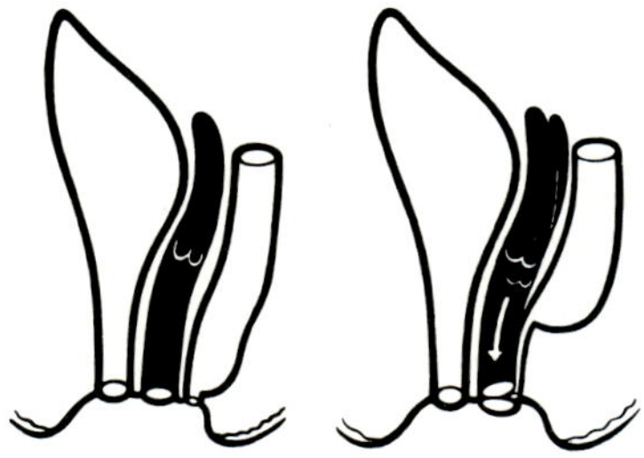

Fig. 77 (left).—Ano-vestibular fistula. Orifice of rectum is stenotic and opens into vestibule.
Fig. 78 (right).—Recto-vestibular fistula. Both the orifice and adjoining rectum are stenotic.

Anal Orifices in the Vestibular Area.—Deformities in the vestibular area are numerous and complex and are described in detail in Chapter 8 and in Figure 75. The lesions encountered are as follows:

(i) Vulvar anus
(ii) Perineal groove
(iii) Perineal canal
(iv) Ano-vulvar fistula
(v) Recto-vestibular fistula
(vi) Ano-vestibular fistula

Superficially, apart from the perineal groove anomaly, these resemble one another in that there is an anal or fistulous opening in the vestibular zone. However, each arises by a slightly differing aberration in embryological development. (i) The *"vulvar anus"* is grouped as a variety of anterior anus and is distinguished by possessing a true anal orifice rather than a fistula (see Fig. 59, *D* and *E*). (ii) A *perineal groove* deformity is encountered in some otherwise normal premature babies, and the anus is functionally normal, requiring no treatment (see Figs. 65 and 66). (iii) A *perineal canal* deformity resembles an ano-vestibular fistula, except that posteriorly it communicates with the anal canal (see Fig. 67). (iv) An *ano-vulvar fistula* is a vulval siting of the forward fistula of the covered anus (see Figs. 60, *B*, and 106, *C*). (v) and (vi) The commonest anomaly in the female is a fistulous opening in the vestibule, immediately behind the vagina. It has been variously described as "imperforate anus with recto-fourchette fistula" (Bill, 1964) and "ectopic vestibular anus" (Nixon, 1961; Partridge and Gough, 1961; Louw, 1959). Stephens (1953 and 1964) attributed the anomaly to a "migratory" defect, in that the rectal opening becomes incorporated into the sinovaginal bulbs and is carried with them into the vestibule. He describes two varieties, the usual type (Fig. 77 and see Figs. 63, 64 and 106, *A*), in which the rectum is normal in caliber but opens by a stenotic orifice in the vestibule, and the unusual type (Fig. 78 and see Figs. 56 and 57), encountered on seven occasions, in which the rectum lies at a higher level and from its anterior wall arises a long fine fistula to the vestibule. Because these two varieties are probably referable to the same aberration of embryological development, Stephens has considered them both as "rectal" in origin and in consequence recto-vestibular fistulae. In further support of this contention is the fact that they are associated with sacral anomalies in a frequency similar to those in other rectal defects, whereas anal anomalies are infrequently so associated. However, in the important respects of sphincter anatomy and treatment, the two varieties are fundamentally different. In the unusual type with a long fine fistula, the normal caliber rectum lies cranial to the pubo-rectalis muscle and requires a complicated rectoplasty, as do other cloacal deformities. The normal caliber rectum of the usual type is surrounded by the pubo-rectalis muscle which can be made to function where it lies by a simple perineal operation, i.e., a low anomaly.

For practical purposes we have now, therefore, separated the two varieties—the rare long fistula-type being called *recto-vestibular fistula* and the more usual type *ano-vestibular fistula.*

The Term "Anal Stenosis"

The term "anal stenosis" is a confusing one and in some classifications is listed as a specific type of anal deformity, e.g., the "microscopic anus" described by Denis Browne. But almost any fistula, e.g., a recto-urethral fistula, might equally be described as a rectal stenosis; however, this term would be quite inappropriate, for it would not convey the essential anatomy of the fistulous connection. We use the term "anal stenosis" for a narrowed channel at the normal anal site but recognize that it may arise by a variety of processes.

Apart from postoperative stenosis by stricture, anal stenosis may appear in three forms:

1. Associated with Covered Anus, Covered Anal Stenosis.—The majority of "anal stenoses" appear to fall into this group. The anal pit, after its formation, becomes covered over at its normal site by excessive development of the genital folds or anal tubercles. The folds may cover the pit from behind or from in front or cross the anus anteroposteriorly, producing a stenotic orifice on either side of a bar of hypertrophied tissue, the so-called bucket handle deformity (see Figs. 39 and 40).

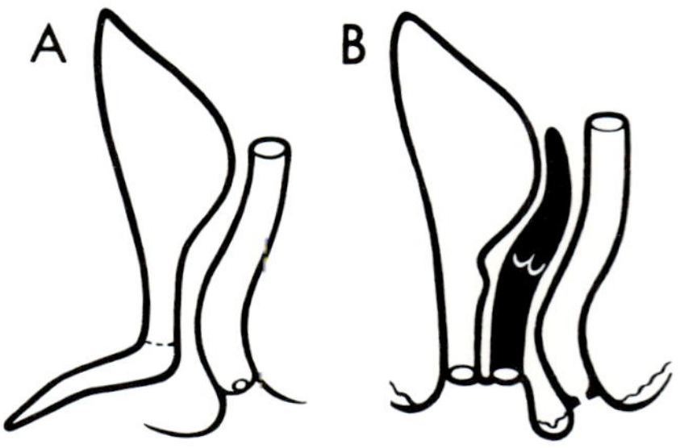

Fig. 79.—Anal membrane stenosis. The anus is at the normal site, but the proctodeal membrane has not completely broken down. **A,** male. **B,** female.

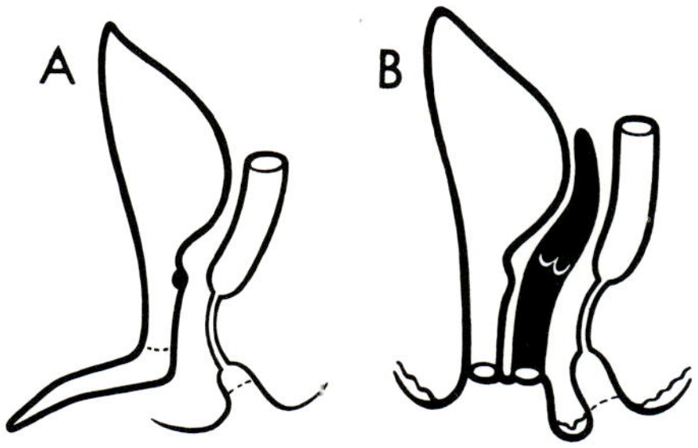

Fig. 80.—Ano-rectal stenosis. A long segment of the anal canal is stenotic; etiology is probably similar to that in rectal atresia. **A,** male. **B,** female.

The latter anomaly was previously described as congenital median band in 6 cases by Bill and Johnson (1953) and in 11 cases by Bill *et al.* (1958). Browne (1951) described 2 cases and Drueck (1925), Saphir (1943), and Perry (1962), each described 1 case. Bill attributed the anomaly to fusion of the anal tubercles and failure of fusion of this structure laterally with the perineum.

2. Anal Membrane Stenosis.—The anal pit may be defective in that the proctodeal membrane has only partially broken down, leaving a circumferential narrowing at the level of the anal valves (Fig. 79 and see Fig. 40, *D*).

3. Ano-Rectal Stenosis.—Rarely the whole pit from anal verge to the valves or beyond the valves into the ano-rectal canal may be stenotic (Fig. 80 and see Figs. 35 and 40, *C*). The lesion may represent an acquired one similar to other areas of stenosis in the bowel or could be a developmental hypoplasia of the gut, including the proctodeal membrane.

In the International Classification, it was decided to use the simple and single term "anal stenosis" for any stenotic orifice *at the normal anal site* and that most of these cases would actually be "covered anal stenosis"; the second process, "anal membrane stenosis," might be recognized by the discriminating surgeon, but no harm would come if the two lesions were confused. Anal stenoses of these two types are low translevator deformities.

On the other hand, the more extensive length of "ano-rectal stenosis" placed the lesion in the intermediate group in the Classification.

Unclassified Types

On rare occasions, complex defects have been described which do not clearly find a place in the above classification, such as vesico-intestinal fissure, duplications of the anus and combinations and variants of the basic deformities. The former rarities are described in Chapter 13, and other variants are described throughout the text under the basic deformity they most resemble.

Comparison of Classifications with Those of Other Authors

The many terms used by writers in this field have caused confusion in interpretation of descriptions of the various malformations of the rectum and anus, a confusion which is exaggerated when male and female deformities are intermixed and considered in the same classification.

At present, lack of agreement in terminology hinders to the point of altogether preventing any true comparison of results in series of case reports of different authors. It is now hoped that the agreement of an International Classification (1970), with the discussions of this chapter, may provide a basis for future critical analysis of results.

To aid the identification of particular groups, the systems used by several authors are assembled in such a way that they may be compared with the new Classification. Appendix C (see inside back cover) includes the page references to the individual abnormalities discussed in this text.

Discussion on Classification

In addition to those of the ten authors listed in Appendix C, many other classifications have been devised over the years. It is now proposed to outline briefly the history of classification and follow with comments on some of the terms used by other more recent writers.

The History of Classification

It is obvious that no system of classification other than one based upon postmortem anatomical studies could have been advanced in the days of blind "cut and thrust" prior to the introduction and advocacy by Amussat of his operation of proctoplasty in 1835. That this original and pioneer surgeon had profited by what must have been a considerable experience in the surgical management of congenital occlusions of the rectum and/or anus is evident from the fact that *Amussat* identified five separate congenital defects affecting this region. In the first, the anus was "preternaturally narrowed"; in the second "closed up by membrane"; in the third, the rectum was "intercepted by a simple septum" at a variable distance from the anal opening; in the fourth, the anus was imperforate and the rectum deficient to a greater or less degree; in a fifth group, the rectum opened into some other organ, such as the bladder, urethra or vagina or at some point in the perineum.

In Amussat's first and second groups may be recognized types 1 and 2 of the widely accepted classification of Ladd and Gross of a later day, and the third, fourth and fifth groups are absorbed in type 3, Ladd and Gross' largest group, and distinguished by its proneness to fistulous openings into neighboring viscera or to the skin. There would seem to be no place in Amussat's sorting out of the different lesions for any corresponding to Ladd and Gross' type 4, a rarely occurring malformation in which a normally developed anus provides entry into a blind proctodeal pouch, associated with occlusion of the terminal rectum above the pouch.

In the years following the original descriptions of Amussat in 1835, no further contribution to classification was made until Bodenhammer, in 1860, in a collection of 287 cases, devised the first systematic classification based largely on postmortem specimens. This system was expanded by Ball (1887) as follows:

Bodenhammer's Classification (1860) modified by Ball (1887)

1. Preternatural narrowing of the anus at the margin.
2. Complete occlusion of the anal aperture by membrane or common integument.
3. No anus whatever, the rectum being partly deficient and terminating in a cul-de-sac at a greater or less distance above its natural outlet.
4. Normal anus, the rectum above being obstructed by membrane or occluded.
5. Anus opens in perineal or sacral area.
6. Rectum issues in the bladder, urethra, vagina or cloaca, and no anus is present.
7. Rectum normal, but ureters, vagina or uterus opens preternaturally into it.
8. No rectum at all.
9. Absent rectum and colon.

Almost all clinical varieties currently recognized are included in this classification.

Stieda (1903), in an important paper, provided a superb survey of anatomy, classification and embryology and described accurately all the types presently recognized, including correct siting of a recto-urethral fistula (so inaccurately drawn in papers of the present decade); he recognized all the varieties of covered anus, including the various sites of fistula opening anywhere from behind the scrotum to the shaft of the penis, even as far forwards as the distal extent of the penile raphe beneath the prepuce; he also distinguished between a recto-vaginal and a recto-vestibular fistula, a point still confused in much modern literature.

Delbet and Brechot (1916) also stressed the sites of fistulae.

Wood Jones (1904) and Keith (1908) classified the lesions on an embryological basis, and Keith (1908), in addition, was particularly accurate in his identification of the various types—Figure 81 indicates his findings in 79 pathological specimens.

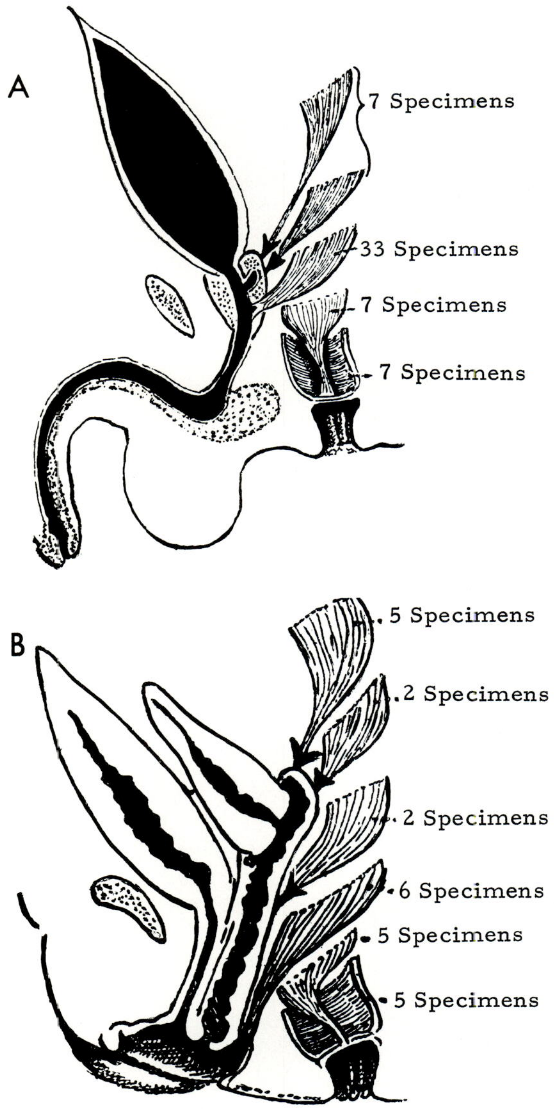

Fig. 81.—Degrees of imperfection of the rectum as depicted by Keith (1908). Deformations found in 54 specimens of male (**A**) and 25 specimens of female (**B**) infants. (Reproduced with permission from Brit. M. J. 2:1736, 1908.)

Keith's Classification (1908)

It is noted especially that Keith, like Stieda, recognized that in the male the urinary fistula opened into the posterior urethra rather than into the bladder, and in the female that a fistula into the fourchette was common and different from those into the vagina.

However, surgeons continued to favor a clinical or anatomical system rather than an embryological one because of its more practical application.

Brenner (1915), for example, suggested the following system:

Brenner's Classification (1915)

(A) *Atresia ani*
1. Partial occlusion or narrowing of the anus.
2. Complete occlusion by a membranous diaphragm.
3. Total absence of the anus, the rectum ending in a blind pouch.
4. Total absence of the anus, the rectum opening into bladder, urethra, uterus, vagina, perineum or sacral region.

(B) *Atresia recti*
1. Partial occlusion or narrowing of the rectum.
2. Complete occlusion by a membranous diaphragm.
3. Complete absence or extensive obliteration of the rectum.

(C) Rectum and anus normal, but ureters, uterus or vagina emptying into the rectal cavity (very rare).

(D) Absence of large intestine, rectum and anus (rare).

(E) Rectal diverticulae (very rare).

Frazer (1926) introduced embryological terms into the clinical classification.

Frazer's Classification (1926)

(A) *Anus*
1. Congenital narrowing of the anal canal.
2. Congenital occlusion of the anal canal by fibrous or membranous tissue, the occlusion being partial or complete.
3. Abnormal location of the anus.
4. Congenital absence of the anus.

(B) *Rectum*
1. Total absence.
2. Atresia or lower end of the rectum.
3. Membranous occlusion of the rectum.
4. Recto-vaginal, recto-urethral and recto-vesical fistulae.

Fitchet (1926), Bacon (1938), and Crowell and Dulin (1940) also published anatomical classifications, but the classification of *Ladd and Gross (1934)*, with its simplified concept of the degree and distribution of the atresia, came to be the established system for many years.

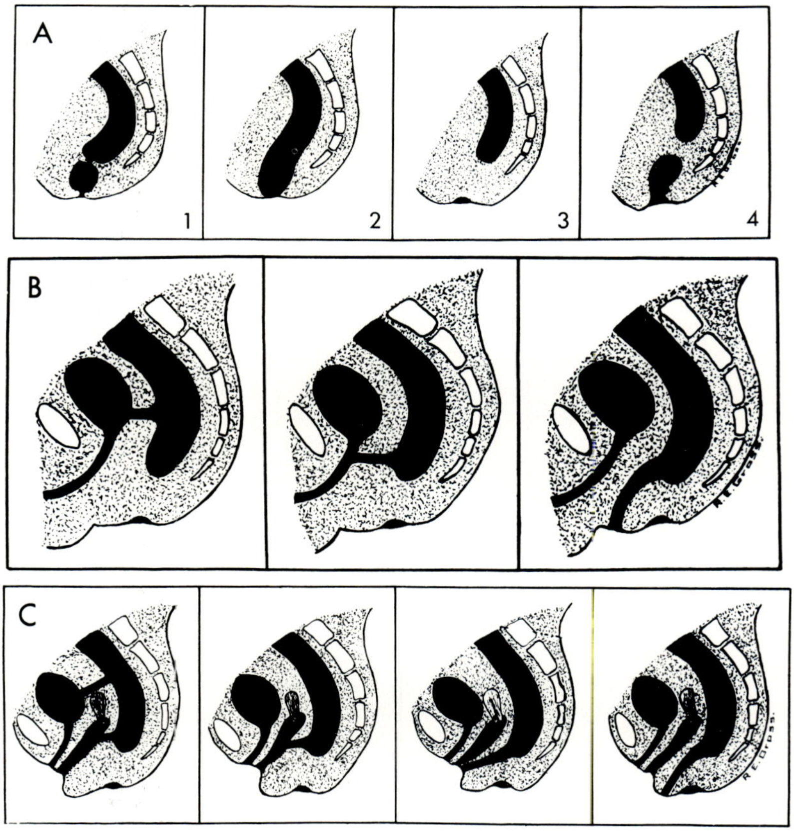

Fig. 82.—Types of anal and rectal abnormalities as depicted by Ladd and Gross (1934). **A,** type 1 deformities, anal stenosis and ano-rectal stenosis; type 2, imperforate anal membrane; type 3, imperforate anus with rectal pouch blind or with fistula as in **B** and **C**; and type 4, rectal atresia. **B,** type 3 deformities with fistulae in males, recto-vesical, recto-urethral and recto-perineal. **C,** type 3 deformities with fistulae in females, recto-vesical and recto-vaginal, recto-fossa navicularis and recto-perineal. (Reproduced with permission from Ladd, W. E., and Gross, R. E.: Am. J. Surg. 23:167, 1934.)

It was based upon clinical studies and did much to facilitate clear thinking in the prevailing confusion.

The Ladd and Gross (1934) Classification (Fig. 82)

Type 1—Anal stenosis and ano-rectal stenosis.
Type 2—Imperforate anal membrane.
Type 3—Imperforate anus with blind rectal pouch or associated with fistulae to the bladder, urethra, vagina or perineum.
Type 4—Rectal atresia.

This classification has been used in many series, especially in North America; (Harken, 1942; Lee, 1944; Dmytryk, 1945; Rosenblatt and May, 1946; Rhoads *et al.*, 1948; Norris *et al.*, 1949; Patton, 1949; Mayo and Rice, 1950; Arnheim, 1951; Santulli, 1952 and 1963; Moore and Lawrence, 1952; Hanley *et al.*, 1954; Potts *et al.*, 1954; Dennison, 1955; Palmer, 1956; Brayton and Norris, 1958; Bradham, 1958; Donovan and Stanley-Brown, 1958; Bradham, 1961; Snyder, 1961; Salzberg and Martin, 1961; Fisher, 1961; Lawler, 1961; Lynn and Ascari, 1962; Trusler and Wilkinson, 1962; Kiesewetter and Turner, 1963; Kiesewetter *et al.*, 1964; Woolam, 1964).

The classification of Ladd and Gross has obviously proved useful, but we, bearing in mind the earlier work of Browne (1951) and Stephens (1953), find the following difficulties:

(a) Types 1, 2 and 4 are all very uncommon, and almost all the malformations (85%) occur in type 3. Type 3 includes simple low anomalies (e.g., ano-cutaneous and ano-vestibular fistulae), which require local perineal operation only and carry a good prognosis, and difficult high anomalies requiring extensive rectoplasty with less satisfactory prognosis. An over-all statement of "results in type 3" is thus relatively meaningless. So broad a grouping, as type 3, provides little guidance in diagnosis or in planning treatment.

(b) Most importantly, the classification does not define the essential relationship of the viscera to the controlling sphincters, especially to the pubo-rectalis muscle. This fact is frequently noted in the complete inaccuracy of the diagrams in many papers, which bear little relationship to the facts as found in anatomical dissections.

The Classification of Denis Browne (1951, 1955), Stephens (1953) and Stephens and Smith (1963)

These authors introduced a classification based upon embryological concepts which related the levels of the visceral malformations to the pelvic floor and the controlling sphincters. It has materially assisted in more accurate diagnosis and defining the type of management which makes best use of the available sphincters. With minor modifications, it is used in the following series of cases: In the United Kingdom: Browne, 1951 and 1955; Forshall, 1960; Nixon, 1959 and 1961; Partridge and Gough, 1961; Swain and Tucker, 1962; McPherson, 1962. In Scandinavia: Winkel-Smith, 1953; Parkkulainen, 1957; Bryndorf and Madsen, 1959; Sommerschild *et al.*, 1964. In South Africa: Louw, 1959; Katzen, 1962; Louw, 1964. In Australia: Stephens, 1953 and 1963. In Poland: Bielowicz, 1965. In the United States: Scott and Swenson, 1959; Swenson and Grana, 1962; Bill, 1964; Lloyd, 1964; Santulli *et al.*, 1965.

The largest series so far reported (323 patients) utilizing this classification is that of Partridge and Gough (1961), from the Hospital for Sick Children, London, where the terms "low" and "high" refer to the level of imperforation with respect to the levator ani. High refers to the bowel ending above the levator ani.

Partridge and Gough, 1961

Low abnormalities

1. Covered anus
2. Ectopic anus
   perineal ectopic (male)
   vulval ectopic
   vestibular ectopic (female)
   vaginal ectopic
3. Stenosed anus
4. Anal membrane
   imperforate
   stenosis

High abnormalities

1. Ano-rectal agenesis, with or without fistulae to urinary or genital tracts
2. Rectal atresia
3. Cloaca
4. Multiple abnormalities

The concept of "high" and "low" anomalies, based upon the level of the agenetic bowel in relation to the levator ani, has proved helpful in planning treatment, and many authors have subsequently based their classifications upon these levels (Nixon, 1959 and 1961; Scott and Swenson, 1959; Sommerschild *et al.*, 1964; Lloyd, 1964). However, to some extent, this has tended to oversimplify the problem, the implication being that low anomalies, having penetrated the levator ani, may be treated by a perineal approach and carry a good prognosis, whereas high anomalies require an extensive rectoplasty, in which the outlook is more problematical. But our experience is that there are anomalies neither high nor low, but intermediate in type, some requiring a simple "low" approach, others requiring management appropriate to a "high" aberration. Examples of these intermediate types are the recto-bulbar fistula and anal agenesis in the male (requiring, in our view, a preliminary colostomy followed by sacro-perineal surgery later), a low recto-vaginal fistula (in which the bowel, but not the fistula, is above the levator, managed by us as a high anomaly but by many others as a low anomaly) and a recto-vestibular fistula (which may be short or long).

This intermediate group has now been recognized in the International Classification (1970), in which the complex relationship of bowel to pubo-rectalis is appreciated and by which surgeons may have varying approaches to this difficult area.

In our earlier writings, to avoid these difficulties, we suggested that the terms "low" and "high" be replaced by the terms "anal" and "rectal," respectively, followed by the description of the fistula; thus the term "recto-vaginal fistula" referred to a deformity of the rectum, communicating with the vagina, but, because it is a "rectal" deformity, the term implies a defect situated *above* the levator, not withstanding how "low" the fistula appears to be in the vagina. This view is supported by the classifications of Bacon and Sherman (1952), Louw (1959), Bryndorf and Madsen (1959), Gans *et al.* (1963) and Santulli *et al.* (1965). These basically embryological considerations have now been satisfactorily incorporated into the realistic and practical International Classification.

Louw (1965) similarly uses the system of anal and rectal deformities in a classification very similar to that originally proposed by us. Within it, he indicates the division between high and low deformities; he includes a low vaginal fistula as a "low" anomaly, with which we would disagree because of the distinctive relation of the fistula and bowel to the levator ani. A minor criticism of this classification is the failure to distinguish between the sexes in some of the terms, although by reading the text these can be identified. Louw's classification, with the incidence in his series, is as follows:

Louw's Classification (1965)

A. *Rectal malformation*		
Atresia of rectum	2	
B. *Ano-rectal malformation*		
1. Ano-rectal agenesis without fistula	2	
2. Ano-rectal agenesis with fistula		
Male – recto-vesical fistula	6	*High*
– recto-urethral fistula	65	*level*
		(42%)
Female – recto-cloacal fistula	3	
– recto-vesical fistula	1	
– high recto-vaginal fistula	5	
C. *Anal malformation*		
1. Vestibular ectopic anus	35	
2. Perineal ectopic anus	10	
3. Covered anal canal		
Male – with ano-bulbar fistula	2	*Low*
– with ano-cutaneous fistula	34	*level*
Perineal 21		(58%)
Scrotal 9		
Penile 4		
Female – with ano-vulvar fistula	6	
4. Anal agenesis	6	
5. Anal membrane		
– imperforate anal membrane	6	
– anal membrane stenosis	4	
Total	187	

Nixon (1959) uses the term "cloaca" for all the high anomalies involving rectal agenesis with recto-vesical, recto-urethral or recto-vaginal fistula. Pannock and Stark (1926) and Stone (1936) originally used the term. The term is readily applicable to a common uro-genito-rectal canal in the female into which urethra, vagina and rectum all open, and we refer to the rectal dysgenesis in our classification as a recto-cloacal fistula. But Nixon also uses it in the male with a recto-urethral fistula ("cloaca, with urethral fistula"), because the genital or mesonephric ducts (vasa) open into a common cavity, the prostatic urethra, near the urethral fistula. However, the common uro-genital conduit so closely resembles the urethra and is, in fact, called the urethra that the descriptive clarity of the term "recto-urethral fistula" is an attractive reason for using the term.

Care needs to be taken that stress on some common embryological derivation for a particular group of defects should not overshadow basic differences in anatomy, with consequent differences in treatment. For example, Nixon (1961) groups together as "failure of migration" a group of "vulval ectopic ani" and includes vestibular fistula, covered anus and low vaginal fistulae in this group; yet each of these, we believe, requires a different surgical approach—a covered anus may not necessarily be in the vulva, and a vaginal fistula, even if low, is "high" with respect to the levator ani. Further, Browne (1951) classifies all the foregoing anomalies as "vaginal," a clinical term which does not correctly describe a vestibular fistula.

The embryological approach has been found useful in clarifying understanding of the various malformations, but it is essential that ideas of development be correlated with accurate anatomical information, especially in relation to the sphincters, if they are to be useful in forming a classification upon which diagnosis and treatment can be based. This, the International Classification has achieved.

The expression "ectopic anus" has also proved a difficulty. Apart from the classifications of Partridge and Gough (1961) and Louw (1965) given above, ectopic anus is so described by Bill *et al.* (1958), Bryndorf and Matsen (1959), Scott and Swenson (1959), Nixon (1961) and Gans and Friedman (1961 and 1963). The term is usually reserved for anal openings in the perineum, vestibule or vagina, indicating a failure of migration of the anus backwards. However, the term "ectopic" simply means "abnormally sited" and could be applied equally to recto-bulbar, recto-urethral or ano-cutaneous fistulae, in all of which the opening is "ectopic." It would seem best to avoid a word so broad in its meaning, or else to accept it as applying to *all* fistulous connections, as do *Gans and Friedman (1961 and 1963)*, who claim on histological evidence that the terminal bowel is always a hypoplastic anal canal wherever it ends. They therefore describe ectopic anus as follows:

Gans and Friedman's Classification (1961 and 1963)

(a) Vesical ectopic anus
(b) Urethral ectopic anus
(c) Vaginal ectopic anus
(d) Vaginal fourchette anus
(e) Perineal ectopic anus

This simple classification fails to recognize, however, the relation of the fistula to the pelvic floor, and, even apart from a possible different interpretation of the histological findings, this lack of sphincter reference gives no guide to therapy.

Other examples of difficult words in the original Browne classification are the terms "stenosed anus" and "microscopic anus" (Browne, 1955) for particular types, because the opening of almost any fistula may be stenosed no matter where it opens; further, stenosis may be produced by many factors—by an incomplete anal membrane, as in anal membrane stenosis, by a process of covering up the anus by the genital or anal folds, as in ano-cutaneous fistula, or by stricture formation. The term "congenital median band," used by Bill (1958), probably represents one variety of stenotic anus of the covered type. We use the term "anal stenosis," but only when defined by its particular type.

Recently, suggestions have been made to amalgamate classifications by introducing the high and low subdivisions, and the terms of Browne and Stephens, into the Ladd and Gross classification, type 3. On the basis of over 300 cases, *Santulli et al. (1965)* proposed the following classification:

Santulli's Classification (1965)

Type 1—Anal stenosis
Type 2—Imperforate anal membrane
Type 3—Anal and rectal agenesis

- A. *Anal agenesis (imperforate anus)*
  - Female
    - (i) With fistula
      - (a) Ano-perineal
        - 1. ano-vulvar
        - 2. ectopic perineal anus
    - (ii) Without fistula
  - Male
    - (i) With fistula
      - (a) Ano-perineal
        - 1. Ano-cutaneous (covered anus)
        - 2. Ectopic perineal anus
      - (b) Ano-bulbar
      - (c) Ano-urethral
    - (ii) Without fistula

B. *Rectal agenesis (imperforate rectum)*
Female (i) With fistula
(a) Recto-vestibular
(b) Recto-vaginal
(c) Recto-cloacal (uro-genital sinus)
(ii) Without fistula
Male (i) With fistula
(a) Recto-urethral
(b) Recto-vesical
(ii) Without fistula

Type 4 – Rectal atresia
(a) Complete
(b) Incomplete

The retention of the "types," however, would seem to us to contribute little guide to diagnosis and management since they do not refer to sphincter levels, except by the breakdown within type 3; further, three of the four types are all rare, and almost all anomalies fit into type 3, so that undue significance is given to types 1, 2 and 4 by giving them a separate type number.

Nevertheless, it can be seen that with the gradual merging of the two schools of thought the time seemed particularly appropriate for an international conference on terminology. As already described, this was achieved in Melbourne, Australia, in March 1970, in a most harmonious and stimulating working group, the result of which is the Proposed International Classification (1970). The new work stresses the basic importance of sphincter level to diagnosis and management. It is consistent with the known embryology, but, because some of the embryology is as yet hypothetical (especially in low anomalies), it avoids controversy by a strictly anatomical layout; it recognizes the difficult "intermediate" group; it uses simple and self-defining descriptive terms; and finally it is a sound guide to surgical approach (by indicating supra- and translevator levels), but with flexibility in the controversial intermediate zone.

Further Problems in Classification

1. Many classifications do not distinguish between the sexes. While some anomalies are common to both sexes (e.g., ano-rectal agenesis without fistula, recto-vesical fistula, imperforate anal membrane, etc.), these represent the least common aberrations, whereas the common abnormalities are distinctive to each sex. In males, the common fistulous connections are to the urinary tract, whereas the intervention of the müllerian system in the female projects these fistulae into the genital tract or external cloaca. These anatomical differences necessitate a different classification for each sex.

2. Classifications which do not recognize the presence or absence of a visceral communication fail to convey suggestions regarding the clinical and diagnostic steps in the newborn period, upon the result of which depend the correct decisions in management. Communicating malformations are revealed by the presence of meconium in the urine or by accurate appreciation of the various orifices in the perineum, whereas noncommunicating defects require inversion radiographs to localize the level of occlusion. This distinction between communicating and noncommunicating anomalies is discussed in more detail in Chapter 8.

3. Many terms in the literature are unsatisfactory because they are inaccurate, nonspecific, too cumbersome, or because they overemphasize one aspect of clinical appearance. For example, "recto-perineal fistula" (Bill and Johnson, 1958) ought to mean specifically the *rectum* opening in the perineum, but it is actually taken to include deformities afflicting the *anus* only, such as ano-cutaneous fistula. "Imperforate anus with no fistula" (Scott and Swenson, 1959) is used to describe a high *rectal* agenesis affecting both anus and rectum. "Vaginal ectopic anus" (Browne, 1951) and "ectopic vulval anus" (Scott and Swenson, 1959) are semantically confusing and somewhat nonspecific when used to describe a fistula into the vestibule, a type with very specific features. In fact, there is frequent confusion in female children when the emergence of feces from the "vagina" may be entered in hospital records as "recto-vaginal," whereas the actual fistulous orifice may be either into the vagina, the vestibule or in the vulva posteriorly. Yet each of these requires a different surgical approach and carries a different prognosis. "Cloacal anomaly with ano-rectal agenesis" (Nixon, 1961) is too long, and "recto-urinary connection" (Bill and Johnson, 1958) is not sufficiently specific as it may include either recto-vesical, recto-urethral or recto-bulbar fistulae.

We suggest that the terms used in the classification be specific and anatomically accurate. Examples of such specificity are in the schemata of Bacon and Sherman (1952), Louw (1959 and 1965), Bryndorf and Madsen (1959), Stephens and Smith (1963), Bill (1964) and Santulli *et al.* (1965). (See above.)

The International Classification proposed in 1970 in Melbourne appears to fulfill the requirements adequately.

CHAPTER 7

Incidence, Frequency of Types, Etiology

Incidence

APPROXIMATELY 1 in 5,000 babies is born with an anal or rectal malformation. There appears to be little variation in different geographical areas, although Louw (1965) reported a higher incidence in South Africa, and Jeffreys and Maxwell (1919) state the condition is "extremely common in China." Few reported series provide an analysis according to race, except those of Louw (1965) (below), and Kiesewetter *et al.* (1964), both commenting on the low incidence in Negroes.

In the United States	Brenner (1915), 1 in 4,800 live births (17 in 81,700 births). Santulli (1952), 1 in 5,000 live births.
	Moore and Lawrence (1952), 1 in 4,500 live births.
	Anderson and Reed (1954), 1 in 5,000 live births.
In South Africa	Louw (1965), white – 1 in 1,740 live births; colored – 1 in 1,770 live births; Bantu – 1 in 2,260 live births.
In Canada	Trusler and Wilkinson (1962), 1 in 5,000 live births.
In India	Shahi and Mishra (1961), 1 in 5,926 live births (5 in 29,633 births).
In Finland	Parkkulainen (1957), 1 in 5,500 live births.
In Israel	Solowiejczyk (1961), 1 in 3,145 live births (18 in 56,625 births).

A few series record widely divergent figures on incidence. Zoehner (1928) stated the incidence as 1 in 25,000 live births and Allen (1932), David (1937) and Neff (1940) as 1 in 10,000; on the other hand, Schapiro (1960) found 1 in 800 (of 77,979 consecutive live births).

TABLE 2.—INCIDENCE IN HOSPITAL ADMISSIONS

AUTHORS	HOSPITAL ADMISSIONS	NUMBER OF CASES	RATIO
Eight authors	591,604	325	1:1820
Schapiro	115,398	97	1:1189
TOTAL	707,002	422	1:1675

Three papers report that congenital "ano-rectal rings" of minor degree may occur asymptomatically in well babies—Harris *et al.* (1954) found that 13.8% of 1,716 consecutive newborns possessed such rings, and Brown and Schoen (1950) found 39 "strictures" in 100 consecutive newborns. Eckerle (1951) suggested that fissures, fistulae, prolapse and hemorrhoids in children may result from minor degrees of anal stenosis. It is possible that such minor degrees of stenosis being treated by the family doctor may not appear in large hospital series.

Expressed as incidence of hospital admissions Schapiro (1960) collected the figures from eight authors and added his own (Table 2).

Sex Incidence

In the present series, a male preponderance prevails, and this fact is in keeping with the combined figures from 35 different series. The following references together with our own cases, in which sex is documented, provide a total of 3,645 cases (Table 3). Keith (1905), Brenner (1915), Starlinger and Richter (1933), Berman (1938), Crowell and Dulin (1940), Harken (1942), Dmytryk (1945), Rosenblatt and May (1946), Mayo and Rice (1950), Moore and Lawrence (1952), Bacon and Sherman (1952), Gross (1953), Winkel-Smith (1953), Hanley *et al.* (1954), Thompson and Hooks (1956), Parkkulainen *et al.* (1957 and 1959), Brayton and Norris (1958), Donovan and Stanley-Brown (1958), Bradham (1958), Scott *et al.* (1960), Salzberg and Martin (1961), Partridge and Gough (1961), Shahi and Mishra (1961), McPherson (1962), Trusler and Wilkinson (1962), Katzen (1962), Swain and Tucker (1962), Swenson and Grana (1962), Santulli *et al.* (1965), Bill (1964), Sommerschild *et al.* (1964), Kiesewetter *et al.* (1964), Bielowicz (1965) and Louw (1965).

TABLE 3.—SEX RATIO

	PRESENT SERIES 260 CASES	36 AUTHORS 3,645 CASES
Male	168 (64.6%)	2,072 (57%)
Female	92 (35.4%)	1,573 (43%)

TABLE 4.—Frequency of Types According to Present Embryological Classification in Melbourne Series (260 Cases) and in Series of 8 Authors (1098 Cases)

Males	Melbourne Series	8 Authors
Rectal Anomalies		
Recto-urethral fistula	44	279
Recto-vesical fistula	4	23
Ano-rectal agenesis (no fistula)	15	41
Rectal atresia	1	7
Total	64	350
Anal Anomalies		
Anterior perineal anus	1	7
Covered anus		
(a) Ano-cutaneous fistula	37	158
(b) Recto-bulbar fistula	13	15
Anal agenesis (no fistula)	7	20
Imperforate anal membrane	6	20
Anal stenosis		
(a) Covered anal stenosis	23	68
(b) Anal membrane stenosis	6	8
(c) Ano-rectal stenosis	2	3
Total	95	299
Unclassified Anomalies		
Vesico-intestinal fissure	8	16
Other rare anomalies	1	1
Total	9	17
Total	168	666

Females	Melbourne Series	8 Authors
Recto-cloacal fistula	8	27
Recto-vesical fistula	1	4
Recto-vaginal fistula (high and low)	8	61
Recto-vestibular fistula	7	7
Ano-rectal agenesis (no fistula)	3	23
Rectal atresia	1	4
Total	28	126
Anterior anus		
(a) Perineal	3	15
(b) Vulvar	2	
Ano-vestibular fistula	22	121
Perineal groove	1	
Perineal canal	3	
Covered anus		
(a) Ano-cutaneous fistula	9	106
(b) Ano-vulvar fistula	3	
Anal agenesis (no fistula)	4	10
Imperforate anal membrane	1	10
Anal stenosis		
(a) Covered anal stenosis	5	21
(b) Anal membrane stenosis	5	7
(c) Ano-rectal stenosis	1	1
Total	59	291
Vesico-intestinal fissure	4	14
Other rare anomalies	1	1
Total	5	15
Total	92	432

Frequency of Types of Malformations

It is difficult to assess the true incidence of the various subgroups in a study of the literature because of the difficulties in comparing series using different classifications. However, seven papers provide figures adequate for abstraction, from classifications based upon the concepts of Denis Browne and Stephens, and are compared with those in the present series in Table 4. In this table, some license in interpretation has been assumed where the information is incomplete, and figures have been extrapolated from the textual description. We apologize for any incorrect interpretation, although any errors will affect the over-all percentiles to a negligible degree. The sources are Keith (1908), Scott *et al.* (1960), Partridge and Gough (1961), Katzen (1962), McPherson (1962), Bill (1964), Louw (1965).

It is noted that throughout this chapter the figures are given on the basis of an embryological classification rather than on the International Classification (1970). This is deliberate, partly because the latter classification is too new to be used to interpret other authors' writings and partly because the significance of a particular incidence is more closely related to a particular developmental process rather than to the anatomical terms of the classification, which may have the same developmental origin yet appear in several places in the list.

A further division may be made of the relative incidence of rectal and anal deformities. In addition to the above series, over 500 cases are recorded in papers in which sex is not identified, but in which "high" and "low" are equated with rectal and anal, respectively—Winkel-Smith (1953), Forshall (1960), Swain and Tucker (1962), Swenson and Grana (1962), Kiesewetter *et al.* (1964), Sommerschild *et al.* (1964), Bielowicz (1965), Swenson and Donnellson (1967). These cases are shown in Table 5, added to those in Table 4, omitting unclassified types.

In over-all numbers, anal anomalies were slightly more common than rectal because of the preponderance of anal defects in females.

From these collected cases, the following conclusions may be drawn:

TABLE 5.—Frequency of Rectal and Anal Cases

Anomalies	Melbourne Series	16 Authors' Series
Rectal ("high")	92 (37.4%)	729 (46.5%)
Anal ("low")	154 (62.2%)	837 (53.5%)
Total	246	1,566

MALES (Table 4)

1. Rectal deformities (350 patients = 53.9%) were slightly more common than anal deformities (299 patients = 46.1%), although in our series the figures are reversed. In the male, therefore, difficult cases will be more frequently encountered than easy ones, and this fact, combined with the slightly higher incidence of serious associated defects in males presages a more unfavorable prognosis in males than in females.

2. Of all deformities in males, only 88 of 649 patients (13.5%) were truly imperforate, i.e., failed to communicate with either the urinary tract or the perineal skin. The high incidence of communicating deformities has long been recognized in both anal and rectal deformities—259 of 299 patients with anal anomalies (86.6%), and 302 of 350 patients with rectal anomalies (86.3%) communicated with urinary, genital or cutaneous structures.

3. The relative incidence of the various subgroups of *rectal deformities* was as follows:

Recto-urethral fistula	79.7%
Ano-rectal agenesis (no fistula)	11.7%
Recto-vesical fistula	6.6%
Rectal atresia	2.0%

In rectal deformities, by far the commonest lesion was a recto-urethral fistula, whereas a communication directly to the bladder was relatively rare. This is in contrast with many series classified in the Ladd and Gross scheme, especially those in earlier papers; Gross (1953), for example, reported 55 recto-vesical fistulae and 59 recto-urethral fistulae in a series of 270 male malformations; Trusler and Wilkinson (1962) described 9 recto-vesical fistulae, 10 recto-urethral fistulae and 38 with no fistulae in 90 male patients. Similar incidences are described by Mayo and Rice (1950), Moore and Lawrence (1952), Hanley *et al.* (1954), Potts *et al.* (1954), Bradham (1958), Swenson and Grana (1962). Perhaps the explanation of the reportedly high incidence of recto-vesical fistulae and "blind" rectum without fistulae in these series derives from dubious evidence gained at the time of neonatal abdomino-perineal procedures. Norris *et al.* (1949), for example, found that 7 of 14 recto-urinary communications were not diagnosed; Brayton and Norris (1958) diagnosed fistulae in only 9 of 31 males preoperatively, and Mayo and Rice (1950), although describing 17 recto-vesical and 27 recto-urethral fistulae, had another 12 patients in whom the connection was only "probably recto-urethral." In contrast, accurate radiological methods used after performance of colostomy (see "Diagnosis," Chap. 8) provides more certain evidence of the fistulae. Similarly, the high incidence of recto-urethral fistulae is demonstrated in series based upon anatomical dissections, such as those of Denis Browne (1951 and 1955), Stephens (1953 and 1963) and even as far back as that of Keith in 1908, in which 40 of 47 dissected male specimens with fistulae into the urinary tract showed such recto-urethral fistulae, only 7 having a communication with the bladder (see Fig. 81).

4. The relative incidence of the various subgroups of *anal deformities* was as follows:

Covered anus Ano-cutaneous fistula	52.8%	75.5%
Covered anus – complete and covered anal stenosis	22.7%	
Imperforate anal membrane	6.7%	
Anal agenesis (no fistula)	6.7%	
Recto-bulbar fistula	5.2%	
Anal membrane stenosis and ano-rectal stenosis	3.7%	
Anterior perineal anus	2.2%	

The high incidence of a communication to the perineum is again emphasized, especially by one or other variety of covered anus, a fact repeatedly stressed in series using Stephens type of classification, e.g., Louw (1959 and 1965), Scott *et al.* (1960), Partridge and Gough (1961), Nixon (1961) and Bill (1964). Again, a contrast may be made with series of case reports using the Ladd and Gross classification, in which the number of type 3 cases with recto-perineal fistula is often surprisingly low.

Females

1. Anal deformities (291 patients = 69.7%) were more than twice as common as rectal deformities (126 patients = 30.3%). As the treatment of the anal group is more simple and satisfactory than that of the difficult rectal group, this fact immeasurably improves the favorable outlook in female children.

2. True imperforation was even less common in female than in male children. Only 47 deformities of 417 patients (11.3%) failed to communicate with either urinary or genital tracts or with the perineum. In *rectal* deformities, 99 of 126 patients (78.6%) possessed a fistulous connection, although the number of fistulae in our series (24 of 28 patients) was even higher. However, in almost all female infants so afflicted, an *anal* deformity may be expected to communicate with either a viscus or the perineal skin; such was the case in 271 of 291 patients (93.1%) in this collected series, a fact also agreed upon in almost all series reported in the Ladd and Gross classification.

3. The relative incidence of the various subgroups of *rectal deformities* was as follows:

Recto-vaginal fistula (high and low)	48.4%	69.5%
Recto-cloacal fistula	21.1%	
Ano-rectal agenesis (no fistula)	18.3%	
*Recto-vestibular fistula	5.6%	
Recto-vesical fistula	3.3%	
Rectal atresia	3.3%	

In this collected series there was a surprisingly high incidence of vaginal communications and also, compared with males, a relatively larger incidence of deformities with no fistula (ano-rectal agenesis). Further, all authors agree on the rarity of recto-vesical communications in female children—there were only 19 cases in a controlled series of 1, 673 females from 29 authors.

4. The relative incidence of the various subgroups of *anal deformities* was as follows:

Covered anus—ano-cutaneous fistula, ano-vulvar fistula and including covered anus complete and covered anal stenosis	43.6%
Ano-vestibular fistula, including perineal groove and canal	41.6%
Anterior anus (perineal and vulvar)	5.2%
Anal agenesis (no fistula)	3.4%
Imperforate anal membrane	3.4%
Anal membrane stenosis and ano-rectal stenosis	2.8%

In our own series, by contrast, there were more patients with an ano-vestibular fistula than with covered anus.

The distinction between a low vaginal fistula and one opening in the vestibule is a constant source of confusion in the literature, especially in series using the Ladd and Gross classification. Denis Browne (1951) included vestibular ani as "vaginal," yet an opening below the hymen into the fourchette is clearly not into the vagina. Gross (1953) listed 143 cases in 237 female children as "vaginal" and Santulli *et al.* (1965) 64 cases in 106 females, without indicating relative numbers opening into the vestibule, yet Gross states "many fistulas open into the fossa navicularis." Trusler and Wilkinson (1962) describe 37 recto-vaginal fistulae yet state in the text that 60% open into the fourchette; Potts *et al.* (1954) state that all except 2 of 22 vaginal fistulae open "near the fourchette"; Hanley *et al.* (1954 and 1965) list 27 vaginal fistulae of which 24 were into the fossa navicularis. Lee (1944), Mayo and Rice (1950), Moore and Lawrence (1952), Bacon and Sherman (1952), Bradham (1958), Donovan and Stanley-Brown (1958), Schapiro (1960), Salzberg and Martin (1961), Swenson and Grana (1962), and Kiesewetter *et al.* (1964) list only recto-vaginal fistulae, and Parkkulainen (1957 and 1959) only 13 vestibular fistulae with 74 vaginal fistulae.

---

*Defined as in Chapter 5, i. e., does not include ano-vestibular fistulae.

On the other hand, Brayton and Norris (1958) list 20 fistulae into the fourchette, as against only 5 into the vagina, and, of 50 girls described by Bryndorf and Madsen (1960), 30 possessed a vestibular anus, and only 1 case of vaginal fistula was encountered. Finally, several very early authors, e.g., Stieda (1903) recognized the common frequency of the vestibular site. Keith (1908) dissected 6 recto-vestibular fistulae in 25 female specimens, Brenner (1915) recognized that the commonest fistula "opens at the fourchette," as also Stone (1936). David (1937) described 6 "vaginal" fistulae, but all were outside the hymen. Berman (1938) drew the lesion, and Winkel-Smith (1953) found only vestibular fistulae in his female patients. Our own experience certainly indicates that the commonest lesion in female children is an orifice at the fourchette, although occasionally it may be difficult to be sure whether this is an ano-vestibular fistula or a covered anus with a vulval opening.

As in the male, lesions of the anal membrane are rare, accounting for less than 5% of all anal anomalies.

INCIDENCE WITH SERIES USING LADD AND GROSS CLASSIFICATION.—Much of the literature is classified in the Ladd and Gross scheme, and 29 authors have been assembled to provide a review of 3,384 cases. These are listed in Table 6.

Table 6 is prepared from the following sources: Harken (1942), Lee (1944), Dmytryk (1945), Rosenblatt and May (1946), Mayo and Rice (1950), Bacon and Sherman (1962), Moore and Lawrence (1952), Gross (1953), Hanley *et al.* (1954), Waite (1954), Potts *et al.* (1954), Brayton and Norris (1958), Bradham (1958), Donovan and Stanley-Brown (1958), Schapiro (1960), Salzberg and Martin (1961), Trusler and Wilkinson (1962), Swenson and Grana (1962), Santulli *et al.*, (1965), Kiesewetter *et al.* (1964). In addition are included the figures

TABLE 6.—3,384 CASES DERIVED FROM 29 AUTHORS, CLASSIFIED ACCORDING TO LADD AND GROSS

TYPE	ANOMALY		
1	Anal stenosis		277
2	Imperforate anal membrane		241
3	Imperforate anus		
	Blind rectum (rectal agenesis)	554	
	Recto-vesical fistula	209	
	Recto-urethral fistula	548	2,756
	Recto-vaginal fistula	816*	
	Recto-perineal fistula	639	
4	Rectal atresia		67
Unclassified			43
	TOTAL		3,384

*Includes recto-cloacal and recto-fourchette fistulae.

TABLE 7.—2,904 CASES DERIVED FROM 23 AUTHORS INDICATING THE RELATIVE FREQUENCY OF LADD AND GROSS TYPES IN EACH SEX

Male		Type		Female
122		1		85
128		2		73
		3		
1,318	340	Blind	85	1,088
	169	Recto-vesical fistula	15	
	486	Recto-urethral fistula	4	
		Recto-vaginal fistula	729*	
	323	Recto-perineal fistula	255	
42		4		15
17		Unclassified		16
1,627		TOTALS		1,277

*Includes recto-cloacal and recto-fourchette fistula.

from other classifications which have been rearranged to conform to the Ladd and Gross scheme, when the information has been sufficient to enable it. These are the present authors (260 cases) and those of Keith (1908), Parkkulainen (1957 and 1959), Scott *et al.* (1960), Partridge and Gough (1961), McPherson (1962), Katzen (1962), Bill (1964) and Louw (1965). Once again, the authors apologize for any inadvertent misinterpretation of the figures where some degree of license has necessarily been used.

Twenty-three of these authors provide sufficient information for analysis by sexes, and Table 7 illustrates the findings in 2,904 patients.

We note the following:

1. The high incidence of fistulae in both sexes, especially females.

2. The higher incidence of recto-vesical fistulae, and examples without fistulae, in males, compared with series listed under our classification, in which recto-urethral fistulae greatly predominate (e.g., Table 4). This contrast is accentuated by a further subdivision of these figures. In Table 7, there were included 644 cases of type 3 deformity from 9 authors using our classification. Of these 644, 312 were recto-urethral and only 24 were recto-vesical. Removal of these 644 cases from the table then indicates 174 recto-urethral fistulae and 145 recto-vesical fistulae.

Some authors do not define the exact site of the recto-urinary communication. Kiesewetter *et al.* (1964) refer only to 30 "high urinary fistulae," Salzberg and Martin (1961) to "recto-urinary fistulae" and Parkkulainen (1957) to 17 of 80 males with "anal atresia and uro-rectal fistulae."

No series, classified in the Ladd and Gross scheme, includes a recto-bulbar fistula, which is presumably listed as type 3 with recto-urethral fistula; we believe this to be a disadvantage, as such an anal lesion may be treated advantageously by a lesser surgical technique than that required for the recto-urethral fistula issuing at a higher level into the verumontanum.

3. Recto-perineal fistulae (ano-cutaneous fistulae in our classification) do not appear to be as common in the collected series, as in the Melbourne series (Table 4). The contrast is increased if, as discussed (2) above, the 9 authors' series using our classification are removed from Table 7. Perhaps this difference is explained by the dispersal of some such cases into types 1 and 2 and by listing some of the large number of "rectovaginal fistulae" as lesions at or near the fourchette, some of which may be ano-cutaneous, ano-vulvar or ano-vestibular fistulae in our classification.

4. The rarity of recto-vesical fistulae in females.

5. The confusion within the hodgepodge group of "recto-vaginal fistulae," which includes recto-cloacal and recto-vestibular (fourchette) fistulae (see Chapt. 6).

6. It is not always clear whether type 1 cases (anal stenosis) also include those with a covered anus type of deformity, which should be more properly grouped with type 3, recto-perineal fistulae, e.g., Mayo and Rice (1950) include 2 males with fistulae in type 1. It is not possible to compare the incidence of such lesions as the varieties of covered anus, anterior anus or anal membrane stenosis. Presumably these are described as varieties of type 1 or type 3, with recto-perineal fistulae.

7. The high incidence of type 2 cases (imperforate anal membrane) is suspect because of the extreme rarity of the condition in females, in our experience and that of many others. The incidence of these type 2 cases is probably much lower than indicated, because of the 73 female patients, no less than 40 appear in one series (that of Mayo and Rice, 1950), a series which only contained 80 females of all types. The same series also contributes 22 of the male patients in type 2. Further, it is difficult to understand the inclusion of cases of fistulae under type 2, in which, by definition, the lesion is imperforate. Norris *et al.* (1949) and Brayton and Norris (1958) include three "recto-perineal fistulae" in type 2, Mayo and Rice (1950), 14 cases in males and 39 in females with fistulae (of a total of 62 type 2), Moore and Lawrence (1952) five fistulae, Santulli (1952) 1 such case and Bradham (1958) 3 cases.

8. The occurrence of fistula cases in type 4, Mayo and Rice (1950) and Moore and Lawrence (1952), must also be unusual, although there is no reason why such atresias should not also have a fistula—instances of fistulae to urethra or forwards to perineum in conjunction with a normal anus are described (see Chapt. 3). In all events, the number of infants falling into type 4 is very small.

9. Cases of anal agenesis (i.e., an anal deformity in our classifica-

tion) cannot be distinguished from rectal agenesis (a high-level lesion) and are included as type 3.

Etiology

The cause of anal and rectal dysgenesis is unknown.

Local destruction of the axial portion of the caudal region between the primitive origins of the pelvic anlage in the chick embryo can produce cloacal malformations (Wolff, 1948). More extensive destruction may produce a sirenomelus monster (symelia – monsters with fusion of the inferior limbs, imperforate anus, anomalies of lumbar and sacral spines, and genito-urinary agenesis), and Duhamel considers that the sirenomelus monster and imperforate anus represent the one comprehensive syndrome, that of an embryonal defect in the formation of the caudal region – the "syndrome of caudal regression" (Duhamel, 1961). However, there is no suggestion in Duhamel's paper as to why caudal development might be defective.

BIRTH ORDER. – Affected infants may appear at any stage of parity. Table 8 indicates the pregnancy which produced the affected infants in our own series.

MATERNAL AGE. – Similarly, no relationship could be established between the birth of an affected infant and the age of the mother at the time. The spread of cases follows the normal pattern in the community, with the greatest concentration between maternal ages 20 – 26 years; there is no evidence that the risk is increased in elderly primiparas.

FAMILY HISTORY. – No mother in this series gave birth to a second affected infant in a subsequent pregnancy. However, isolated instances of more than one sibling being affected appear in the literature. Norris *et al.* (1949) include two sisters in 52 patients, Seitz and Bäntze (1951) reported a mother and two daughters with perineal

TABLE 8. – AFFECTED INFANTS IN RELATION TO PARITY

PARITY	NO. OF CASES
1st	41
2nd	34
3rd	26
4th	9
5th	5
6th	6
7th	3
12th	1

This span of incidence parallels the size of average Australian families, and no inference can be drawn as to relative risk with increasing parity. There is, perhaps, a slight preponderance amongst first-born infants.

anus, Kaijser and Malmström-Groth (1957) describe a mother and two daughters with recto-vaginal fistulae (3 other children being normal), and Partridge and Gough (1961) three families with more than one member affected. Anderson and Reed (1954) comment that the risk that a subsequent sibling of a child with anal atresia will have the same anomaly is less than 1 per 100, calculated "after evaluation of many reports," but the basis of their calculation is not documented.

On the other hand, identical twins, each with identical anal lesions, have appeared twice in our series of 260 patients. All 4 infants had a covered anus deformity and were males, the first twins being the first-born of an 18-year-old mother, the second twins being the fifth-born of a 32-year-old mother. Feggeter (1939) also reported uniovular twins with identical imperforate anus.

Only very infrequently has a family history of these anomalies been reported in members other than siblings. Suckling (1949) found 3 patients in four generations of a family, Bryndorf and Matsen (1959) had 3 patients whose mother, half-sister and father's cousin, respectively, were affected, Moore and Lawrence (1952) found a family history in 1 patient in 120 cases, and Santulli *et al.* (1965) 3 in 220 patients. Van Gelder and Kloepfer (1961) summarized the reported cases with positive family history and found five families. They concluded that two families represented a possible autosomal recessive, two an autosomal dominant with incomplete penetrance, and one autosomal dominant. In a recent review, Weinstein (1965) described three families in which two could be explained as instances of sex-linked recessive inheritance of the disease. His study of 1,919 cases showing slight male preponderance supports this rather than autosomal recessive inheritance with selection against the female.

There is an interesting association of a syndrome of coloboma (of iris and choroid), microphthalmia, hypertelorism and imperforate anus, first described by Haab (1878). Schachenmann *et al.* (1965) described 3 patients and found that all three, and the mother of one of them, possessed an extra chromosome, which was very small, smaller than group 21–22.

It is apparent that heredity plays only a minor and obscure role in etiology. Some authors would deny its significance altogether (Oeconomopoulos, 1961; De Staerke, 1962).

THALIDOMIDE.—There is a correlation between imperforate anus and maternal ingestion of thalidomide, although the risk is small (Ives, 1962; Indahl *et al.*, (1963). Two of our babies have phocomelia, but the mothers had not taken thalidomide.

CHAPTER 8

Diagnosis and Investigations

DECISIONS concerning initial management of a newborn baby affected by one or other variety of imperforate anus or rectum can only be made after accurate determination of the exact type and level of the anomaly. With such information, a decision can then be made whether to perform a primary perineal operation in the neonatal period, as in most anal anomalies, or to perform colostomy only, deferring definitive repair till a later period, as in most rectal anomalies. In addition to determination of level and exact anatomical type, further facts may influence the primary management, such as the integrity of the neural and muscular components of the pelvis, the presence of serious associated visceral malformations and especially the state of the urinary tract. Much of this information can be derived from clinical observation and radiographic study before any operation, but, in high rectal anomalies when colostomy has been performed, more detailed assessment can be made at leisure by additional investigations, such as colography through the colostomy, pyelography and endoscopy of the urinary tract.

The surgeon must not operate until he is quite certain about the exact type of malformation present. With the means of diagnosis now available, it is inexcusable to explore the perineum to increasing depths in the mistaken notion that the lesion is a "low" one; irreparable damage may result to the controlling muscles. Conversely, accurate documentation of level, site of fistula and neural supply may avoid the needless morbidity from abdominal exploration, colostomy or rectoplasty, when the lesion is, in fact, a low one or is associated with a neurogenic state and certain incontinence. In earlier papers, several authors refer to the "missed fistula" as assessed on clinical or radiological evidence but found subsequently at operation. Norris *et al.* (1949) reported that 7 of 14 recto-urinary fistulae were not diagnosed; Brayton and Norris (1958) reported 22 fistulae "missed" preoperatively in 31 males; Mayo and Rice (1950) reported 17 recto-vesical and 27 recto-urethral fistulae and an additional 12 which were only "probably recto-urethral." These authors with Rhoads and Koop (1955) and Rehbein (1967), because of the alleged inaccuracies of the inversion x-rays, omitted them and advocated abdomino-perineal reconstruction for all type 3 lesions (Ladd and Gross classification), the site of occlusion or fistula being then determined at operation. We cannot agree with this advice, for it results in a number of unnecessary abdominal explorations for essentially anal malformations. Except in occasional patients with late presentation and gross distention, several hours are available for good x-ray studies, the pitfalls of inversion x-rays are now better understood, and the injection of water-soluble radiopaque dyes into fistula and urethra is a simple matter in a modern radiology department. Knowledge before operation of level of lesion and of fistula is of incalculable value in the surgical approach and is obligatory for prevention of sphincter damage. Bacon and Sherman (1952) and Bradham (1961) have similarly stressed the accurate preoperative documentation of the anatomy.

The chief object of investigation prior to operation is to amass sufficient evidence to complete the whole picture of the deformity, each piece of evidence representing part of a jigsaw puzzle. It can be anticipated that the fewer gaps in the puzzle the more correct will be the planning of the steps in management.

As a guide to initial management in the newborn period, therefore, three assessments must be made:

1. The level of the malformation in relation to the muscular sphincters and the site of any fistulous communications.
2. The integrity of the sphincters and their nerve supply.
3. The associated visceral malformations which may affect survival.

After initial management in the newborn period, either by primary perineal operation or by colostomy, these three facts may be further clarified by additional tests, and, in this period, especial importance is given to the elucidation of associated urinary tract anomalies.

Diagnosis in the Newborn Period

1. Assessment of Level of Anomaly and of Fistula in Relation to Sphincters

The internal anatomy is analyzed by the following:

(i) The clinical examination
(ii) Inversion x-rays
(iii) The presence of gas in other viscera
(iv) Radiopaque medium studies of the fistula, urinary tract, and bowel
(v) Endoscopy

The emphasis varies a little in each sex, and will be separately described. The detailed clinical appearances of the perineum are described in Chapters 3 and 4.

A. Male.

(I) Prediction from Clinical Appearance.—As a basis for future comparison and accurate documentation, the perineal appearances should be recorded by sketch or photography.

An orifice visible externally in the perineum predicts an anal translevator anomaly, except in the single anomaly of rectal atresia. There may be what is obviously a normal anus, although displaced anteriorly in the perineum, as in *anterior perineal anus.* But the fistulous opening of an *ano-cutaneous fistula* (see Figs. 44, *A* and 45, *A*) may be more difficult to locate, especially if there are associated genital fold abnormalities. A careful search must be made with the aid of a magnifying glass if necessary for a minute orifice along or beside the perineal raphe, from behind the normal anal site to the tip of the penis. A "flyspeck" of meconium or a bubble of gas may direct attention to the minute orifice. The fistulous tract may be suggested by a fine bluish line, a bulge of meconium or white epithelial pearls along its course. In the variants of *anal stenosis of the covered anus* type (see Figs. 40, *A* and *B* and 126, *A*), the anal opening must be sought amongst the folds or raphe, at the normal anal site. In *imperforate anal membrane* (see Fig. 38), *ano-rectal stenosis* (see Fig. 40, *C*), *anal membrane stenosis* (see Fig. 40, *D*) and *rectal atresia* (see Fig. 27), the superficial appearance of the anus may be normal, but the presence of intestinal obstruction or the passage of ribbon stools should lead to a digital examination and discovery of the membrane, atresic septum or stenotic canal.

When no patent anal orifice can be identified in the perineum, it is not possible to predict the level of the anomaly with certainty, although most will be rectal (supralevator or intermediate) lesions. There is nothing distinctive about the shape of the perineum, which may possess a raphe, hypertrophied genital folds, a dimple, a pigmented patch or show obliteration of the natal cleft. The diagnosis of a *covered anus—complete* will be suspected in the presence of hypertrophied genital folds or median band over the normal anal site, especially if a tinge of meconium staining can be seen; nevertheless, in the absence of such staining, this cannot be assumed because we have seen hypertrophied folds, even when the lesion is a high one.

In many patients with *recto-bulbar fistula* (see Fig. 33), the diagnosis may be suspected because of associated genital fold defects in the anterior part of the perineum, such as atypical hypospadias, cleft scrotum, a slender perineum or a flimsy floor to the urethra.

When no patent anal orifice is found in the perineum, massage of the urethra may produce meconium at the meatus, and the urine must be collected and examined for the color of meconium, bits of meconium jelly or squamous epithelial cells. Voided urine is more significant than a catheter specimen because, in recto-urethral fistulae, the bladder neck sphincters may prevent meconium from entering the bladder. However, if urine has not been passed, a catheter should be inserted (and left in place for the x-ray studies).

(a) If no meconium is present in the urine, either a fistula is blocked with meconium, or a noncommunicating anomaly is present, such as *ano-rectal agenesis (without fistula), anal agenesis (without fistula), a completely covered anus* or *imperforate anal membrane.* Inversion x-rays are essential for further identification of type, because the two former lesions require colostomy, the latter two only a perineal procedure.

(b) If meconium is present, the rectum communicates with the urinary tract, either as a *recto-vesical, recto-urethral* or *recto-bulbar fistula.* In our view, these three lesions require initial colostomy, and further identification is not essential at this stage. However, accurate information is still desirable because of an occasional unexpected anomaly, and because of the need to document the urinary tract at the onset of treatment (see Fig. 137). We therefore perform inversion x-rays and radiopaque studies through the urethra (micturition cystourethrogram). A further rule may, therefore, be stated: *the presence of meconium in the urine indicates the need for a defunctioning colostomy* in the neonatal period.

When a recto-bulbar fistula is suspected because of meconium in the urine in an infant with anterior genital fold defects, a probe passed up the urethra may pass through the fistula and be felt in the perineum.

(II) INVERTOGRAPHY AND RADIOGRAPHIC ANATOMY.—In 1930, Wangensteen and Rice first described the use of plain radiographs with the baby in the inverted, head-down position to indicate the distance of the gas bubble (in the terminal blind pouch) from the perineal skin. Subsequent writers defined the critical distance as 1.5 cm., less than which a surgical approach could be safely made from the perineum, and greater than which was a high lesion requiring an abdomino-perineal approach. Authors relying on measurement of distance were Berman (1938), Crowell and Dulin (1940), Mayo and Rice (1950), Palmer (1956), Bradham (1958), Trusler and Wilkinson (1962), Gans *et al.* (1963), Santulli *et al.* (1965) and Kiesewetter and Turner (1964).

Measurement of distance alone, however, does not provide the essential information required, namely, the relation of the blind pouch to the bony landmarks of the pelvis, which in turn indicate the relation to the levator ani muscle. It is the latter fact which fundamentally determines whether the level is "high" or above the levator or "low" and translevator and hence determines the surgical approach. Further, measurement of distance to the natal cleft is unreliable because in high anomalies the ischio-rectal fat pads meet in the midline below the bowel and fill out the natal cleft (Nixon, 1961). Winckel-Smith (1953) similarly found distance measurement unreliable in high lesions.

Identification of the gas bubble *with respect to the bony pelvis* provides the relevant information regarding the likely relation of the rectal deformity to the sphincter muscles, a concept first developed by one of us (Stephens, 1953). The pelves of both normal and abnormal stillborn babies were hemisected in the sagittal plane (25 normal pelves), and, in each, three radiopaque wires were stretched across the pelvis. The relationships of the pelvic viscera to both the

Fig. 83.—Topography of normal pelvis. **A,** male and, **B,** female with corresponding radiographs **A**[1] and **B**[1]. *P/C* denotes the pubo-coccygeal lines. The lowest markers lie on the level of the anal valves, and the middle markers denote the junction of membranous urethra and bulb in the male and the urethral outlet in the female. (The 5th half vertebra of the sacrum is not shown on the radiographs.)

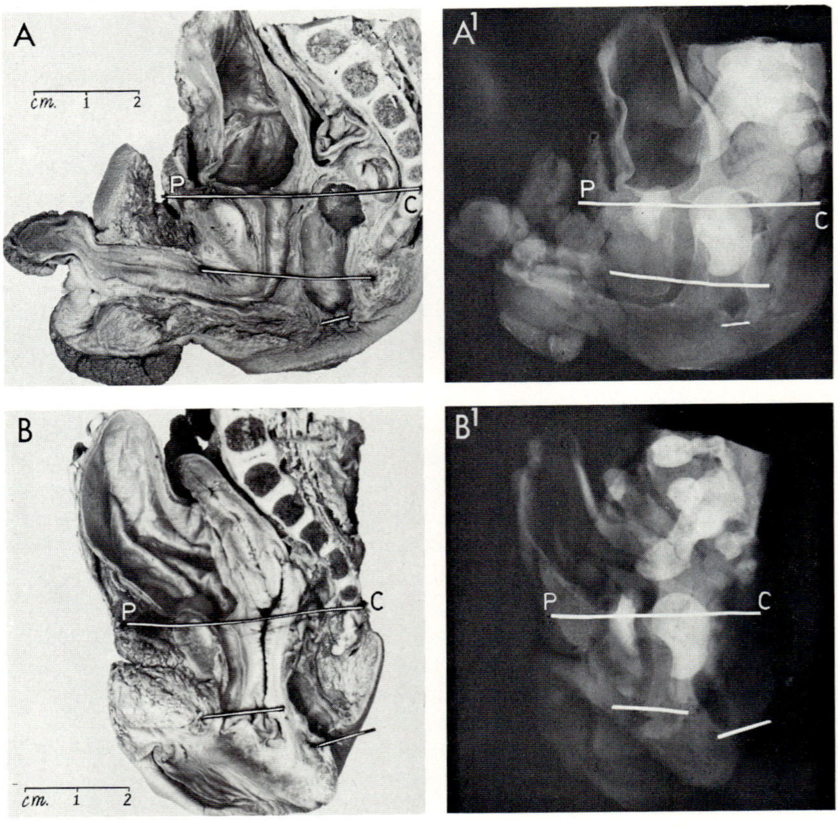

wires and the lines produced by them on the radiograph in the lateral view were studied (Fig. 83).

The three wires and their radiographic lines were as follows:

(i) The Pubo-Coccygeal Line (P/C line).— This was the uppermost wire, stretching from the upper border of the symphysis to the sacro-coccygeal junction. At the symphysial end, it is important that this line be taken at the centre of the "boomerang" shape of the os pubis, and not at the upper border of the shadow, as the latter is the superior pubic ramus. The angle of junction of the "boomerang" is the pubic point ("P" point). It is shown in Figures 83 and 84. The ossification of the pubis begins at the 2d fetal month, under the acetabulum, and extends along the superior ramus to the body, its situation at birth being as seen in Figure 84.

At the coccygeal end, the "C" point is just caudal to the last (5th) ossific center of the sacrum. The center for this 5th piece appears at approximately the 4th month of fetal life and at birth shows as a small ossific ring. The coccyx does not begin to ossify until the 2d to the 5th year and is, therefore, not visible at birth (Fig. 85).

The pubo-coccygeal line cuts through the upper crescentic margin of the ossified ischium, i.e., the junction of the cranial one-quarter with the caudal three-quarters of the ischial shadow (Fig. 86). If

Fig. 84.—Denuded pelvis to show relative proportions of bone to cartilage in the full-term baby, and the sitings of the *P/C* line and *I* point. **A,** x-ray. **B,** diagram. (Reproduced with permission from Kelly, J.: J. Pediat. Surg. 4:432, 1969.)

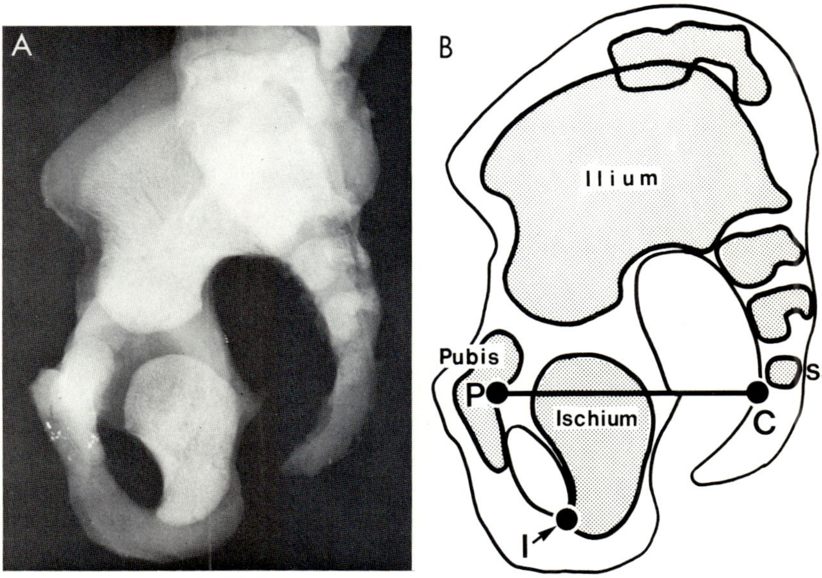

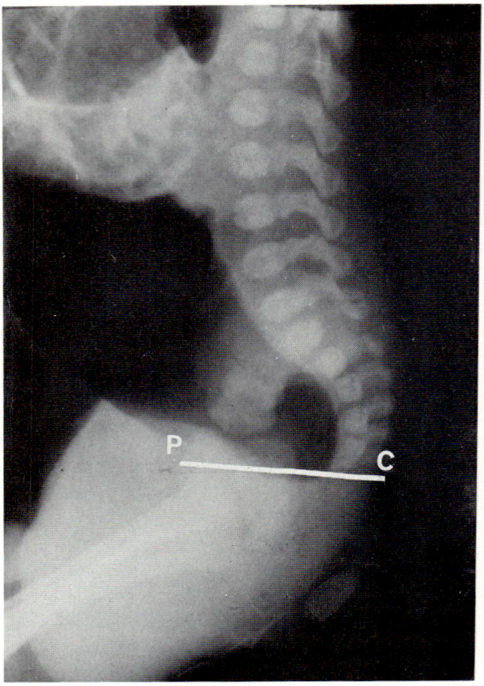

Fig. 85. – Invertography. Gas in rectum lies on the pubo-coccygeal line in patient exhibiting recto-urethral fistula.

Fig. 86. – *P/C* line and absence of sacral vertebrae. **A,** *P/C* line drawn from pubic ossific center through the ossified ischium at the junction of the cranial one-fourth with the caudal three-fourths. Line *PX/CX*, and incorrect projection, joins pubis to the last sacral vertebra, S3. **B,** *P/C* line correctly drawn. Note absence of S5.

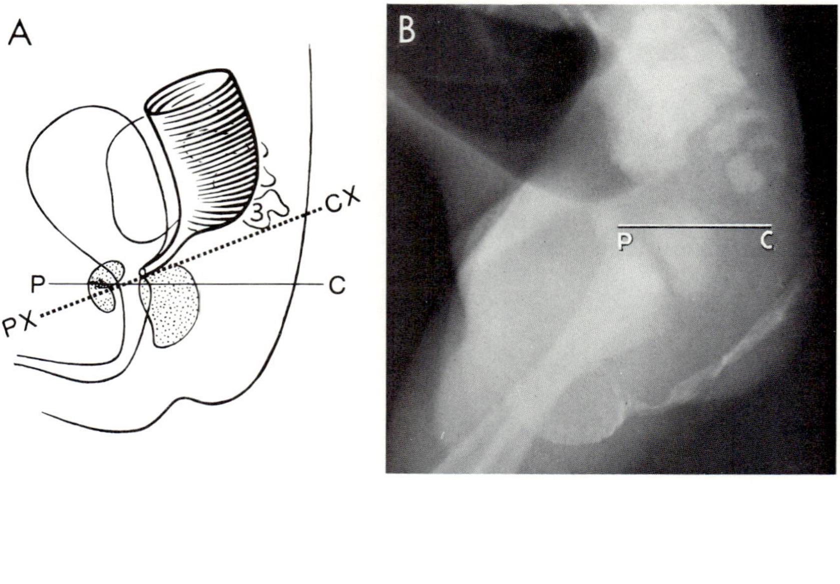

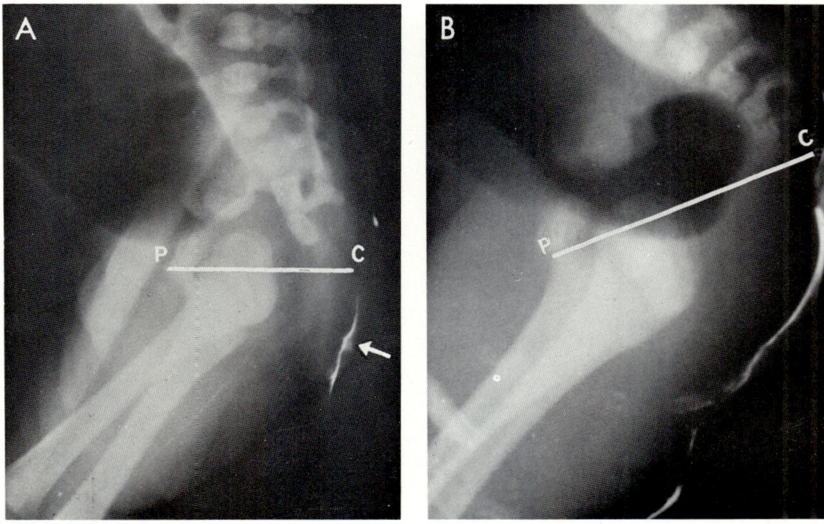

Fig. 87.—Invertography in ano-rectal agenesis (no fistula). In **A,** agenesis at a high level, the gas shadow lies cranial to the *P/C* line (arrow indicates anal dimple). In **B** the gas shadow overlaps the line, indicating a lower level of agenesis or overdistention of the rectum.

the caudal segments of the sacrum are deficient, the line can be developed by projection from the pubis through the same site on the ischium, which serves as a reliable alternative landmark (Fig. 86). In these circumstances the "P/C" line lies well caudal to the last ossified vertebra of the defective sacrum.

The soft tissues lying at the approximate level of this line are bladder neck, the verumontanum, the peritoneal reflexion from the rectum to the prostate and the external os of the cervix uteri. Of 12 female specimens dissected, the pouch of Douglas lay on the line in 9, cranial to it in 1, and caudal in 2. More importantly, the dissected pelves indicated that in the contracted state both the lateral regions of the pubo-rectalis sling and the diaphragm part of the levator ani lie caudal to the pubo-coccygeal line (see Figs. 90 and 91).

In assessing the gas bubble in an anal or rectal anomaly, its relation to the pubo-coccygeal line thus defines the essential fact as to whether the blind pouch is above or below the levator ani. In recto-urethral fistula, the hindgut gas shadow is usually at the pubo-coccygeal line (see Fig. 19); in a high fistula near the bladder neck, the hindgut shadow is above the line; rarely, the rectum may issue lower down in the urethra, but above the bulb, and the bowel shadow is then below the line. In ano-rectal agenesis (no fistula), the shadow is usually identical with that for recto-urethral fistula but may be higher in the pelvis (Fig. 87). In recto-vesical fistula, the shadow is above the line.

All these lesions in which the blind pouch lies at or above the P/C line are above the levator and require a defunctioning colostomy in the neonatal period.

(ii) The Ischial Line and Ischial Point.—In the dissections, a wire marker was placed at the level of the lowest part of the ossified ischial bone. The I point is demarcated on the radiograph as the inferior end of the ischial comma. The I line is drawn through the I point, parallel to the P/C line, and corresponds with the upper surface of the bulb of the urethra in the male and, in the female, the upper limit of the perineal body and the level of the triangular ligament. The urethral orifice lies caudal to the I point.

In anal agenesis and in recto-bulbar fistula, the gas shadow reaches to the ischial line, and this is the lowest point of the levator in these deformities (Figs. 88 and 89 and see Figs. 28, *C* and 34, *C*).

(iii) The Anal Pit Line.—This line passes through the normal anal pit, approximately parallel to the P/C and I lines. It is 1–2 cm. caudal to the lowermost level of the ossified ischium (see Fig. 83). It corresponds with the posteroinferior part of the bulbo-cavernosus muscle. An imperforate anal membrane lies on this line, and the gas shadow reaches to it (see Fig. 97, *B″*).

Scott and Swenson (1959), Snyder (1961) and Robertson *et al.* (1965) utilize the pubo-coccygeal line but describe the symphysial marking as the lower border of the pubis. Santulli (1965) was unable to correlate the pubo-coccygeal line with either the surgical approach or the anatomic type and performs an abdomino-perineal rectoplasty for all lesions above the "ischial line," as described above. However, this would seem unnecessary for two essentially intermediate or low lesions at the ischial line, viz., anal agenesis and recto-bulbar fistulae, both of which may be safely approached from the sacro-perineal route alone, without opening the abdomen.

Kelly (1969), working in our department, has extended these anatomical studies and provided important information on the actual origin and insertion of the levator complex. He first demonstrated the extent of the unossified cartilaginous pelvis in the neonate, which overlaps considerably the ossified centers seen on the lateral radiograph (see Fig. 84). After accurate dissection of the normal neonatal pelvis, he outlined with fine wire the actual attachments of the levator (Figs. 90 and 91). The upper transverse wire indicates the *origin* of the pubo-rectalis and pubo-coccygeus muscles, anteriorly from the back of the symphysis and extending across the lateral wall of the pelvis along the "white line" of the obturator membrane and then posteriorly and medially to the coccyx. In the normal neonate, the pubo-coccygeal line ("P/C") is parallel and a little cranial to this origin.

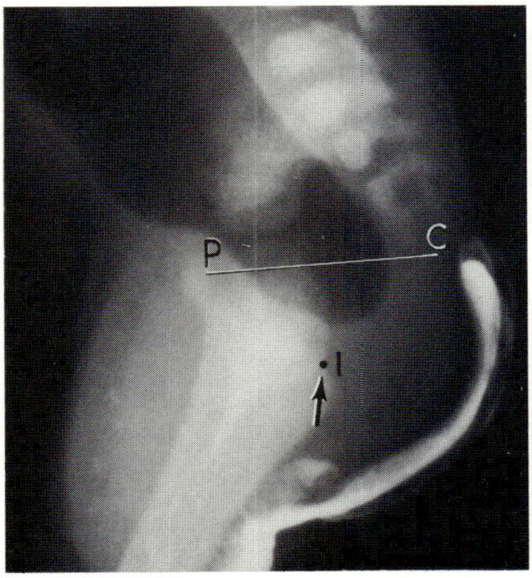

Fig. 88.—Invertogram of recto-bulbar fistula. The gas shadow extends caudal to *P/C* line, approaching the I point.

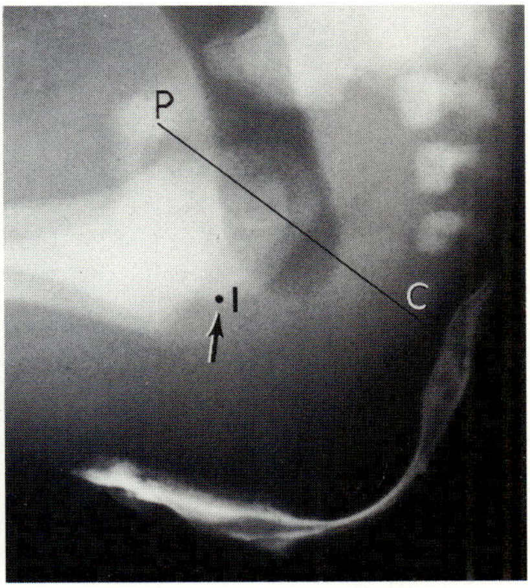

Fig. 89.—Invertogram in anal agenesis (no fistula). Gas extends beyond *P/C* line towards the I point (*arrow*) (similar level to that in recto-bulbar fistula).

Fig. 90.—Landmarks of bony pelvis and levator ani muscle—normal male. Dissection of specimen shown in Figure 83, *A*, with wire sewn accurately along the upper surface of origin of levator ani and down the ano-coccygeal raphe. A transverse wire is sewn along the anal valves. **A**, radiograph showing the wire in relation to ossific centers and the urethra and rectum. **B**, composite diagram, indicating the relation of the muscular attachments to the *P/C* line, *I* point and the viscera.

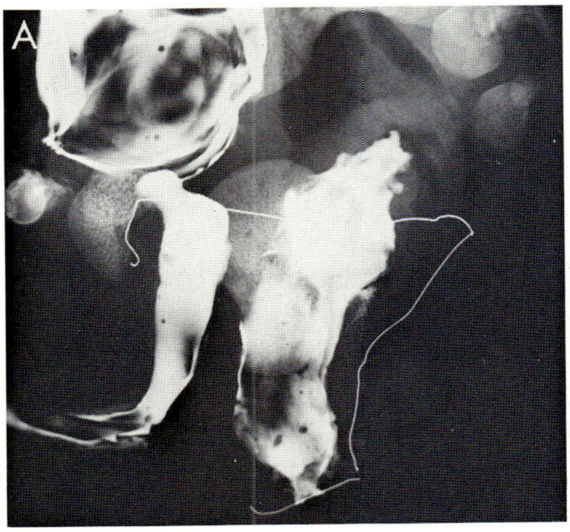

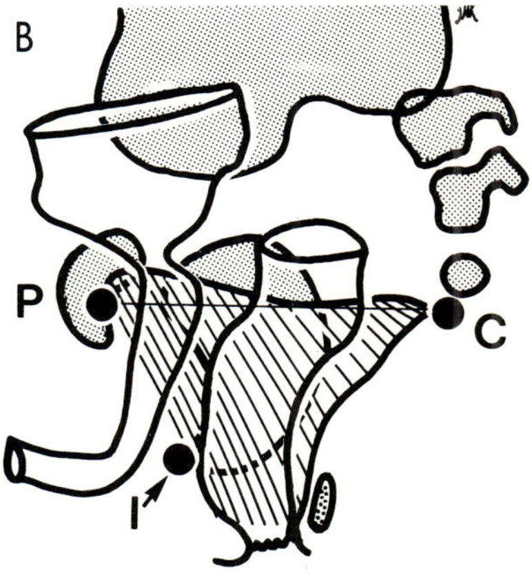

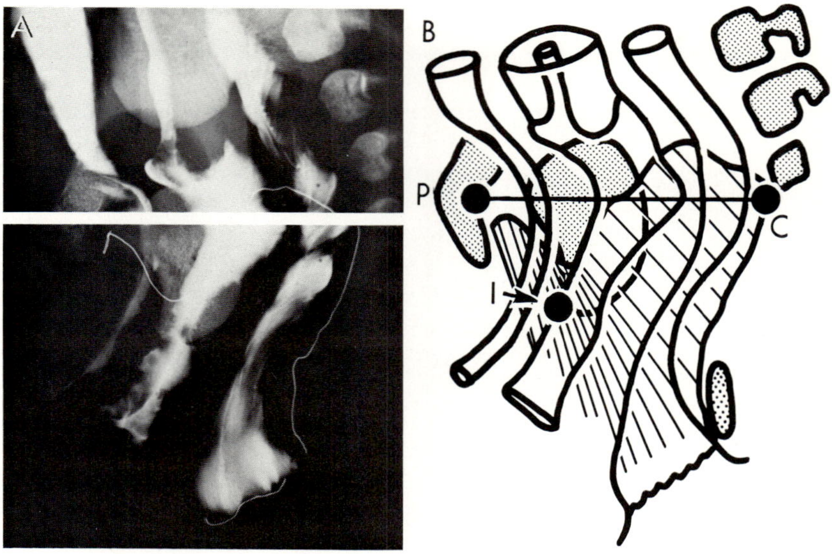

Fig. 91.—Landmarks of bony pelvis and levator ani muscle—normal female. Dissection of specimen shown in Figure 83, *B,* with wire sewn accurately along the upper surface of origin of levator ani and down the ano-coccygeal raphe. **A,** radiograph showing wire in relation to ossific centers, the P/C line, the urethra, vagina and rectum. **B,** composite diagram indicating the relation of the muscle (*hatched*) to the *P/C* line, *I* point and the viscera.

The vertically oriented course of the wire outlines the central fusion line of the converging pubo-coccygei as they meet in the midline and with the longitudinal muscle coat of the rectum. The third and lowest transverse course of this wire demarcates the pectinate line or the line of the anal valves. It can thus be seen that, although the "P/C" line outlines the origin of the pubo-visceral sling anteriorly and laterally, the actual normal attachment to the rectum is very much lower in the pelvis, in fact 2–3 cm. below even the ossified ischium.

In relation to the bony landmarks, the lowermost tip of the ischium is of importance because it defines the location of the perineal body and the lower and most anterior attachment of the pubo-visceral sling to it. This point on the inferocaudal tip of the comma-shaped ischial ossific center is the "ischial point" or "I" point. It is the most anterior point of Stephens' ischial line. If points "P" and "I" are joined on the lateral radiograph and projected caudally an equal distance, another point, "A," is identified. It indicates the site of the anus and the pectinate line and is on Stephens' anal-pit line. The line "P/I/A" is thus the lower border of the pubo-rectalis and pubo-coccygeus; and "C/A" is approximately the insertion of the levator components as the midline raphe.

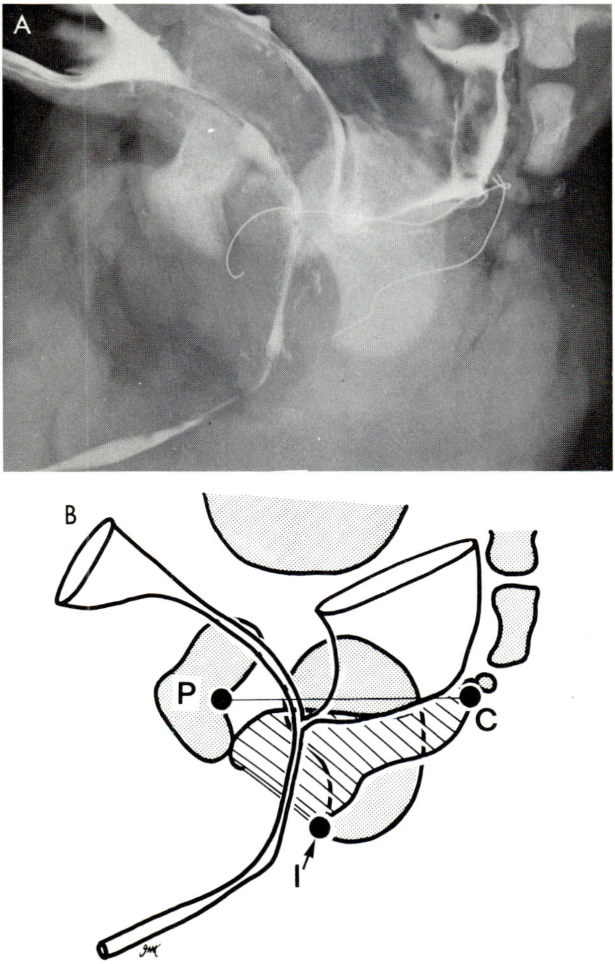

Fig. 92.—Recto-urethral fistula. Landmarks of bony pelvis and levator ani muscle. Dissection of specimen shown in Figure 15, *B*, with wire sewn accurately along upper surface of origin of levator ani and down the ano-coccygeal raphe. **A,** radiograph showing wire in relation to ossific centers, the urethra, rectum and fistula. **B,** composite diagram. Note small area of levator ani muscle compared with the normal in Figure 90, *B*.

Kelly then dissected the pelves in neonates with rectal and anal anomalies at various levels and related the bony landmarks and points "P," "C," "I" and "A" to the visceral and muscular anatomy. In general, the levator complex accommodates to the malformation and lies higher in the pelvis compared with the normal disposition as outlined by the triangle "P/C/A." It was found that the origin of the levator muscles was constant and followed closely the P/C line in

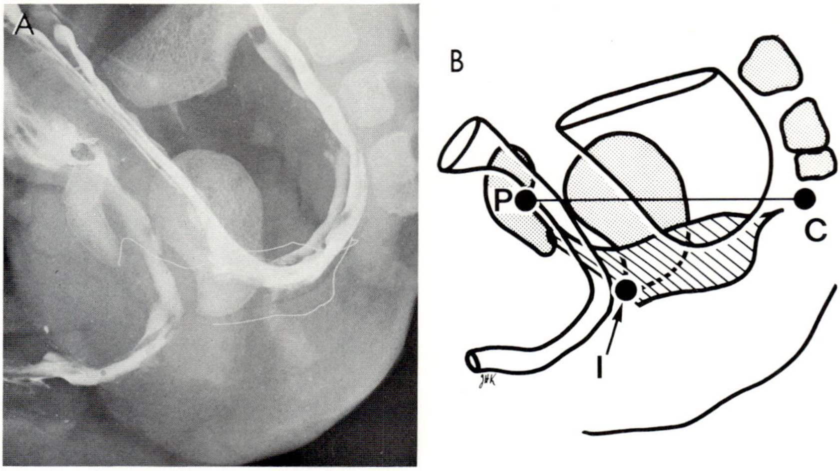

Fig. 93.—Anal agenesis in the male (no fistula). Landmarks of bony pelvis and levator ani muscle. Dissection of specimen shown in Figure 28, *A,* with wire sewn accurately along upper surface of levator ani and down the ano-coccygeal raphe. **A,** radiograph showing wire in relation to ossific centers, the urethra and rectum. **B,** composite diagram. Note smallness of area of levator ani muscle compared with the normal in Figure 90, B.

Fig. 94.—Covered anus in male. Landmarks of bony pelvis and levator ani muscle. Ano-cutaneous fistula issuing onto the back of scrotum has been cut back to the anal dimple. Dissection of specimen with wire sewn accurately along upper surface of levator ani and down to ano-coccygeal raphe. **A,** radiograph showing wire in relation to ossific centers, the urethra and rectum. **B,** composite diagram. Note relatively normal-sized area of levator ani muscle, the lower part of which is more anterior than normal (compare with Fig. 90, *B*).

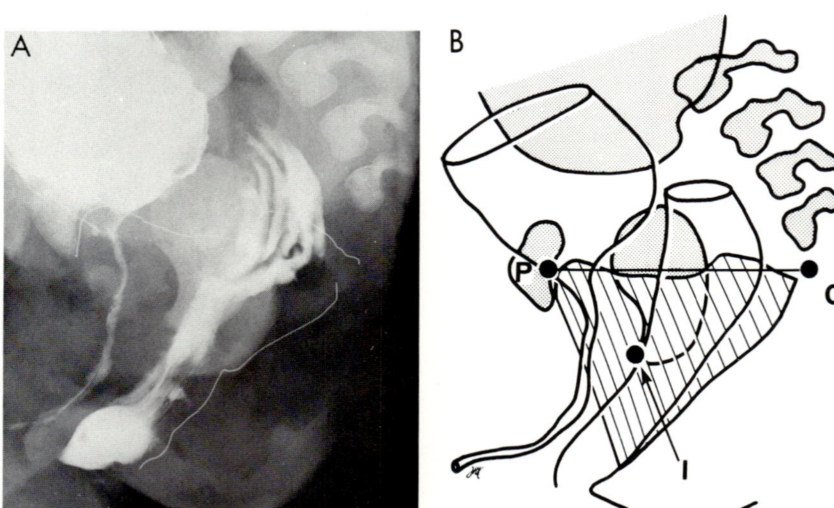

both normal patients and those with malformations of the rectum; that the insertion of the levator muscles varied in level between site "A" in the normal and the "I" point in malformations of the anus and rectum; that the effective contraction of these muscles as judged from these "wire" and other cineradiographic studies can occlude the lumen of the rectum to a level intermediate between the I point and the P/C line; and that the lumen of the rectum of patients exhibiting recto-urethral fistula at the usual level of the verumontanum or higher in the urinary tract is out of reach of the action of the levator ani. It is these facts which provide validity to the interpretation of the gas shadows in relation of the P/C line, as previously described.

The Radiographic Points and Levator Triangles in Relation to the Anomalies.—Triangle "P/I/C."—This triangle denotes the radiographic markings of the levator complex of babies exhibiting anorectal agenesis without fistula, recto-urethral fistula, anal agenesis and recto-bulbar fistula. Here the pubo-rectalis is shorter than normal, and its origin and course are on a more cranial plane. In a patient with recto-urethral fistula (Fig. 92), the wire marker outlining the extent of the pubo-rectalis and pubo-coccygeus indicates that no muscle extends below the "I" point, i.e., the muscle lies above the level of the bulb of the urethra and intimately surrounds the urethra below the fistula. The barium outline of the rectum, which corresponds to the gas shadow, lies near the P/C line, adjacent to the upper fourth of the ossified bone. In a patient with anal agenesis without fistula (Fig. 93), the wire marker again indicates the shortened and compressed nature of the levator, which similarly lies above the I point within the triangle "PIC." P/C again represents the cranial limits of the levator origin, "P/I" the pubo-visceral sling and "C/I" the line of the raphe in the diaphragm of the levator muscle. The barium outline of the rectum, which corresponds to the gas shadow, lies well below the P/C line but still above the I point and through the lowest fourth of the ossified ischium.

In all the rectal deformities lying at or above the I point, the bowel fails to penetrate the levator ani muscle.

Triangle "I/A/C."—In perineal deformities, such as the covered anus with or without ano-cutaneous fistula or imperforate anal membrane, the wire markers outlining the muscles (Fig. 94) extend well down into the pelvis into the triangle I/A/C. Normal caliber bowel in such lesions extends a variable distance caudal to the I point. The pubo-rectalis grasps the most distal limit of the normal bowel and only extends along the fistula for a few millimeters. In a covered anus, which issues by a fistula to the peno-scrotal raphe or urethra, the segment I/A is shortened, whereas the farther back the orifice of the fistula the more I/A approximates to the normal length.

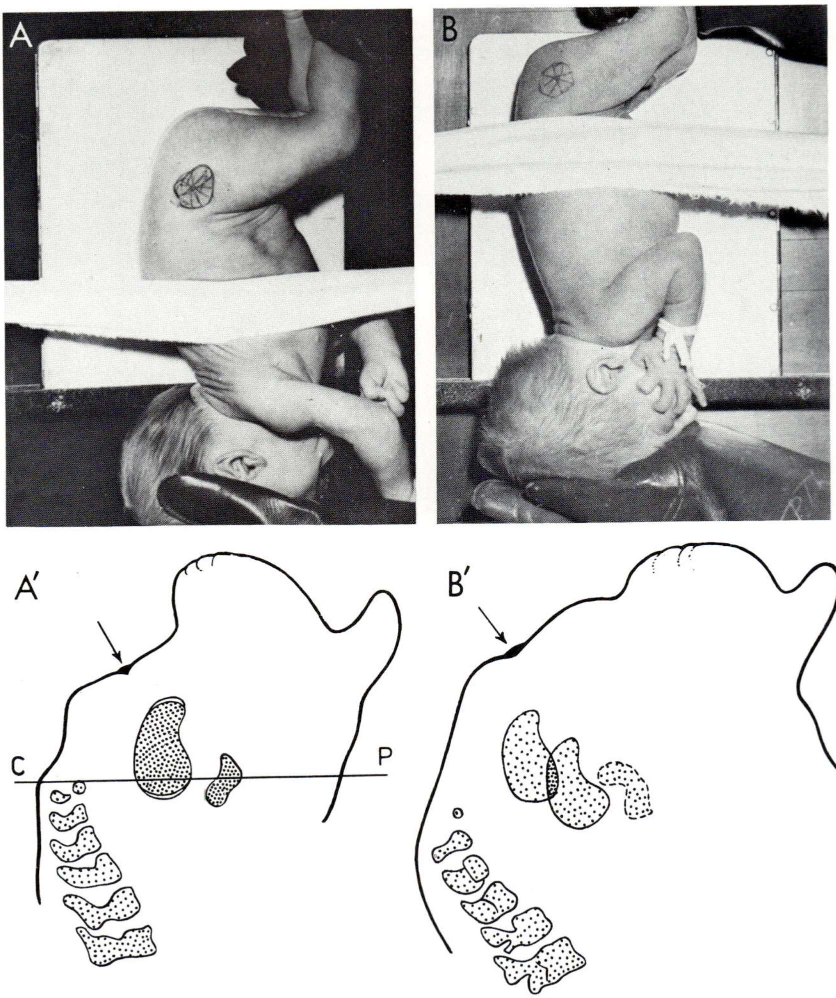

Fig. 95.—"Inversion" radiography. **A** and **A′**, the pelvis is correctly centered in the middle of the x-ray field, and the ischial shadows are superimposed. **B** and **B′**, the pelvis is incorrectly placed in the periphery of the field, causing dislocation of the shadows of the pelvic bones, inaccuracies in the tracing of the diagnostic lines and confusion in the assessment of the levels of contrast media in the bowel. Surface guide to the center of the pelvis is the greater trochanter which should be the clearly marked bull's-eye of the radiographer's target. The hips should be extended beyond the right angle (see Fig. 96, *A*).

Only those deformities lying caudal to the I point in males actually traverse the levator muscles; the I point is the key to the levator anatomy.

Technique.—1. Accurate Centering.—A true lateral view with accurate centering on the greater trochanter is essential. It ensures that the two shadows of the faintly ossified centers of the pubes are superimposed and readily recognized; that the two ischial bones are accurately superimposed, appearing as one; and that the anal dimple and the natal cleft, when outlined by barium cream, are correctly aligned (Fig. 95). Under these circumstances, the pubo-coccygeal line can be accurately drawn and the visceral anatomy interpreted. The common error, the centering on the middle of the abdomen, results in angled projections of the right and left ischiac bones, which appear on the skiagram widely separated and tilted and displaced to the far corner of the picture, the less important abdominal shadows occupying the area of direct projection. The pubo-coccygeal line and its relation to the gas shadows of the rectum are, under such conditions, difficult or impossible to assess. The hips should be slightly extended, as in this position the femoral shadows are clear of the pubic ossific centers, which are then more readily identified (Fig. 96).

Rhoads (1946) and Wilson (1945) felt that in the inverted position gravity might pull the terminal bowel ½–1 inch away from the perineum and advised taking the lateral films with the infant on its side, with the knees firmly flexed, and counterpressure on the anal site. However, there would seem a greater danger of gas escaping into more proximal rectum in this position.

Fig. 96.—Invertograms. **A,** correct positioning of hips; extension of hips exposes the pubic ossific centers. **B,** flexion of hips obscures pubic ossific centers.

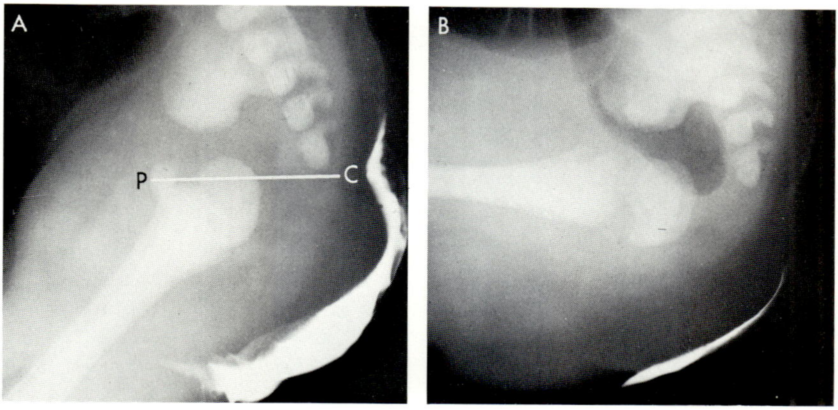

2. Timing.—The baby should be held upside down for 3 minutes before taking the film, to allow gas to displace meconium and to rise to the termination of the pouch. Swenson and Donnellan (1967) precede this position by 30 minutes in the Trendelenburg position.

3. Outlining the Anal Site.—A thin smear of barium paste in the natal cleft is more accurate than a metal marker.

4. Catheter in Urethra.—Recently, Gans *et al.* (1963) suggested the value of a catheter in situ to relate the gas shadow to the urethra. It may be conveniently inserted for the collection of urine as well and, after the invert film, is already sited for the performance of micturition cystourethrography.

5. Repeat Films.—Unless the gas shadow is already below the ischial line, the procedure should be repeated at least once after a 3-hour interval or until some degree of abdominal distention has developed so that sufficient gas has collected to displace all the meconium, lest an erroneous diagnosis of a high lesion be made (Fig. 97, *A*). Further, at each procedure, two or more lateral films should be taken, as a precaution against the possibility of the film being taken at the time of active contraction of the pubo-rectalis, which may cause deceptive obliteration of the lower rectum, again fallaciously suggesting a rectal lesion (Fig. 97, *B′*, and see Fig. 34, *B*).

Errors in Interpretation.—In general, a gas shadow arrested at or above the I point indicates a supralevator lesion and one below the I point, a translevator lesion. However, certain fallacies may cause a misleading interpretation at both sites.

Winslow *et al.* (1961), Shopfner (1965), Robertson *et al.* (1965) and Berdon and Baker (1967) have reviewed some of the pitfalls which may ensue in inversion radiographs. Shopfner, for example, in a series of 48 patients with good radiographs found that only 60% were accurate in assessing the length of the atresic segment when correlated with the operative or autopsy findings. Kelly (1968) has amplified the study of gas shadows in relation to the I point, and showed some of the fallacies. Kurlander (1967) also gives a good review of the radiological features of these anomalies.

1. Gas Shadows Erroneously Suggesting a Supralevator Rectal Lesion.—(i) Insufficient time for gas to reach the terminal bowel. Although Paine and Nessa (1942) showed that gas may reach the rectum in normal newborns as early as 6 hours after birth, nevertheless, until some degree of abdominal distention commences, the gas level may be misleadingly high (Fig. 97, *A*). In fact, Berman (1938) indicated that gas rarely reaches beyond the hepatic flexure by 24 hours after birth. As there is seldom urgency in the first 24 hours, this period, at least, should pass before executing the radiographs. The gas shadow must be smooth and rounded, and the terminal gut fully distended. The precaution of repeating further films at 3-hour intervals minimizes the error. Rhoads and Koop (1955) showed that

gastric aspiration does not affect the validity of the rectal gas shadows.

(ii) Meconium may remain stuck in the terminal gut and give an erroneously high shadow (see Fig. 103, *C*). Wilkinson (1944), Ehrenpreis (1945), Arnheim (1951), Solowiejczyk (1961) and Shopfner (1965) have all documented low-level lesions with high gas shadows so caused. In Wilkinson's case with a high shadow at 36 hours, the meconium was too thick to be aspirated through a wide-bore needle, but he suggested that aspiration is still a valuable check on the depth of the pouch, as such meconium may stick to the end of the needle. However, the index for suspicion that an accumulation of meconium may be present should be aroused by the observation that the gas

Fig. 97.—Possible radiological misinterpretations. **A,** invertogram of anal agenesis. Film taken too early. Interpretations of level of occlusion fallacious when rectum not fully expanded by gas content. **B′** and **B″**, imperforate anal membrane. **B′**, levator ani muscle contracted, causing deceptive occlusion of rectum. **B″**, relaxed, showing true patency of gut to a low level.

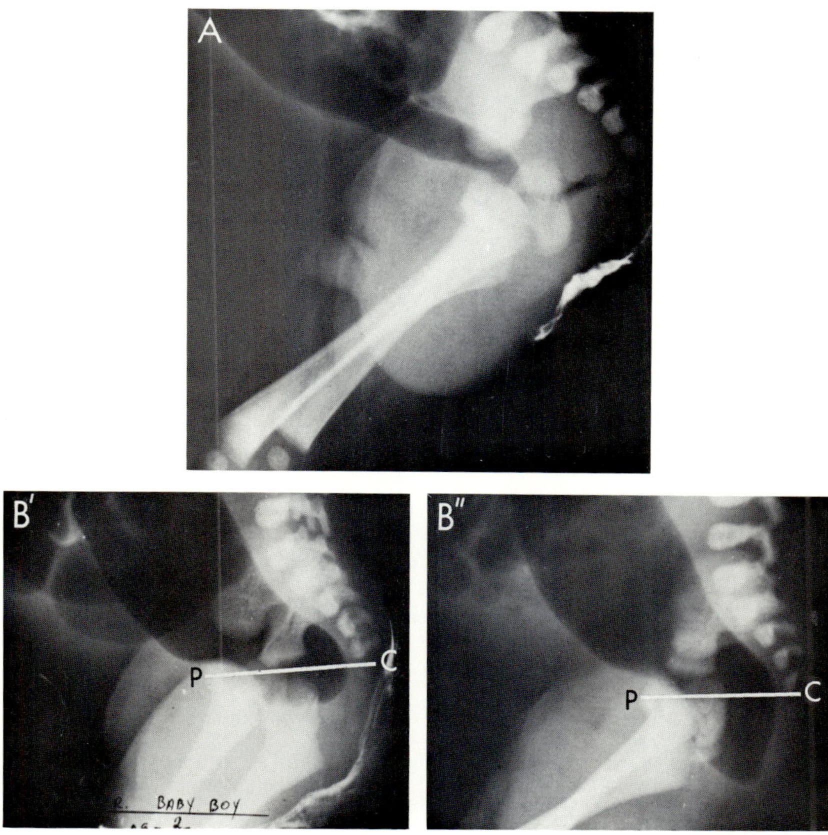

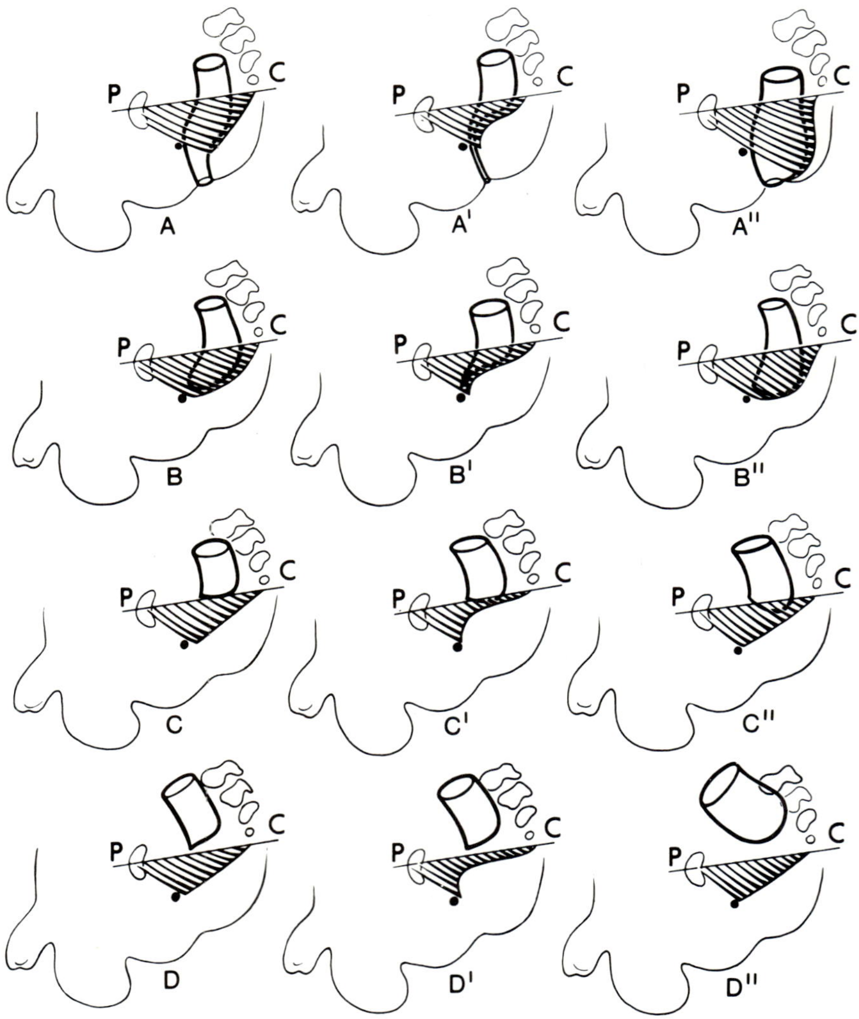

Fig. 98. — Effects of levator ani muscle contraction on gas level in rectal and anal deformities as demonstrated by invertography in males. (*P/C* = pubo-coccygeal line and · = I point. **A,** imperforate anal membrane — pubo-rectalis relaxed; **A′,** contracted; **A″,** stretched; gas level correspondingly altered. **B,** anal agenesis and recto-bulbar fistula — pubo-rectalis relaxed; **B′,** contracted and gas level higher; **B″,** overstretched and gas level more caudal. **C,** ano-rectal agenesis or recto-urethral fistula — rectum lies too far cranially to be influenced by contraction of pubo-rectalis (**C′**) or to permit stretching of the muscle by overdistention (**C″**). **D,** ano-rectal agenesis or rectovesical fistula — level of gas in the rectum not influenced by the levator ani muscle (**D′** and **D″**). Repeated lateral invertograms should be studied to detect the true level, which may need further confirmation by colonograms after colostomy.

shadow is not smooth and rounded. Holding the infant in the inverted position for up to 10 minutes may succeed in displacing the meconium (Robertson *et al.*, 1965).

(iii) Active contraction of the pubo-rectalis. As discussed above and in Figure 98 (see Figs. 34, *B* and *D*, 57 and 97, *B′*), repeated films should prevent this confusion. Further, the deception should be suspected if the outline of the rectum overruns the pubo-coccygeal line, or if other clinical features indicate a more caudal anomaly.

(iv) Gas escape through a fistula to skin, vagina or urethra (see Fig. 45). Such fistulae are recognized on clinical grounds, and their presence invalidates the interpretation of the gas shadows. However, in recto-urethral fistulae, the fistula is usually so small that meconium easily blocks it, preventing the escape of gas; the gas outlines in this lesion are reliable.

(v) Distortion by x-ray magnification resulting in the appearance of a longer gap between gas and skin. This applies only to the measurement of distance which we believe to be unreliable in any case. It will not affect the relationship to the various radiographic lines.

(vi) Improper placement of an anal marker. A large metal marker may not lie in the natal cleft. We advise barium paste, which fills the pit and defines the cleft. A large marker held out from the depth of the cleft may erroneously suggest a long distance of gas shadow from the skin.

2. Gas Shadows Erroneously Suggesting a Translevator Anal Lesion. – (i) Berdon and Baker (1967) and Berdon *et al.* (1968) have pointed out that the pubo-rectalis sling may descend markedly when relaxed and when abdominal pressures are raised by straining and crying. The rectal pouch, e.g., that associated with a recto-urethral fistula, may be filled with gas and lie below the I point, thus simulating a translevator anal anomaly. This downward movement of the levator ani muscle (as with the upward movement when contracted, simulating a high lesion) necessitates repeat radiographs when the infant is not straining (Fig. 98). The phenomenon reported by Berdon *et al.* has rarely been encountered in our experience but is recognized by the closeness to the skin of the gas-filled bowel in a patient exhibiting recto-bulbar fistula (Fig. 29). While admitting the validity of the point, in practice there is usually some additional clue that makes one suspect the erroneous appearance – especially the appearance of a "beak" anteriorly at the site of the urethral fistula (see Fig. 34, *E*). The beak is frequently present, even in the absence of a fistula, as in ano-rectal agenesis without fistula (see Fig. 30, *A*), or when a fistula is plugged or obliterated. In a translevator abnormality, the levator sling may compress the lower bowel and lead to a similar "beaked" appearance (see Fig. 97, *B″*), but, in these lesions, there will nearly always be some other external evidence of the true anal derivation, e.g., an external fistula.

(ii) Inaccurate placement of the pubo-coccygeal line in the presence of sacral agenesis, which may place the line too high and result in a mistaken diagnosis of a low level lesion. The line must pass through the upper one fourth of the ischium, and this precaution should be especially noted in the presence of sacral agenesis (see Fig. 86). Similarly the pubis may be too faintly outlined, in which case the radiographic penetration should be adjusted.

(iii) Error in interpreting gas in vagina or a low-lying loop of small bowel as being in the rectum, and hence considering the lesion to be lower than it should be.

(III) GAS IN OTHER VISCERA. – Evidence for recto-vesical or recto-urethral fistula may be occasionally deduced by the presence of gas in the bladder in a lateral view, provided this is taken before the insertion of a catheter (Winslow *et al.*, 1961; Shopfner, 1965; and Robertson *et al.*, 1965. It is obviously diagnostic (Fig. 99 and see Fig. 104, *B*).

(IV) RADIOPAQUE DYE STUDIES. – (a) Direct Injection of a Fistula or Anus. – As early as 1938, Berman had advocated the value of injection of the fistula with sodium iodide in defining the anatomy of the anomaly. Crowell and Dulin (1940), Arnheim (1951), Bacon and Sherman (1952) and Bradham (1958) similarly injected an external fistula.

Because of the pitfalls in the invert gas films (only 48 of 80 patients, with adequate x-rays, showed adequate assessment of the true level of atresia when correlated with surgical or autopsy findings), Shopfner (1965) has developed a "flushing technique" of introducing an opaque medium into the fistula. The assessment was correct in 15 of 16 patients. When an anal or fistulous opening was visible, the dye was introduced rapidly by a syringe with its nozzle held

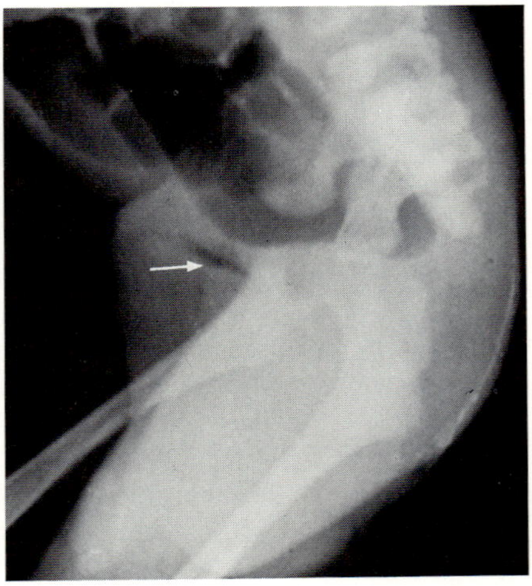

Fig. 99. – Recto-urethral fistula. Inversion radiograph showing gas shadow in the rectum and in the bladder (*arrow*), the latter indicating proof of the fistulous communication.

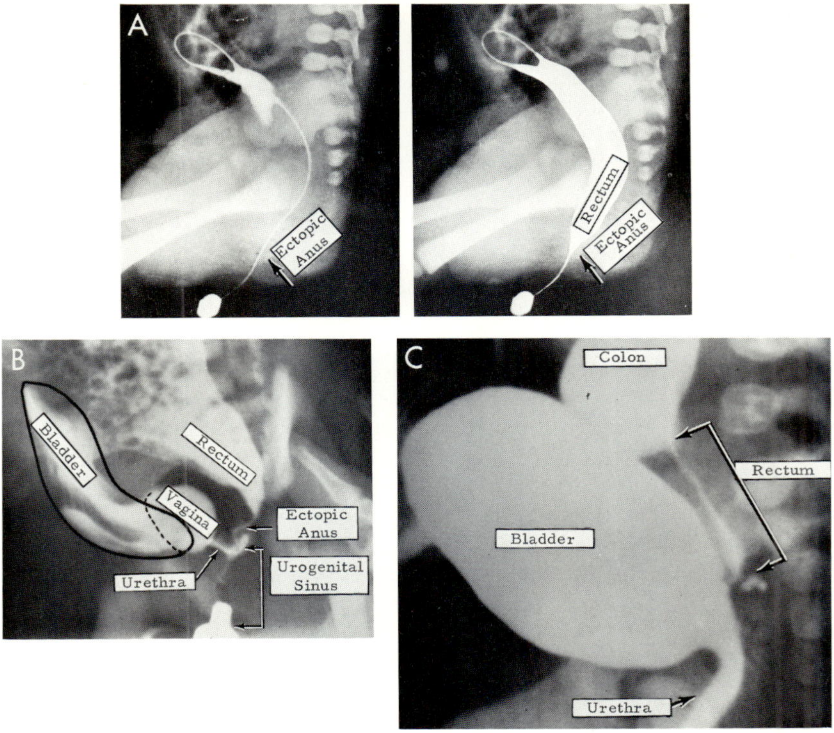

Fig. 100.—Flushing technique as depicted by Shopfner (1965). **A,** anteriorly sited perineal orifice is catheterized, and the rectum is flushed with opaque material. The rectal lumen is demonstrated in its expanded state to the level of the orifice. **B,** recto-cloacal fistula in newborn female baby. Tip of syringe is in the cloacal canal just inside the perineal opening; radiopaque material was flushed into the canal, displaying bladder, vagina and rectum. **C,** recto-urinary fistula—flushing retrograde urethrogram demonstrated the urethra, bladder, rectum and rectal fistula. (Reproduced with permission from Shopfner, C. E.: South. M. J. 58:712, 1965.)

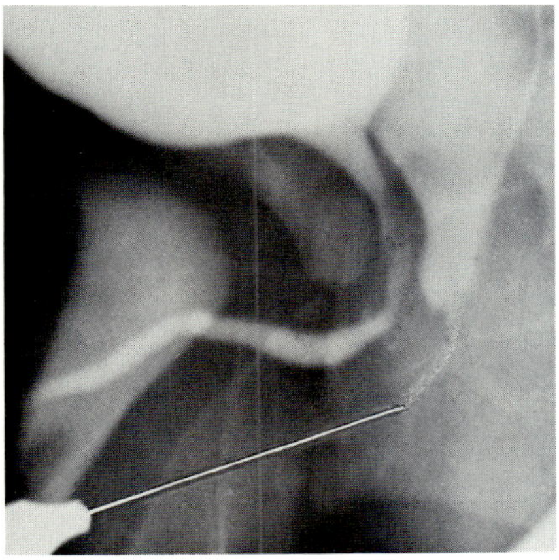

Fig. 101.—Ano-cutaneous fistula outlined by retrograde injection. Iodide in tract and rectum; bladder and urethra filled separately and outlined during simultaneous voiding cystourethrography; rectum ends at level of bulb.

in the fistulous orifice or by a small catheter. In males without visible fistula, the urethra was similarly flushed in a retrograde manner to define a urethral fistula. In these patients, dye was prevented from entering the bladder by a Foley catheter pulled down into the bladder neck, the dye being injected beside the catheter. In females without visible fistula, the vagina was similarly filled with dye (Fig. 100). Ham and Harlin (1953) had more simply filled the urethra via a catheter as it was being withdrawn.

We have not used the injection technique on more than a few occasions, because when the orifice is visible the anatomy can be predicted in any case. Figure 101 indicates the anatomy of an ano-cutaneous fistula. The injection technique does, however, provide valuable confirmatory data and is especially useful in defining the length of an ano-rectal stenosis (see Fig. 35). In the case of a possible urethral fistula, however, the technique may be invaluable in distinguishing between recto-bulbar and recto-urethral fistulae. This information may be obtained at the time of the micturition cystourethrogram (see below); if not, retrograde urethral injection should be performed (Fig. 102).

(b) Direct Percutaneous Needle Aspiration and Injection of the Rectal Pouch.—Most surgeons at some time or other have tried to ascertain the depth of the rectal pouch by insertion of a needle into the perineum. If meconium or gas is found within 1–2 cm. of the perineal skin, it may suggest an anal lesion, but failure to find meconium should not be interpreted as a rectal lesion. It is notoriously

Fig. 102.—Recto-bulbar fistula. Cystourethrogram and cologram depicting the level of the fistula. Arrow indicates the level of the anal dimple.

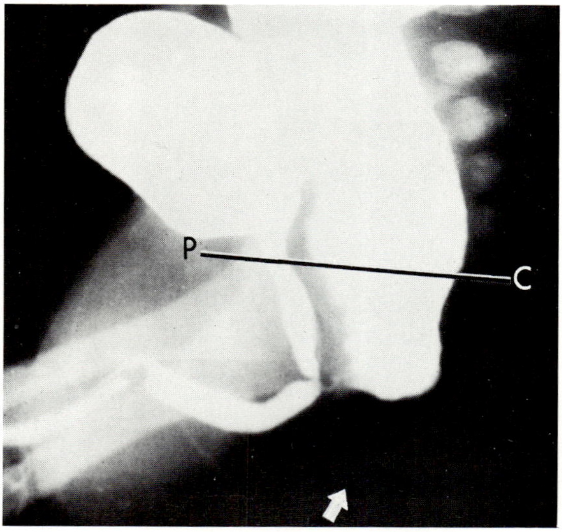

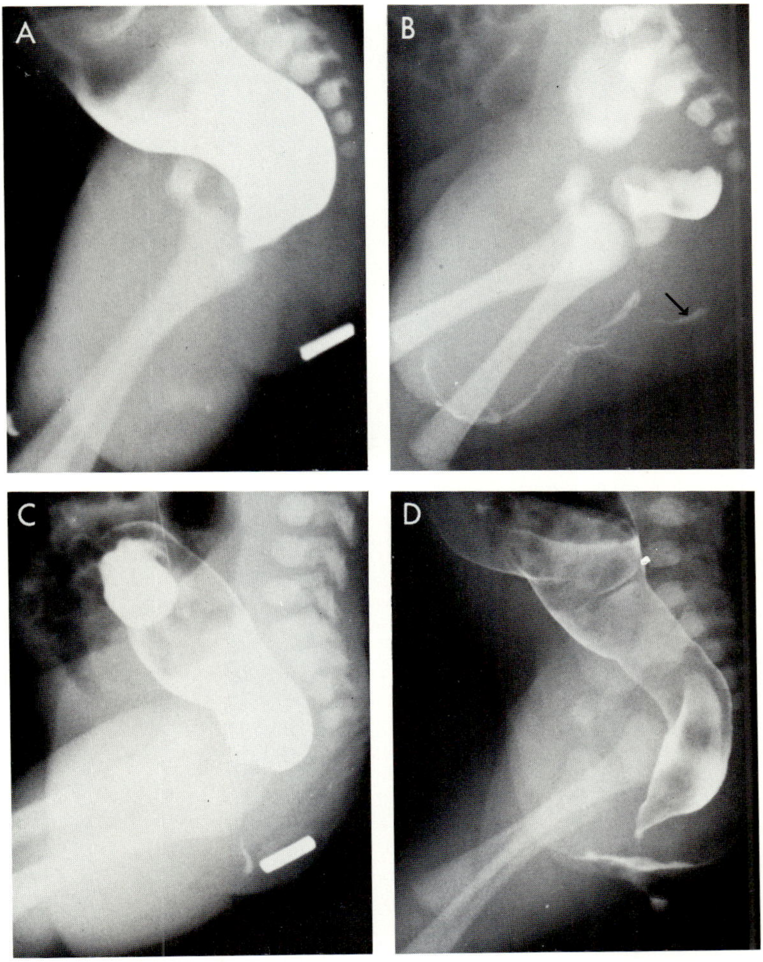

Fig. 103.—Percutaneous injection of iodide into rectum or fistula. Dense contrast medium demonstrates fine fistulae, and the lumen of the bowel can be distended by the injecting pressure. **A,** recto-bulbar fistula showing a "beak" at the I point; note fleck of iodide at urethral meatus, detected after voiding and indicating proof of the urinary communication. **B,** ano-cutaneous fistula; injection of orifice shows fine fistula in raphe of the scrotum and dye pool in the rectum. Arrow depicts a smear of iodide on the anal pit. **C,** ano-cutaneous fistula; percutaneous injection of rectum shows fine fistula near anal dimple, not suspected prior to this injection, the gas shadows previously indicating a high lesion. **D,** ano-cutaneous fistula in female; injection of fistula shows expanded bowel lying close to skin of perineum. (Reproduced with permission from Murugasu, J., Singapore General Hospital.)

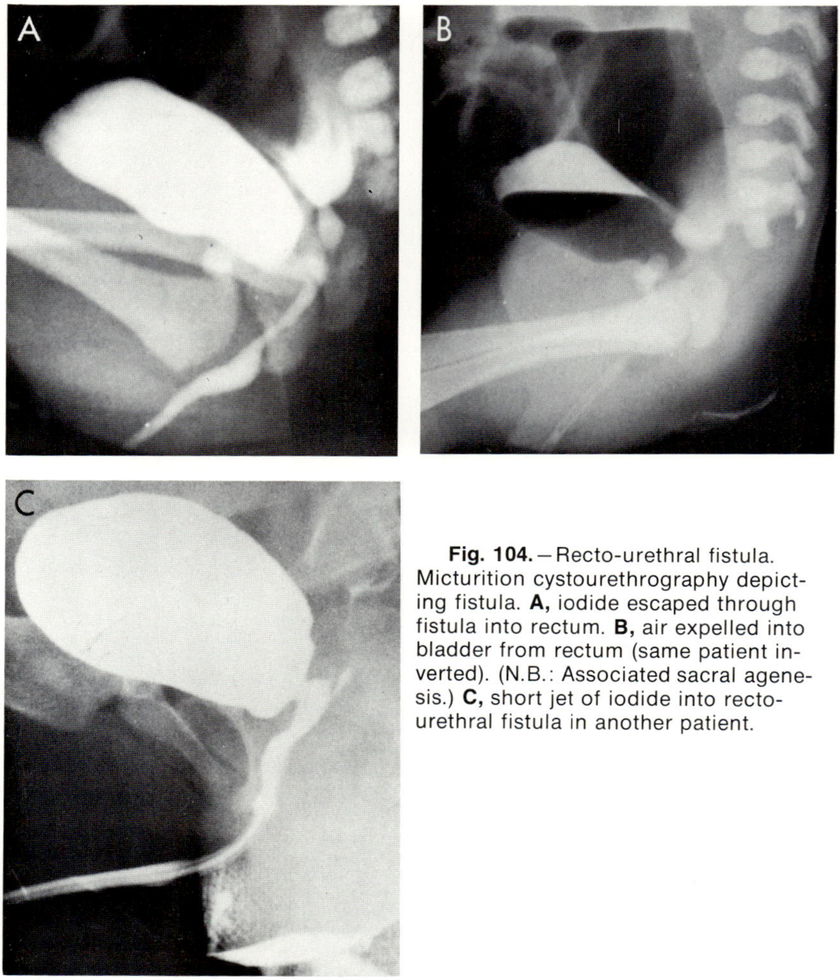

Fig. 104.—Recto-urethral fistula. Micturition cystourethrography depicting fistula. **A,** iodide escaped through fistula into rectum. **B,** air expelled into bladder from rectum (same patient inverted). (N.B.: Associated sacral agenesis.) **C,** short jet of iodide into recto-urethral fistula in another patient.

easy to "miss" a pouch, and, if a "high" lesion is thus fallaciously interpreted, a needless colostomy may be performed. Needle aspiration is simple and always worthwhile.

Recently, Murugasu of Singapore (personal communication, 1968) has displayed the fistula and bowel in a very accurate and graphic manner by injecting radiopaque medium into the terminal bowel per perineum. He used a 19-gauge needle to puncture the dilated pouch, and after confirming the correct site by the aspiration of meconium (with or without the introduction of saline), 8–10 cc. of 30–60% urografin is injected. Posteroanterior and lateral views are then taken. He has had no complications or morbidity and finds the method reliable in demonstrating the exact distal end of the bowel and in outlining a fistulous connection to the genito-urinary system. Figure 103 reproduces four such studies from Murugasu's own series. By this technique, he has demonstrated the presence of a fistula unsuspected on other grounds.

We have no experience of attempts to outline the rectal pouch and fistula from within the intestine by the instillation of 10–15 cc. of Gastrografin (meglumine diatrizoate) via a naso-gastric tube (Kiesewetter *et al.*, 1964).

(c) Micturition Cystourethrogram.—In males without visible external anal orifice or fistula, we now regularly perform this investigation at the time of the invert film. A catheter in situ aids interpretation of the invertogram, and through it the bladder can be conveniently filled with radiopaque medium. Voiding films may provide two valuable clues (1) the site, if any, of a recto-urethral or ano-urethral fistula. Even if the fistula should not be filled, there is usually some characteristic angulation or tenting at the site of the fistula or a telltale streak from the urethra directed posteriorly near the ischial line (Fig. 104 and see also Figs. 22 and 23, and, for recto-bulbar fistula, Fig. 34). (2) It may document an associated urinary abnormality, especially vesico-ureteral reflux (see Fig. 137), which alerts the surgeon to special vigilance in the prevention and treatment of urinary infection (see Chapter 12).

Berdon *et al.* (1966) and Kurlander (1967) also advocate intravenous pyelography and micturition cystourethrography in the neonatal period.

B. Female

(I) Prediction from Clinical Appearance.—Even more than in the male, the internal anatomy of the female anomalies can nearly always be predicted from a careful study of the visible orifices in the perineum. Noncommunicating anomalies are rare in the female, so that some clinical evidence for a fistulous communication can nearly always be elicited, by the emission of meconium or gas.

A sketch or photograph is highly desirable to record accurately the perineal appearances and as a basis for future comparison.

In some females, there may be some fusion of the labial folds preventing adequate inspection of the vulva and its orifices. Such a "closed" vulva must first be opened (Fig. 105), if necessary by division under anesthesia.

The site, number and configuration of all orifices must then be carefully documented by inspection and with a probe, with especial attention to the vestibular area, where a small orifice may be easily overlooked beneath an overhanging fourchette. Classification then depends upon the number of orifices found.

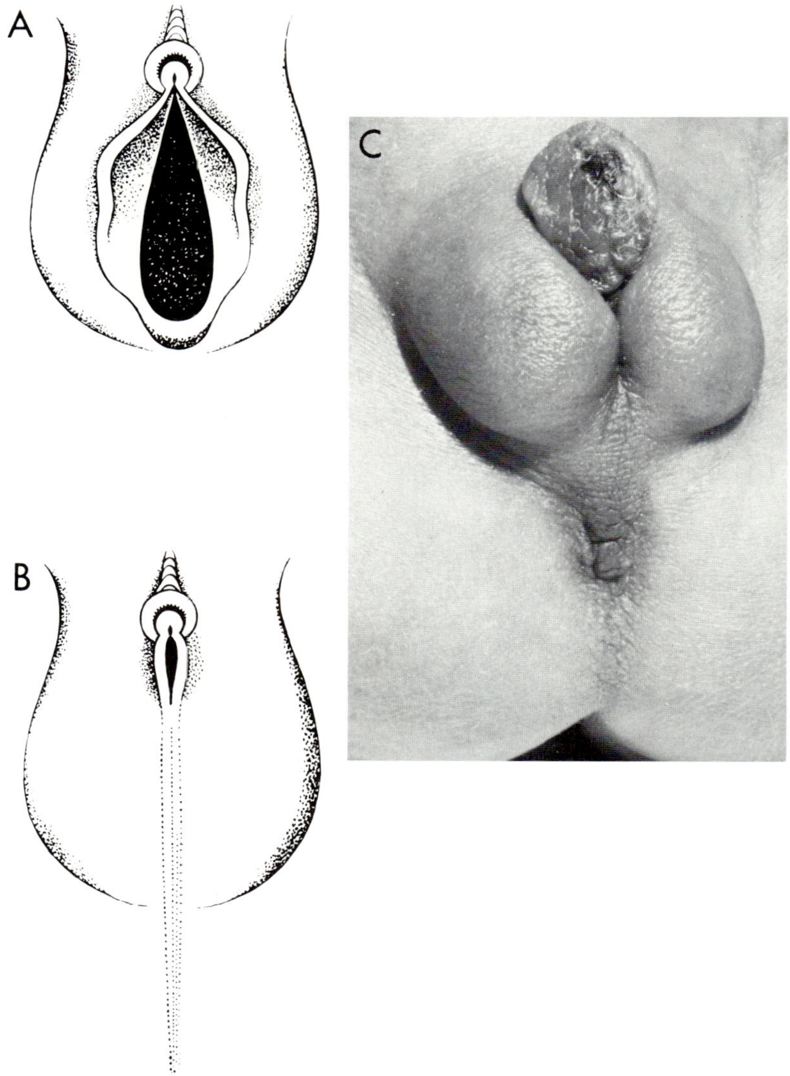

Fig. 105.—Open and covered vestibule. **A,** open. **B,** closed or covered by fusion of genital folds, which project the anal, vaginal and urethral orifices into a common canal issuing beneath the clitoris. In this situation, it is not possible to assess the true position of the anal orifice until the folds are separated. **C,** female infant with some clitoral hypertrophy and fusion of the genital folds. The fused folds obscure any orifices beneath them.

1. *Only one orifice* in the vulva. Such an orifice implies a common cloaca for urethra, vagina and rectum, and the internal anatomy will be that of *recto-cloacal fistula* or *recto-vesical fistula.* Meconium and urine issue from the common orifice. Colostomy is required.

2. *Two orifices* in the vulva and no anal orifice. One orifice is the urethra, while meconium issues from the second orifice, that of the vagina. The internal anatomy is that of a *recto-vaginal fistula,* although, if the rectal orifice cannot actually be seen, it is not possible to predict by inspection alone whether the recto-vaginal communication is high or low in the vagina. As all recto-vaginal fistulae require colostomy in the newborn period, in our view, the actual level of the fistula is of no significance to the immediate decision of treatment, provided the fistula is truly vaginal, and not vestibular, the latter being so commonly, and erroneously, called "vaginal."

Two orifices in the vulva, no passage of meconium, and the anal site covered by hypertrophied folds may suggest *covered anus—complete,* but this lesion has not been seen by us in the female.

3. *Three orifices* in the vulva and perineum. Urethral and vaginal orifices are normal, but a third orifice is present, either in the shape and site of a normal anus or as a fistulous opening at an abnormal site. Further diagnosis then depends upon the actual anal site—whether it be at the normal anal site, further forward in the perineum or in the vulval area.

(i) *At normal anal site*: Seven deformities may present an anal pit at the normal anal site (perineal groove, perineal canal, imperforate anal membrane, anal membrane stenosis, covered anal stenosis, anorectal stenosis and rectal atresia). In six of these, the anus may superficially appear normal or near normal.

(a) *Perineal groove* (Chapt. 4 and see Figs. 65 and 66). The anus is not stenotic but exhibits ectropion anteriorly in continuity with a red, moist perineal groove between anus and fourchette. The labia minora are normal, and the minoral tails flank the groove and are often hypertrophied. The fourchette is sunken and lies at the anterior end of the groove. The labia majora extend backwards to flank the anus.

(b) *Perineal canal* (Chapt. 4 and see Fig. 67). The anus may or may not be stenotic anteriorly but is patent and normal if at the normal site. Deep in the fourchette is a fistulous orifice, and a probe demonstrates a fistulous tract from the vestibular orifice to the anterior wall of the anal canal.

(c) *Imperforate anal membrane* (Chapt. 4).

(d) *Anal membrane stenosis* (Chapt. 4).

(e) *Anorectal stenosis* (Chapt. 4).

(f) *Rectal atresia* (Chapt. 4 and see Fig. 54).

These last four lesions may present an apparently normal anus, but intestinal obstruction or ribbon stools lead to digital or probe examination to discover the membrane, atresic septum or stenotic canal.

The seventh lesion (g) *covered anal stenosis* (Chapt. 4) has a stenotic hole overhung by a hypertrophied raphe at the normal anal site.

(ii) *At perineal site:* That is, at some point between the normal site and the fourchette. Two deformities may be seen, one an anus, the second a fistula.

(a) *Anterior perineal anus* (Chapt. 4 and see Fig. 59, *A, B* and *C*). The anus is normal in caliber and appearance but is sited forwards in the perineum at or near the vulva. It is surrounded by dry skin of the perineum.

(b) *Ano-cutaneous fistula* (Chapt. 4 and Fig. 106, *B*). The appearances resemble the male covered anus, with the fistulous orifice at a forward site, anywhere in the perineum up to the posterior border of the vestibule. The orifice is stenotic and beveled and projects the meconium anteriorly. Unless the orifice reaches to the vestibule, the skin around the orifice is dry and flat; if it is on the vestibular border, the anterior margin is wet.

A probe passes readily and preferentially backwards beneath the perineal skin but also possesses mobility cranially (cf. ano-vestibular fistulae).

(iii) *At vulvar site*: Four deformities occur (vulvar anus, ano-vulvar fistula, ano-vestibular fistula and recto-vestibular fistula). Identification of the exact type depends upon careful examination of the site and size of the orifice and its surrounding mucosa and by the direction taken by a probe into the orifice. Identification is important because the vulvar anus usually requires no treatment, a recto-vestibular fistula requires defunctioning colostomy, whereas ano-vestibular and ano-vulvar fistulae usually only require a perineal "cutback" in the neonatal period.

(a) *Vulvar anus* (Chapt. 4 and see Figs. 59, *D* and *E*). The anus is normal in caliber, but lies within the vulva in the vestibule behind the vaginal orifice. It is surrounded by red, wet, vulvar epithelium. Occasionally, the orifice will lie at the junction of the vulva and perineum, being surrounded by wet mucosa in front and dry skin behind. In these cases, the minoral tails split to pass both in front and behind the orifice.

(b) *Ano-vulvar fistula* (Chapt. 4 and Fig. 106, *C*). This orifice is sited in the posterior margin of the vestibule and superficially resembles an ano-vestibular fistula. It is distinguished from the latter by (1) the skin behind the ano-vulvar orifice is raised up and dry, (2) the lateral borders of the vestibule project posteriorly beyond the vestibule, around the orifice of the anal fistula and (3) the direction of the

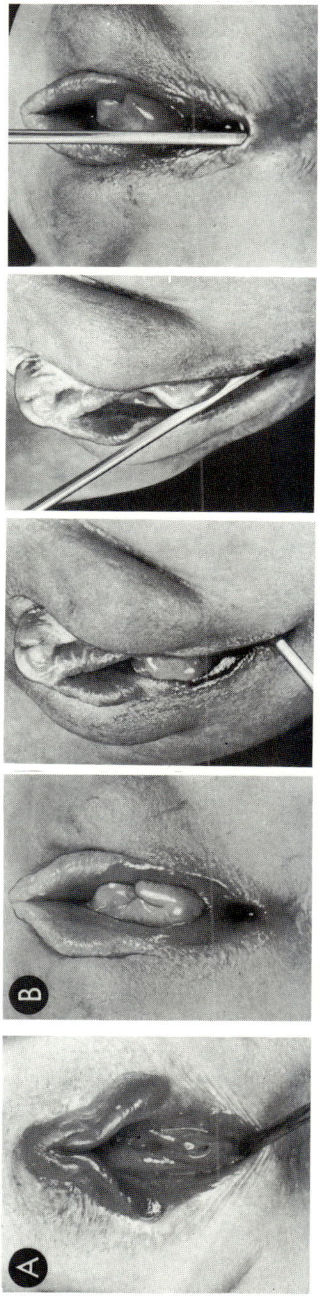

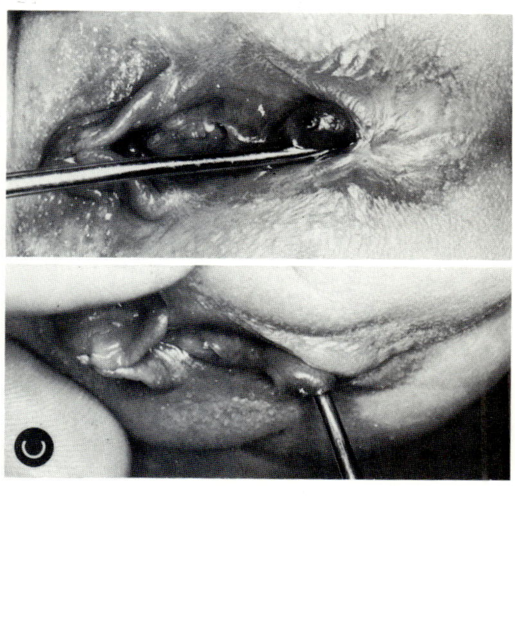

Fig. 106.—**A,** ano-vestibular fistula (and recto-vestibular fistula)—probe passes cranially but is restricted posteriorly. **B,** ano-cutaneous fistula; orifice is behind fourchette—probe passes freely in both cranial and posterior directions. Probe pouts skin of perineum. **C,** ano-vulvar fistula—probe test showing free passage cranially but preferentially under the skin of perineum posteriorly.

probe is as in ano-cutaneous fistulae, i.e., preferentially backwards along the line of the fistula in the perineum.

(c) *Ano-vestibular fistula* (Chapt. 4 and Fig. 106, *A* and see Figs. 63 and 64). The anterior part of the vulva appears normal, and the labia and borders of the vestibule show no signs of hypertrophy. The fistula opens by a stenotic orifice tucked up into the fossa navicularis and may be hidden from view by the overhanging fourchette. The orifice is completely within the vestibule and is surrounded by wet, red mucosa all around; occasionally it may encroach a little onto the posterior rim of the vaginal orifice. The vagina is usually single but occasionally septate. A probe passed into the orifice passes preferentially *upwards* parallel to the vagina, but the degree of backward play is very much limited (Fig. 106, *A*).

(d) *Recto-vestibular fistula* (Chapt. 4 and see Figs. 55 and 56). The external appearances are identical with those described in ano-vestibular fistula, but three tests may suggest the distinction. In recto-vestibular fistula, a probe passes strictly caudocranial immediately behind the vagina, and the length of the fistula inhibits the mobility in a backward direction or in the rectum. Secondly, a Foley catheter marked at 1 cm. intervals can be passed into the rectum, and the inflated balloon pulled down against the termination of the rectum. The length of the fistula can then be measured on the catheter, this length being at least 1 cm. in recto-vestibular fistula but shorter in ano-vestibular fistula (see Fig. 56). Thirdly, the vagina may be double, in which case the fistula lies in the posterior part of the septum between the two vaginae.

(II) INVERTOGRAPHY.—Noncommunicating anomalies are rare in the female infant. In imperforate anal membrane and rectal atresia, a superficially normal anus may be seen but without meconium. In ano-rectal agenesis (no fistula) and anal agenesis, no clue to identification can be obtained from inspection, as in both lesions there is no distinguishing mark in the blind perineum, and the vaginal and urethral orifices are normal and do not emit meconium. Identification requires inversion x-rays, the technique and interpretation being identical with that described above for the male infant. In complete covered anus, the hypertrophied raphe may suggest the lesion, and the gas shadow will be very low near the skin, below the I point.

(III) GAS IN OTHER VISCERA.—As in the male, gas in the bladder as seen in a lateral x-ray is diagnostic of a recto-vesical fistula, although this lesion is very rare in the female. Gas in the vagina probably indicates a recto-vaginal or recto-cloacal fistula but is not diagnostic because air may enter the vagina externally.

(IV) RADIOPAQUE DYE STUDIES.—(a) Direct Injection of a Fistula or Anus.—This technique and its usefulness in the male was discussed earlier, and it may be helpful in distinguishing recto-vestibu-

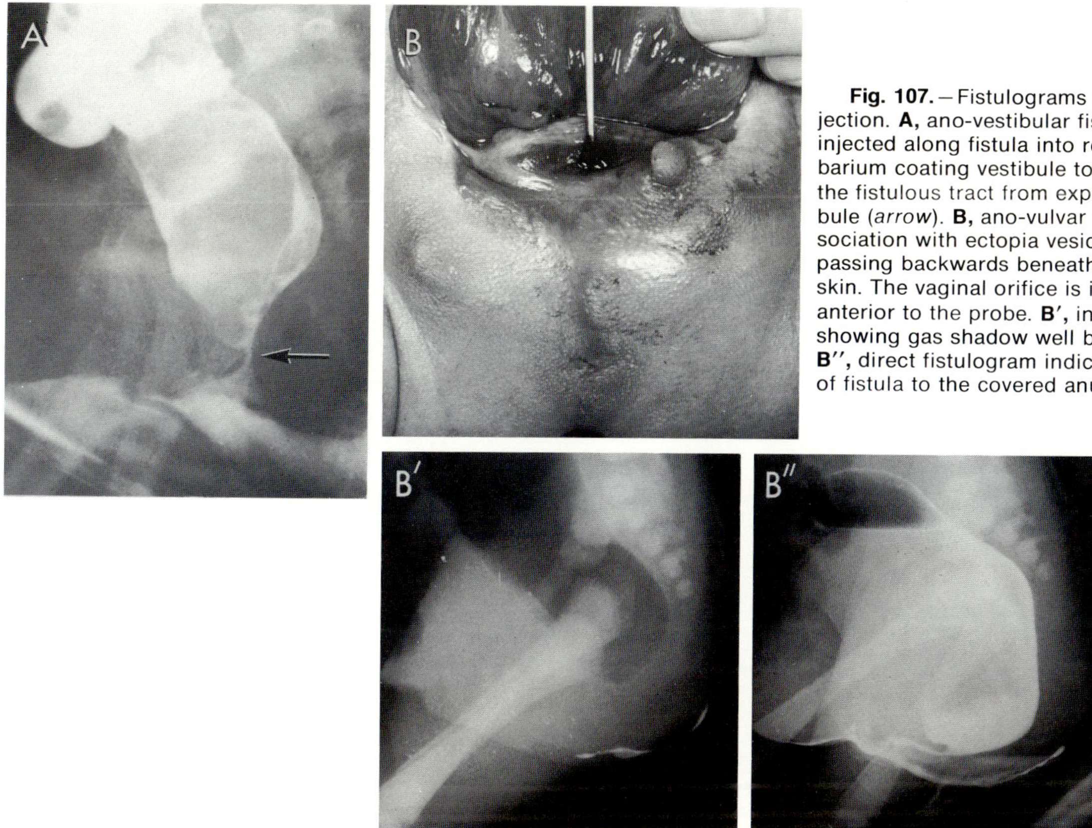

Fig. 107.—Fistulograms by direct injection. **A,** ano-vestibular fistula; barium injected along fistula into rectum, and barium coating vestibule to demonstrate the fistulous tract from exposed vestibule (*arrow*). **B,** ano-vulvar fistula in association with ectopia vesicae; probe passing backwards beneath perianal skin. The vaginal orifice is immediately anterior to the probe. **B′,** invertogram showing gas shadow well below 1 point. **B″,** direct fistulogram indicating course of fistula to the covered anus.

lar, ano-vestibular and ano-vulvar fistulae and in assessing the depth of an ano-rectal stenosis (Fig. 107 and see Fig. 57). As in the male, we believe the tests are not essential, however, because the differences are discernible on clinical grounds with careful examination and with a probe.

(b) Direct Percutaneous Needle Aspiration and Injection of the Rectal Pouch.—The remarks concerning these procedures in the female are the same as in the male.

(c) Micturition Cystourethrogram.—Because of the rarity in the female of recto-urinary communications, the cystogram is of less immediate importance from this point of view; however, we believe that, as in the male, within a few days of treatment it is still advisable to document associated urinary disorders.

(v) VAGINOSCOPY.—When only two orifices (urethra and vagina) are visible, the internal anatomy of a recto-cloacal or recto-vaginal fistula can be simply and accurately defined. The examination can be conveniently performed at the time of the colostomy, and we use a panendoscope.

2. ASSESSMENT OF THE INTEGRITY OF THE SPHINCTERS AND THEIR NERVE SUPPLY

INTEGRITY OF THE LEVATOR ANI MUSCLE.—There is a close relationship between the development of the sacrum and the extent of formation of the levator ani muscle. *Radiographs of the sacrum and lumbar spine* (anteroposterior and lateral views) are essential in the neonatal period (Fig. 108 and see Fig. 132). A normal spine and sacrum portends a well-developed levator muscle. A defective spine presages imperfections of the muscle or adaptations of the posterior attachments. However, a deformed sacrum on the x-ray is not the final criterion of integrity of the muscle and its nerve supply and must be evaluated together with the sacral outflow tests described below. The following conclusions generally apply:

(i) Deficiencies of the 4th and 5th sacral vertebrae usually allow normal innervation of the bladder and levator and adequate development of the levator.

(ii) Deficiencies of the 3d, 4th and 5th sacral vertebrae are accompanied by variable innervation and muscle development, but most patients are incontinent.

(iii) Deficiencies involving the 1st or 2d segments have always been associated with incontinence in this series, and the levator ani poorly developed and defective in innervation.

(iv) Innervation and muscle development accompanying hemisacral defects are unpredictable, but if only one or two vertebrae show the hemisacral defect, the innervation and muscle development are adequate.

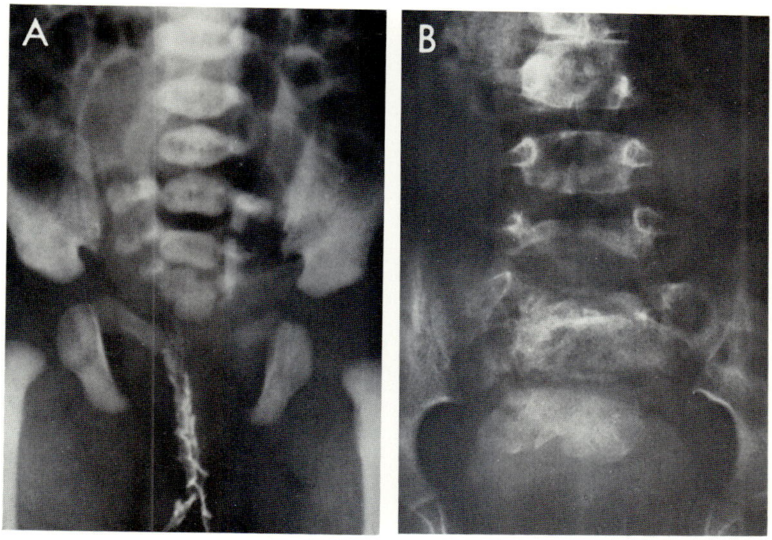

Fig. 108.—Sacral defects and rectal malformations. **A,** hemisacrum—3d and 4th sacral vertebrae are defective on the left side. **B,** sacral agenesis—absence of 3d, 4th and 5th vertebrae.

(v) The presence of a lumbo-sacral myelomeningocele almost always involves a serious defect in innervation. The levator is usually well developed but lacks the central neural connections in the dysplastic cord.

The radiological appearance of the deformed sacrum is not the sole criterion of muscle and nerve integrity because of the occasional presence of sacral innervation, even in the absence of corresponding bone segments. On the other hand, Smith (1959), in dissections of specimens of sacral agenesis, found that in four of these the sacral roots failed to develop caudally to the lowest formed vertebra and there was close correlation between absent sacral nerves and deficient sacral bone segments as shown in Figure 109.

In these subjects, the levator ani muscle, which was poorly developed, lacked its nerve supply. On the other hand, in two specimens lacking sacral bony segments, a full complement of sacral roots was present, together with the levator ani muscles, although the course of these nerves through the lumbar theca was abnormal (Fig. 110). The possibility of normal innervation to the levator ani in the presence of sacral agenesis is thus demonstrated.

Sacral Outflow Tests for Sphincter Innervation.—Radiographs showing sacral defects put the surgeon on guard regarding probable defects in the levator ani and the sphincter nerve supply, but the final criteria are those depending upon clinical tests of the

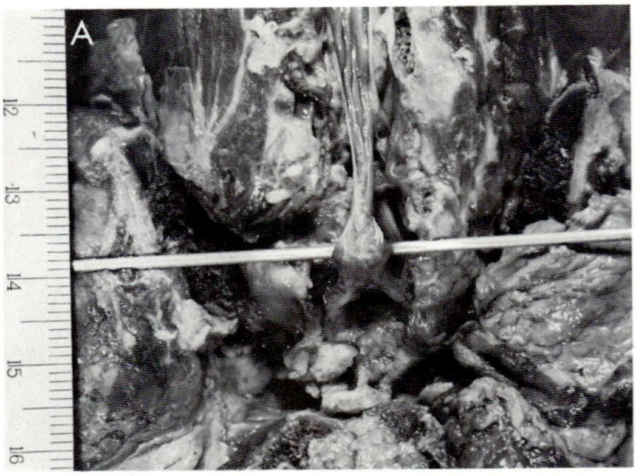

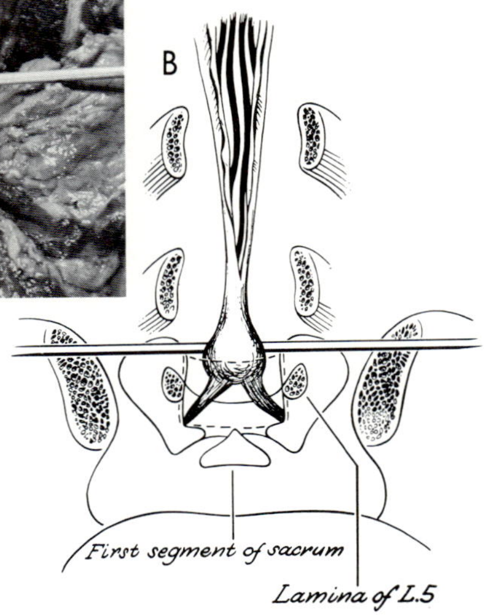

Fig. 109. – **A,** dissected specimen with a sacrum of one segment only. The cauda equina terminates in a nodule over L5 from which emerge the last two lumbar roots. There are no sacral nerve roots and no sacral canal. This is the usual finding in severe sacral agenesis. **B,** drawing to show the termination of the cauda equina.

sacral outflow of nerves. The same sacral segments (2d, 3d or 4th) innervate levator ani, anal sphincters, bladder parasympathetics and perineal dermatomes; analysis of the bladder and perineal skin provides information about the hidden pelvic floor innervation.

(i) History of Urinary Control. – In the first day or two, it may be difficult to be sure about urinary control, but, in older children and infants, the history seldom leaves doubt. Wetting from neurogenic defects is constant and permanent, with not a single day of normal control. There are two classical voiding patterns: (1) Almost continuous dribbling of small volumes through a patulous urethra and, in older children, absence of sensation of fullness or voiding and inability to stop the stream. (2) Overflow leakage; the bladder is firm and tense, and leakage occurs at irregular intervals in episodes up to 1 – 2 hours; in older children, there is no sensation and no ability to stop the stream.

(ii) Bladder Expressibility. – The most constant and useful confirmatory sign of the paretic bladder is its expressibility by manual pressure. Even in the neonate, urine cannot be expressed from the normal bladder. Two expressibility patterns are found: (1) Freely expressible, with little pressure required, and the bladder impalpable. (2) Nontender, palpable bladder for which considerable force is required to achieve expression, often only during the transient relaxation of the abdominal muscles during inspiration.

(iii) Perineal Sensation.—If absence of response to pinprick stimulation of the perineal skin indicates anesthesia, the sacral outflow is defective. However, normal sensation does not always necessarily mean normal sphincters. The details of the analysis of perineal sensation are amplified in Chapter 12.

As a result of these sacral outflow clinical tests, it is almost always possible, even in the neonatal period, to predict the innervation to the levator ani. Defective innervation of perineal skin, urinary leaking and an expressible bladder indicate defective innervation of the levator ani. In such a situation, the prognosis for rectal continence is virtually hopeless, and, in the case of rectal anomalies, a permanent colostomy must be planned.

Fig. 110.—An unusual finding in sacral agenesis. Despite sacral agenesis (one segment only), there is a full complement of sacral roots. **A,** dissection of cauda equina showing sacral roots. **B,** drawing of same specimen following laminectomy and dissection of buttock. Seven sacral roots emerge on the right side. Both pudendal nerves appear on the right, one subsequently crossing to the left side. Sacral innervation may therefore be present despite the radiological appearance of sacral bone agenesis.

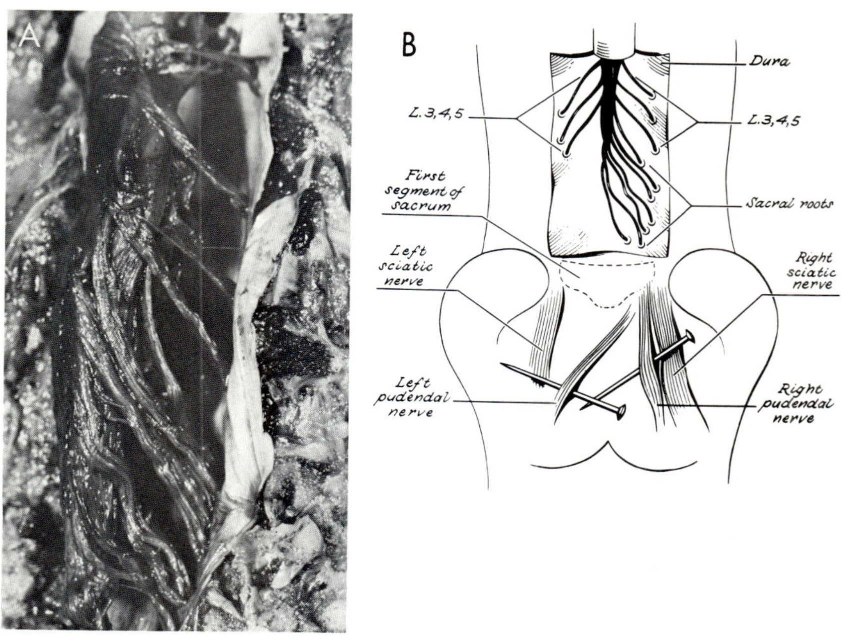

3. Assessment of Associated Visceral Malformations

Urinary Tract.—In the immediate neonatal period, the micturition cystourethrogram is the only investigation required. Subsequent follow-up and other investigations are, however, important and are discussed in the following section.

Other Visceral Anomalies.—In the diagnostic assessment, many of these lesions will be suggested or obvious on clinical examination (e.g., cardiac lesions, myelomeningocele, Down's syndrome, exomphalos, etc). Because of the relatively common association with esophageal atresia, a firm rubber catheter should be passed into the esophagus. Other alimentary obstructions will be suggested by early bile-stained vomiting.

The influence of these associations on early decisions about rectal management can be important, and are discussed in Chapter 11.

Diagnosis Beyond the Neonatal Period

In many patients, if all these steps outlined in the foregoing section have been taken, most of the information desired about the internal anatomy will have been established. However, a colostomy provides access to the bowel for further radiological studies important in confirming or amplifying the previous information. Further, the age and size of the child now permits more refined and detailed assessment of the urinary tract and of the sphincter anatomy and its nerve supply. Finally, there will be some infants and children seen for the first time at this age, treated elsewhere without all the foregoing tests. In these children colographic studies, micturition cystourethrography, radiographs of spine, injection of fistulae, sphincter assessment, etc., become essential.

1. Colography

Keiller (1924) was the first to use a barium suspension into the distal limb of the colostomy to demonstrate the site of the fistula. Other authors followed (Crowell and Dulin (1940), Bacon and Sherman (1952), Palmer (1956) and Bradham (1961) but probably because of the stress in the Northern hemisphere on one-stage rectoplasty without colostomy few centers have advocated the procedure. Colography, in our opinion, still further documents the internal anatomy, thus aiding the surgeon in his decision on surgical approach.

Gastrografin (meglumine diatrizoate), being water soluble, is preferable to barium sulphate, which tends to dry and impact in the distal colon. The colon is thoroughly evacuated of its meconium or fecal contents, and 10–20 ml. is run into the distal colon via a catheter, the child being held erect. Following colostomy in the newborn, we generally perform colography before the child goes home, 2–3 weeks after operation, but in any case in the first 2 or 3 months of life.

The dye may actually run into a fistula; if not, the dye shadows, indicating the level of occlusion, are related to the bony landmarks, as in the invert film (see Figs. 27, 29, 30, 34, *E*, and 102).

Occlusion of the rectum and rectal fistula occur commonly at the following three levels in each group.

MALES.—1. Noncommunicating Lesions.—Level of occlusion at or above P/C line = ano-rectal agenesis (no fistula).

Level of occlusion at ischial line reaching to just above the "I" point = anal agenesis.

Level of occlusion at pit line, below the "I" point = covered anus complete and imperforate anal membrane, although in most cases such lesions will not require a colostomy.

2. Communicating Lesions.—Fistula above the "P/C" line = recto-vesical fistula.

Fistula at verumontanum, at or below "P/C" line but above the "I" point = recto-urethral fistula.

Fistula at bulb, at ischial line, just above "I" point = recto-bulbar fistula.

FEMALES.—1. Noncommunicating Lesions.—As in male.

2. Communicating Lesions.—Colography is not so essential in these lesions because the internal anatomy can be confidently assessed on clinical grounds, but it is still worthwhile to determine the caliber of the terminal gut for the presence or absence of secondary megacolon, especially in those children who have continued to defecate for weeks or months through the fistula.

Fistula at or above "P/C" line = recto-cloacal fistula or recto-vesical fistula.

Fistula between "P/C" line and "I" point = recto-vaginal fistula, but the level will depend upon whether it is high or low in the vagina.

Fistula at or below the "I" point = recto-vestibular fistula.

2. MICTURITION CYSTOURETHROGRAPHY

Whether or not this has been performed in the neonatal period, we may repeat this investigation at the time of the cologram in search of further important clues. If combined with the cologram in males with communicating lesions, the rectal fistula can be more accurately defined in relation to the bladder or urethra. Even if the full course of the fistula is not seen, a suggestive angulation of the urethra pointing towards the rectal end of the fistula strongly suggests a recto-urethral or recto-bulbar fistula. In noncommunicating male lesions, cystourethrography is still worthwhile, if only for its negative findings, and occasionally has demonstrated a fistula when one was thought not to exist. In the female, because of the rarity of urinary communications with the rectum, cystourethrography is not important from the point of view of the bowel lesion, but we still perform it in both sexes because of the information it provides about associated urinary anomalies, such as vesico-ureteral reflux, and for its value in assessing a neurogenic bladder (see Chapter 12 and Figs. 22, 23, 24, 34, 102, 104 and 137).

3. Urethroscopy

Further information about the site and size of the urethral communication in males may be obtained by cystourethroscopy. Although a small fistula may be difficult to see, the knowledge that the fistula is large is a help at the time of operation. Prior knowledge of a large fistula alerts the surgeon to the possible risk of excising a portion of the urethral wall with the fistula.

It is usually sufficient to defer the endoscopic examination until the day of definite rectoplasty, which it precedes. If, however, the investigation of urinary infection in either sex necessitates cystoscopy and retrograde pyelography prior to the rectal procedure, then this opportunity is used for visualizing the fistula.

4. Vaginoscopy

In female children with communicating lesions, vaginoscopy, like urethroscopy, should immediately precede the rectoplasty for the same reasons as in the male. We use a panendoscope and water irrigation and allowing free efflux of irrigating fluid out through the vaginal orifice. High fluid pressure may force fluid into the peritoneal cavity. Vaginoscopy may provide necessary information about the genital tract (vaginal malformations, etc.) as a basis for future management.

5. Assessment of Sphincters and Their Nerve Supply

In addition to the above tests, in patients not previously seen, it is essential to assess the sphincter anatomy and nerve supply prior to further decisions. Radiological examination of the spine and pelvis and the clinical tests for urinary control described for the neonatal period above are vital.

Even in those patients seen and assessed at birth, the passage of time provides more definitive historical information about urinary control and from it further confirmation of the neural pathways.

6. Assessment of the Urinary Tract

In addition to the information provided by the *micturition cystourethrogram* (see above), the high frequency of associated urinary anomalies necessitates adequate urological analysis in the first 2 or 3 months of life.

Regular *microscopy and culture* of urine specimens are desirable. A practical problem is the method of collection of adequate specimens of urine to prove or disprove urinary infection in the presence of a recto-urinary communication. In a recto-bulbar fistula, a catheter may enter the fistula at the bulb rather than pass up to the bladder and is then obviously contaminated; further, both in this lesion and in recto-urethral fistula, the urethra may already be contaminated with fecal organisms, and it may be difficult to interpret the vesical specimen. Suprapubic needle puncture of the bladder may be necessary and is safe and satisfactory.

Intravenous pyelography and *blood urea nitrogen estimation* should also be completed in the first few days after birth in rectal lesions, and later in anal anomalies. The radioisotope *renogram* provides an important method of estimating renal function in both kidneys and of stasis in the pelvis or ureter. *Retrograde pyelography* will be necessary when the urine findings, pyelogram, or renogram suggests upper urinary tract stasis.

In these ways, the plan of treatment of both the malformations of the bowel and the urinary tract can be mapped to best advantage in advance. Serious urinary tract disease may necessitate consideration preceding any major operation upon the rectum (see Chapter 12).

Relatively few surgeons have stressed the urinary assessment in the early months, but Thompson and Hooks (1956), Palmer (1956), Kiesewetter *et al.* (1964), Kiesewetter (1966) and Swenson and Donnellan (1967), all stress the need for intravenous pyelography and voiding cystograms, and Bradham (1958 and 1961) advises pyelography and cystoscopy.

CHAPTER 9

Operative Management of Rectal Deformities

(Supralevator Lesions)

THE RATIONALE of the choice of the various operations for each specific rectal deformity has been discussed in Chapters 3 and 4, which should be referred to in reading this chapter. The present chapter deals with operative decisions in general in the rectal group and specifically with operative technique and pre- and post-operative care.

The target in treatment is maximal continence of the newly fashioned anal canal. No amount of finesse in the construction of a cosmetically pleasing anal opening, or in performing heroic surgery in the newborn, is of any avail if the child is committed to a life of fecal incontinence. Accurate preoperative assessment, precise knowledge of the anatomy and meticulous and delicate surgical technique are essential requirements for success. The experience of Willis J. Potts (1959) led him to the following conclusion:

> In general, atresia of the rectum is more poorly handled than any other congenital anomaly of the newborn. A properly functioning rectum is an unappreciated gift of greatest price. The child who is so unfortunate as to be born with an imperforate anus may be saved a lifetime of misery and social seclusion by the surgeon who with skill, diligence and judgement performs the *first* operation on the malformed rectum.

By far the most important factor in continence is the integrity of the sphincter mechanisms, and a constant consciousness of their protection before, during and after surgery must ever be in the surgeon's mind.

(i) Which sphincters are present, and are they developed adequately for the purpose?

(ii) Are they innervated correctly?

(iii) Are they preserved intact by the operative technique?

(iv) Are they subjected to forces beyond their control after operation, e.g., stricture, scar formation or secondary megacolon?

The answers to these questions govern the choice of operative procedure and the postoperative care.

In the rectal deformities (supralevator and intermediate) considered in this chapter, the only effective sphincter available for subsequent fecal control is the levator ani and, in particular, the pubo-visceral sling, which intimately surrounds the urethra, cloacal canal or vagina caudal to all the rectal anomalies. The internal anal sphincter is absent, and the external sphincter is frequently represented only by superficial, sagittal strands of voluntary muscle, situated beneath the perineal skin and of little functional value.

In the operation "rectoplasty," common to all these rectal malformations, with or without fistulae, the rectum must be manipulated down to the perineum *within this undamaged sling*, if continence is to be preserved to the maximal extent.

The first decision is whether the rectoplasty should be performed in the newborn period in one stage or performed later as a staged procedure after initial colostomy. The second decision concerns the actual technique to be used.

One-Stage Rectoplasty Versus Colostomy and Delayed Rectoplasty

In all rectal dysplasias, except recto-vaginal and recto-cloacal fistula, the baby presents with intestinal obstruction in the neonatal period, and clearly some form of decompression is required. Since the application of rectoplasty for infants advocated by Rhoads, Piper and Randall (1948), the majority of surgeons have preferred a one-stage rectoplasty in the neonatal period, the principal papers being by Norris *et al.* (1949), Moore and Lawrence (1952), Butcher (1953), Gross (1953), Potts *et al.* (1954), Rhoads and Koop (1955), Palmer (1956), Thompson and Hooks (1956), Forshall (1957), Brayton and Norris (1958), Ravitch (1958), Louw (1959) (but not in 1965), Scott and Swenson (1959), Nixon (1961), Partridge and Gough (1961), Salzberg and Martin (1961), Snyder (1961), Solowiejczyk (1961), Swain and Tucker (1962), Trusler and Wilkinson (1962), Gans and Friedman (1963), Nicolai and Rehbein (1963), Sommerschild *et al.* (1964), Woolam (1964), Bielowicz (1965), Swenson and Donnelson (1967), Rehbein (1967) and Soave (1969).

As we support a staged program of preliminary colostomy and later rectoplasty at 12–15 months, we propose to set out the various arguments advanced in support of one-stage neonatal rectoplasty and the counter arguments.

ARGUMENTS TO SUPPORT ONE-STAGE NEONATAL RECTOPLASTY AND COUNTER ARGUMENTS.—These arguments are listed below.

(i) It is claimed that in the newborn period the dilated bowel is more easily freed, with minimal division of blood vessels and nerves, and greater preservation of sensation to the bowel (Scott and Swenson, 1959; Scott *et al.*, 1961; Partridge and Gough, 1961; Nixon, 1961; and Woolam, 1964). At an older age, the bladder moves from its abdominal position into the pelvis, the pelvis deepens, and the fistula becomes less accessible from above (Nixon, 1961). One of the principal reasons which stimulated Rhoads *et al.* (1948) to develop neonatal rectoplasty was the high morbidity and mortality rates attending the multiple procedures consequential to the perineal approach (overlooked fistulae, recurrence of fistulae, retraction of the rectum, stenosis, peritonitis and incontinence). The advantages of the abdomino-perineal approach over the perineal approach in completing the reconstruction in a single operation were immediately apparent.

The argument really rests on the functional results of neonatal rectoplasty compared to those obtained after delayed rectoplasty. Our results, with those of Trusler and Wilkinson (1962), Kiesewetter *et al.* (1964), Louw (1965), Kiesewetter (1966) and Cozzi and Wilkinson (1968), suggest that bowel control is better and mortality lower when rectal reconstruction is performed at a later time. We believe that the access is improved by the increased pelvic dimensions at a later age. Further, in the sacro-perineal route, proposed below, the fistula is defined from the posterior approach, and this access is also improved by pelvic growth. Lynn and Arcari (1962) also find the access easier, and Santulli *et al.* (1965), who previously advocated a neonatal reconstruction, now believe that the rectum can be more accurately sited through the pubo-rectalis sling at the later period. Louw (1965) now takes the same view, which contrasts with his preference, in 1959, for neonatal reconstruction.

(ii) The defunctioned sigmoid colon and rectum (after colostomy) is said to shrink, and at a secondary operation there may be difficulty in retaining an adequate blood supply after mobilization (Scott and Swenson, 1959; Scott *et al.* 1960; Nixon, 1961; and Partridge and Gough, 1961). Further, there may be adhesions from the original laparotomy, which add to the difficulties of bowel mobilization.

Apart from change of lumen because of the decompression, we have not observed any failure of development in the gut. Nonviability may occur in a delayed rectoplasty, although not in our experience, but this is a technical failure of inadequate mobilization reported in all series, including one-stage repairs.

At the original colostomy, we do not explore the lower left side of the abdomen, and the colostomy is made in the transverse colon, so that adhesion formation is not a barrier to subsequent mobilization. In addition, in our view, it is essential for proper postrectoplasty management to be conducted while the new anal canal is defunctioned by the colostomy.

(iii) The colostomy itself carries risks in the infant—serositis, stenosis, prolapse, retraction, fistulae, intestinal obstruction, skin excoriation, sucrose intolerance with diarrhoea, and infection (septicemia, meningitis, etc.).

The risks of colostomy in infants are well documented. MacMahon *et al.* (1961), for example, in 129 colostomies in 122 infants and children, found that 88 (66%) patients developed complications due to the colostomy, 3 (2.3%) of whom died. Cain and Kiesewetter (1965), in 120 infant colostomies found a 20% complication rate, 4 (3.3%) of whom died. Brenner and Swenson (1967) found technical complications in 16 of 70 colostomies in infants and children, and Cozzi and Wilkinson (1968) a similar complication rate. There is thus a definite morbidity and mortality risk related to colostomy, and this is a serious disadvantage of the staged program. Further, a third stage (namely, closure of the colostomy) is added to the program, and every hospital admission involves some risk of anesthesia, infection, etc., apart from the psychological and financial disadvantages. Several authors include colostomy complications among their reasons for choosing one-stage neonatal rectoplasty, Rhoads *et al.* (1948), Norris *et al.* (1949), Moore and Lawrence (1952), Thompson and Hooks (1956), Partridge and Gough (1961), Katzen (1962), Woolam (1964) and Swenson and Donnellan (1967).

We admit to complications arising from transverse colostomy, but we consider that the technique used (described subsequently) overcomes many of these hazards, and in the first year of life, the stoma is easily managed by the parents.

(iv) After colostomy, the persistence of a rectal fistula into the urinary tract may predispose to urinary infection, especially in rectovesical fistulae. Apart from the effects of infection on the upper urinary tract, calculi may form in the defunctioned colon, although not in our series, and hyperchloremic acidosis may develop from the absorption of urinary chlorides through the bowel mucosa (Poth, 1956; and Shepherd and Kiesewetter, 1966). These risks of infection influence several authors against colostomy (Butcher, 1953; Palmer, 1956; Nixon, 1961; Partridge and Gough, 1961; Sommerschild *et al.*, 1964; Bielowicz, 1965; and Swenson and Donnellan 1967). Urinary infection has certainly occurred in some of our infants whose colons have been defunctioned, but it can generally be avoided by careful cleansing of the distal limb of colon and by the treatment of associated urinary anomalies. Rarely is disconnection of the fistula necessary.

(v) In performing neonatal rectoplasty, the postoperative dilations are performed in a period which is less disturbing to the infant and parents than at a later time (Potts *et al.*, 1954; Nixon, 1961; Partridge and Gough, 1961; and Katzen, 1962). This is probably true; however, even in the staged program, dilations are mostly completed by the age of 18–21 months, and furthermore they cause minimal disturbance to the child if done by the parents.

(vi) The older infant is more likely to develop excoriated buttocks during bowel training than the neonate, leading to perianal sepsis and anal fistula (Partridge and Gough, 1961; and Katzen, 1962). However, neonates are not free of this complication either, and, in our experience, the excoriation is self-limiting, lasts about 4–6 weeks and is free from fissures and fistulae.

(vii) With neonatal reconstruction, the infant learns normal evacuation early (Potts *et al.*, 1954). However, the normal infant, although continent, is not ready for toilet training until 12–18 months of age and hence is not deprived of training by deferring rectoplasty till this age.

THE INDICATIONS FOR COLOSTOMY BY THOSE WHO GENERALLY FAVOR ONE-STAGE NEONATAL RECTOPLASTY.—Under certain conditions, all surgeons advise a preliminary colostomy. Those who normally advocate neonatal rectoplasty reserve colostomy for the following situations:

(i) In premature infants or those under 4½ lb.
(ii) In the presence of other life-threatening anomalies, e.g., tracheo-esophageal fistula and in seriously ill infants
(iii) When there is gross distention of the abdomen with embarrassment to respiration

Following such a colostomy, most of those surgeons choose to hasten fairly quickly to the subsequent rectoplasty, e.g., Nixon (1961), at 3 months; Snyder (1961), from 10 days to 6 months, depending on physical state, and Gans and Friedman (1963), at 3–6 months.

PRELIMINARY COLOSTOMY AND RECTOPLASTY AT 12–15 MONTHS.—Authors in favor of neonatal colostomy and a later rectoplasty are Bacon and Sherman (1952), Stephens (1953), Bradham (1961), Katzen (1962), Lynn and Arcari (1962), Kiesewetter *et al.* (1964), Lloyd (1964), Louw (1965), Santulli *et al.* (1965), Sauvage and Bill (1965) and Kiesewetter (1966 and 1967).

We favor this policy for the following reasons:

(i) The principal consideration is to choose a technique which most effectively preserves the vital pubo-rectalis sling. The objective of one-stage rectoplasty is to permit the unimpeded passage of feces immediately. To achieve this, a functional rectal canal must be constructed of adequate size and must be dilated immediately; this entails rushed or immediate dilation of the pubo-rectalis sling. We believe that the delicate pubo-rectalis, so intimately bound to the urethra or vagina, must be first tunneled to a dimension only large enough to admit the collapsed and defunctional bowel, and the tunnel subsequently dilated through the anus *slowly* and *gently* over several months, thus obviating damage by laceration and overstretching of its fibers (Fig. 111). Preliminary colostomy permits such gentle, unrushed dilatation of the pubo-rectalis sling. It is for this reason also that we favor preliminary colostomy, even for a non-

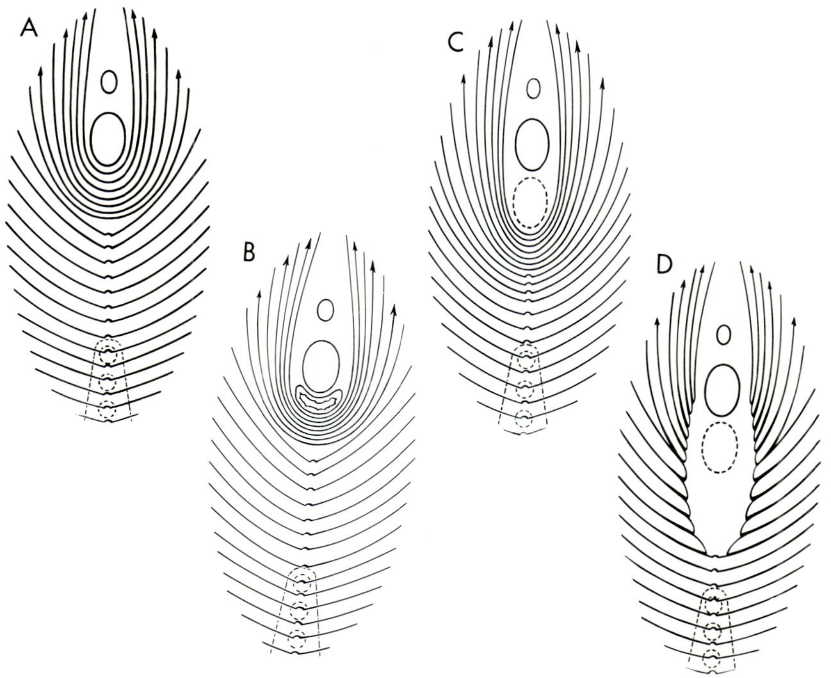

Fig. 111.—Diagrammatic representation of the methods of tunneling the pubo-rectalis sling in reconstruction of the anal canal—recto-vaginal fistula. **A,** pubo-rectalis fibers embracing the urethra and vagina. **B,** posterior retraction of the sling sufficient only to "squeeze" the rectum through the tunnel. **C,** (correct), the sling unharmed after gentle dilatation subsequent to operation. **D,** (wrong), overstretching of the pubo-rectalis at operation, to provide comfortable accommodation of the rectum, harms the sling.

urgent rectal anomaly such as low recto-vaginal fistula, rather than one-stage rectoplasty at whatever age. Prior to closure of the colostomy, the surgeon can predict, with reasonable accuracy, the future status of continence in many children who have undergone rectoplasty, by the contractility of the pubo-rectalis sling detected by his finger when he assesses the adequacy of dilatation. This accent on the pubo-rectalis is not to imply that other surgeons have not appreciated its vital importance or that it is not now preserved in modern techniques of one-stage rectoplasty. Nevertheless, it is a remarkable fact that in operative descriptions from 1948 to 1960 this portion of the levator ani muscle, or indeed any of the muscle, received scant, if any, mention, and all stress was laid upon the "external sphincter." This is all the more remarkable when it is realized that, even with all the disadvantages of perineal exploration for high anomalies performed up until 1949, the surgeons of this cut-and-thrust era constantly stressed the reconstruction of the levator after its division in these extensive explorations (Dieffenbach, 1826; Rizzoli, 1874; Matas, 1897; Brenner, 1915; Stone, 1936; Crowell and Dulin, 1940; and Harken, 1942). Denis Browne (1951 and 1955) and Stephens (1953) emphasized its importance as did Scott and Swenson (1959). Since 1960, most surgeons have accepted its essential role (Lawler, 1961; Snyder, 1961; Swenson and Grana, 1962; Gans and Friedman, 1963; Nicolai and Rehbein, 1963; Lloyd, 1964; Kiesewetter *et al.*, 1964, 1966 and 1967; Woolam, 1964; Edwards and Phillip, 1965; Hanley, 1965; Louw, 1965; Santulli *et al.*, 1965; Sauvage and Bill, 1965; Swenson and Donnellan, 1967; and Cozzi and Wilkinson, 1968).

(ii) The larger pelvic dimensions in the older infant make the rectoplasty technically easier, thus ensuring more careful localization of the pathway inside the pubo-rectalis sling, a point of view now shared by Santulli *et al.* (1965). Other technical advantages are that operation is performed in a clean field, healing of the mucocutaneous suture line occurs without infection (and subsequent stenosis), and the surgery can be performed under planned elective conditions rather than as a neonatal emergency at the end of a rigorous and perhaps incomplete investigational program, after hasty decisions, and at times when staff and other facilities may not be so readily available. We, therefore, perform transverse colostomy soon after birth for all infants, of either sex, in whom a rectal malformation calls for an eventual rectoplasty, and certainly advise all surgeons who meet the emergency only rarely and any who are unsure of the diagnosis and proper management to do likewise.

(iii) Colostomy provides "time" for a proper assessment of the sphincteric integrity and nerve supply. A sacral agenesis may be apparent on the plain radiograph, but only careful clinical assessment of urinary control, combined with micturition cystourethrography, defines the presence or absence of sacral innervation to the bladder and, in consequence, to the levator ani. Rectoplasty through a denervated sphincter with consequent certain incontinence is therefore avoided. Marked bulging of the perineum in the newborn may suggest pelvic floor paralysis (Gross, 1959) but a neurogenic bladder, and lesser degrees of sphincteric weakness, may be present without such bulging.

(iv) Postcolostomy colography using air or Gastrografin permits accurate diagnosis of the type and site of fistula, from which information the sphincter anatomy can be predicted. This aids in planning the surgical approach to a rectal malformation and it avoids the mistake of subjecting a child to a complicated rectoplasty when, in fact, the deformity is of the anal type. The original inverted radiograph has occasionally been misleading because of pubo-rectalis contraction, which obliterates the most distal part of the lumen, or because the gas has not reached the end of the bowel or has escaped through the fistula or more rarely because meconium is not dislodged by the gas. On the other hand, performance of a colostomy by a surgeon who is in doubt as to the exact abnormality is a far safer policy than is his attempting reparative surgery of any kind, even if subsequently the colostomy is found to have been unnecessary.

Some surgeons, Rhoads and Koop (1955), Brayton and Norris (1958) and Rehbein (1967), feel that one advantage of the one-stage abdomino-perineal operation is that it is not necessary to identify the type of fistula in type 3 (Ladd and Gross) anomalies, as it will be found more positively at the time of operation. Provided the defect lies high in the pelvis, this view is justified, but if it lies nearer the perineum, as in anal agenesis or recto-bulbar fistula, a needlessly complicated abdomino-perineal operation would be performed.

For these several reasons we favor a preliminary colostomy and staged rectoplasty at 12–15 months for all rectal deformities, including low recto-vaginal fistulae and, in addition, for anal agenesis and recto-bulbar fistula. To this list, Santulli *et al.* (1965) would now add ano-vestibular fistula, although we approach this from the sacroperineum. For special reasons where expedience is indicated (e.g., urinary infection), we are prepared to perform the rectoplasty earlier, especially in view of the satisfactory results obtained by Louw (1965).

Other surgeons who also utilize a staged program choose to do the rectoplasty as follows: Bacon and Sherman (1952), at 3–5 years; Palmer (1956), at 1–4 years (except for urinary fistulae in which he performs neonatal rectoplasty, because of the risk of urinary infection); Bradham (1961), at 12–18 months; Katzen (1964), at 10–12 lb. weight; Louw (1965), at 3 months; Lynn and Arcari (1962), at 25 lb. weight or more; Lloyd (1964), at 12–15 months; Santulli *et al.* (1965), at 9–12 months; Sauvage and Bill (1965), at 12 months; and Kiesewetter (1966), at 6 months.

Management Before Colostomy (Newborn)

1. Preliminary Investigations.—Reference should be made to the individual lesions discussed in Chapters 3 and 4 and to Diagnosis and Investigations, Chapter 8, from which the maximal information about the internal anatomy should be obtained. These investigations are summarized as follows:

(a) Careful inspection of the perineum, especially in females, by clinical examination, probe or scope of all orifices for a telltale speck of meconium or for visible or audible bubbles of gas escaping from an orifice of the upturned baby to be certain that the bowel communicates with the exterior. This may necessitate surgical division of a "covered vulva" and further inspection of the laid-open introitus. The perineal appearances should be recorded by sketch or photography prior to or at the time of the first general anesthesia.

(b) The urine is examined for meconium, gas or epithelial cells, if necessary by insertion of a catheter or by suprapubic puncture.

(c) Documentation of other malformations, including results of the passage of a naso-gastric tube down the esophagus when checking for an accompanying tracheo-esophageal fistula.

(d) At least two lateral radiographs in the inverted position, repeated if necessary in 4–6 hours if it is suspected that the true termination of the bowel is obscured by muscular compression, or lack of gaseous distention. In at least one lateral radiograph, a radiopaque urethral catheter should be in position and radiopaque paste applied in the natal cleft to define the anal site.

(e) An anteroposterior radiograph to indicate the presence of vertebral, especially sacral, anomalies.

(f) Micturition cystourethrography.

(g) Fistulography.

(h) Clinical assessment of the sacral nerve supply. If there is unequivocal evidence of a totally neurogenic state (e.g., a bulging perineum, expressible bladder and perineal anesthesia in the presence of severe sacral agenesis or myelomeningocele), a permanent colostomy may be planned, in which case left iliac colostomy using the terminal colon or rectum is preferable, at a site suitable for the wearing of an appliance. If the sacral nerve supply appears normal or is equivocal, a transverse colostomy is planned so that it does not impair mobilization of the colon in the neighborhood of the rectal malformation at subsequent rectoplasty.

2. Preoperative Preparation.—The usual steps prior to any neonatal operation are instituted, and are summarized without discussion.

(a) Recording of weight

(b) Isolette nursing at controlled temperature, humidity and oxygen concentration

(c) Aspiration through indwelling naso-gastric catheter, after investigations completed

(d) Vitamin K

(e) Blood cross-matched and ready; intravenous infusion commenced

(f) Antibiotics

(g) Prevention of heat loss prior to and during operation.

Colostomy Technique

Several points are stressed and illustrated in Figure 112.

(i) We prefer a short upper left paramedian incision and approach the peritoneum via a rectus muscle split, leaving only a 0.5-cm. strip

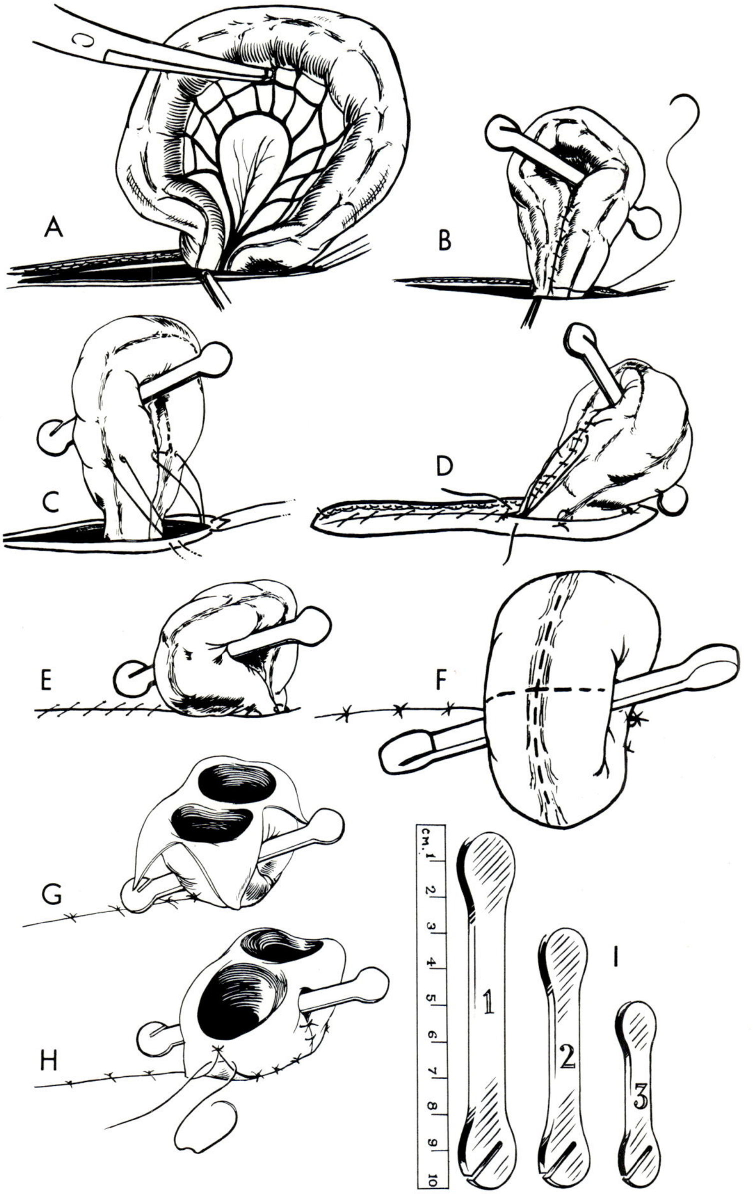

Fig. 112.—Defunctioning colostomy. *A–H,* five steps in the technique. **A,** selection of window for colostomy rod protecting arterial arcades. **B,** creation of a spur external to abdominal skin. **C** and **D,** fixing of limbs of colostomy to peritoneum by four equally spaced sutures 1.0 cm. apart. **E,** colostomy rod lies free and away from skin level. **F, G** and **H,** cruciate incision of antimesenteric wall of colon and anastomosis of mucosa to skin. **I,** home-made Perspex colostomy rods. Three sizes for use in children, infants and neonates, and premature babies, respectively. Note the cut in one end which permits ready snap and easy removal of the rod.

of muscle medially. It is easier to disconnect the colostomy later through this incision, with clean restoration of both layers of the rectus sheath, than through one involving transverse section of the rectus muscle, as advocated by Louw (1965).

(ii) The two limbs of the colostomy are arched over a colostomy rod, which separates the two stomas (Fig. 112, *B*). One of us (E. D. S.) prefers to suture the skin between the limbs of the colostomy in addition to using the colostomy rod. A colostomy planned for 12 months or more is semipermanent, and in order to minimize infection and stenosis the everted mucosal edges of the colon are sutured to the skin edges of the incision.

(iii) It is important to prevent spillover of feces into the distal limb (which contributes to urinary infection through the fistula); to do this, the adjacent edges of the two limbs are sutured together for approximately 1.5 cm. The limbs of the colostomy are sutured to the peritoneum at such points as will ensure that the spur protrudes well beyond the skin level. The colostomy rod is passed through a window in the mesocolon between the marginal vessel and the bowel wall in the loop at the end of the spur. This technique produces two pouting orifices tilted on the spur which minimizes spillover and allows function as an end colostomy. The method of suturing and the narrow caliber of the stoma reduce the risk of prolapse. To achieve the same end, other surgeons divide the colon completely (Mayo and Rice, 1950; Bradham, 1961; Kiesewetter *et al.*, 1964; and Louw, 1965) with a 1–2 cm. skin bridge between the stomata.

(iv) Except when a permanent colostomy is planned (see above), in which case the site should be left iliac, we prefer a midtransverse colostomy to allow the left colon to be adequately mobilized at subsequent rectoplasty. We are, therefore, not in favor of a sigmoid colostomy, and we do not favor closing over the distal end and replacing it in the peritoneal cavity (Santulli 1965), because it prevents adequate cleansing of the colon and rectum and any subsequent colographic studies.

(v) If the general condition of the infant permits, a limited inspection of the abdominal viscera for other associated anomalies should be made, but no exploration is made in the area of the left lower colon and rectum other than to assess the length of the sigmoid colon, so that adhesions may not be encouraged.

(vi) Again, if the general condition permits, a start should be made on the operating table to evacuate both limbs of the colon of meconium by washouts with normal saline, using a 20-cc. syringe and a soft rubber catheter. It is worth spending an extra 15 minutes or more irrigating the meconium away. If a fistula is present, thorough cleansing over the next 2 weeks is vital in preventing urinary infection.

Postcolostomy Management

1. Immediate.—As in preoperative preparation, these steps are common to any neonatal operation and are summarized without discussion.

(a) Isolette nursing at controlled temperature, humidity and oxygen concentration

(b) Naso-gastric aspiration of the stomach until evidence of bowel activity

(c) Intravenous fluids until fluids tolerated by mouth

(d) Colostomy dressings

(e) Estimation of serum electrolytes

Of special concern, however, is the continued clearance of the distal limb of the colostomy, not only to prevent the formation of rock-hard meconioliths but also to prevent urinary infection via a urethral or vesical fistula, if present. This limb is washed out daily from the 3d to the 14th day, with saline through a soft rubber catheter. Before the baby's discharge, the segment of bowel should be checked radiographically with radiopaque medium (not barium) for filling defects of meconium masses in the iodide column, and if the lumen is not clear, further washouts are required (Fig. 113).

2. Later.—In the following 2–3 months, a series of investigations is carried out to determine the following features:

(i) Assessment of the exact visceral anatomy by (*a*) micturition cystourethrogram, (*b*) Urografin or Gastrografin cologram through the distal stoma of the colostomy and (*c*) endoscopy of bladder, urethra and vagina.

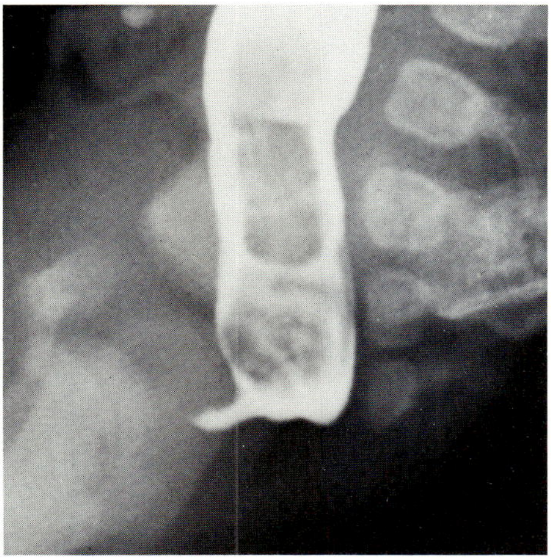

Fig. 113.—Cologram to demonstrate inadequate clearance of colon and rectum. Meconium concretions appear as filling defects in the column of contrast medium.

(ii) Assessment of the urinary tract by (*a*) the above tests, (*b*) intravenous pyelography and ureterograms if necessary and (*c*) renal function tests—renograms, and chemical tests as indicated.

(iii) Assessment of other anomalies, e.g., cardiac anomalies.

(iv) Assessment of nerve supply of the potential sphincters because a paralytic sphincter would indicate a change in plan and the need for a permanent iliac colostomy.

These essential clinical and investigational details for each malformation are discussed in Chapters 3 and 4 and Diagnosis and Investigations in Chapter 8. The management of urinary anomalies is described in Chapter 12.

Techniques of Rectoplasty

To fulfill the requirements of a satisfactory rectal reconstruction designed to achieve maximal continence, the following objectives are suggested:

1. The mobilized rectum should lie precisely within the entire pubo-rectalis sling.
2. The sling muscle must be undamaged by the operative technique and by the subsequent dilatations.
3. There should be minimal interference with the pelvic nerve supply of the bowel and bladder.
4. The anus must be supple and adequate in size, free of stenosis and redundancy of mucosa and appropriately sited for hygienic cleansing.
5. The operative morbidity rate should be low.

Opinions differ as to how these criteria can best be met. The following section discusses the available methods (apart from perineal rectoplasty), the detailed techniques of each and their advantages and disadvantages.

A. Perineal rectoplasty.

B. Abdomino-perineal "pull-through" (Rhoads *et al.*, 1948) or its subsequent modifications.

C. Abdomino-perineal rectoplasty through a buttock-reflecting incision (Sauvage and Bill, 1965).

D. Submucosal resection and abdomino-perineal or abdomino-sacro-perineal rectoplasty (Rehbein, 1959, 1965 and 1967).

E. Sacro-perineal rectoplasty (without abdominal exploration) or sacro-abdomino-perineal rectoplasty (with abdominal exploration) (Stephens, 1953 and 1963).

F. Sacro-abdomino-perineal rectoplasty (combined sacro-perineal approach with Rehbein procedure) (Kiesewetter, 1966 and 1967).

A. Perineal Rectoplasty

Historically, the approach from the perineum was the established procedure until 1948. We have reviewed the progress of the numerous modifications in technique in Chapter 1. Since the advent of abdomino-perineal reconstruction, almost every surgical group has pointed out the serious deficiencies in the perineal route to high anomalies.

The papers by early surgeons reported the disadvantages (Matas, 1887; Brenner, 1915; Berman, 1938; Crowell and Dulin, 1940; and Lee, 1944), as also the papers in the first few years after the advent of Rhoads' operation in 1948 (Norris *et al.*, 1949; Mayo and Rice, 1950; Bacon and Sherman, 1952; Moore and Lawrence, 1952; Winkel Smith, 1953; Gross, 1953; Butcher, 1953; Thompson and Hooks, 1956; and Brayton and Norris, 1958). The technique will not therefore be described.

The serious disadvantages are as follow:

(i) The special sleevelike disposition of the pubo-rectalis, so intimately related to the urethra or vagina, prevents access to the fistula and rectum without harm to the sling. *The space available in the perineum provides no reasonable access to mobilize the rectum unless the sling is divided or stretched markedly*—both of which lead to irreparable damage to its sphincteric action and incontinence (Fig. 114, *C*).

(ii) The inadequate access frequently resulted in not locating a urethral or vagina fistula and consequent multiple operations subsequently in search of it. The morbidity and mortality rates from multiple procedues were high.

(iii) Incomplete mobilization of the rectum (because of the difficulties mentioned above) causes retraction of the mucosa, with consequent infection, dense scarring into the pelvis, recurrence of fistulae to urethra or vagina and secondary megacolon. Subsequent procedures to close such fistulae or repeat the rectoplasty through dense scar have proved extraordinarily difficult. Our most difficult cases have been those presenting after efforts "to reach the rectum" in the course of a perineal reconstruction.

(iv) The inadequate access to the fistula and rectum deep in the wound may result in damage to the bladder neck and urethral sphincters. Victims of such accidents have presented to us with urinary incontinence.

(v) Forcible dilatation through the scarred pelvis has resulted in a fistula into the bladder neck in one patient referred to us.

Although almost everyone has abandoned the perineal approach for rectal anomalies, mention should be made that both Potts *et al.*

(1954) and Snyder (1961) advocated a perineal transplantation operation for high recto-vaginal fistula. Furthermore, Solowiejczyk (1961) suggests that with a high gas shadow, it is reasonable to commence with a perineal dissection for 1 cm., but if bowel is not encountered, an abdomino-perineal rectoplasty or colostomy should be done. He stresses that this is, in no sense, a perineal exploration.

Gans *et al.* (1963), in cases of recto-urethral fistula, go farther. Because they fear nerve damage in the abdominal approach, "in questionable cases a reasonably extensive attempt should be made to transplant the urethral ectopic anus via the perineal approach, but that this should be abandoned and approached abdominally if it becomes evident that satisfactory mobilisation cannot be accomplished from below alone." For reasons stated above, particularly the fact that any attempted mobilization from below must first dislocate the pubo-rectalis, we cannot agree with this suggestion; later, in the same paper, Gans and his associates indicate that the dissection must be very delicate, strictly in the midline, and in front of the pubo-rectalis sling.

B. Abdomino-Perineal Pull-Through

The early history of the abdominal route as a two-stage procedure is described in Chapter 1.

Norris in 1943 and Rhoads in 1944 first reported the one-stage operation of abdomino-perineal rectoplasty in neonates, and Gross reported the same operation as a secondary procedure in 1944. Potts *et al.* (1954) recorded performing the operation in 1947.

The first description of this operation was published by Rhoads, Pipes and Randall in 1948, in 2 patients, and a few months later by Norris, Brophy and Brayton in 1949 on 4 patients. It has been the adopted operation for high anomalies by most surgeons. Many surgeons have added minor modifications and in a recent authoritative textbook on pediatric surgery, Santulli (1969) describes a procedure which is representative of several techniques available (see footnote).

The principal points in Santulli's technique are as follow*:

> In selected cases we have divided the rectourethral fistula (or high rectovaginal or rectocloacal in females) at the first operation in the newborn period and brought out the bowel at this level as an end colostomy. This procedure has several advantages, including early division of the urinary fistula, a single colostomy stoma, and preservation of the entire available bowel for the later pull-through procedure. The pelvic adhesions and scarring that may follow this more extensive operation have not created undue difficulties in the subsequent abdominoperineal operation.

---

*Reprinted with permission from Mustard, W. T., *et al.* (eds.): *Pediatric Surgery* (2d ed.; Chicago: Year Book Medical Publishers, Inc., 1969), p. 1000.

For the *abdominoperineal repair* the infant is placed supine at the end of the operating table with the thighs partly flexed and abducted to allow for the combined abdominoperineal approach. A number 8 or 10 F. urethral Foley-type rubber catheter is passed into the bladder. In those cases in which it is impossible to insert a urethral catheter because of a stricture, or where the catheter repeatedly enters the bowel through the fistula, a suprapubic cystostomy is done at the beginning of the abdominal procedure. A catheter is then passed from inside the bladder outward through the urethra. Some surgeons prefer to leave a suprapubic tube in the bladder for post-operative drainage.

The precise location of the external anal sphincter muscle is ascertained with the help of the electrical Faradic muscle stimulator. By this means one can be sure of placing the perineal incision directly over the sphincter muscle. A 1.0 to 1.5 cm. cruciate incision is made in the skin and the wound deepened through the subcutaneous layer to the level of the external sphincter. Skin flaps are sharply dissected with care to avoid making them too thin. The underlying sphincter is then gently dilated in a ventral and cephalad direction until the resultant opening will admit a size 10 Hegar dilator or 32 F. rubber catheter.

The abdomen is entered through a left lower oblique or a lower midline incision. The sigmoid colon and rectum are mobilized by dividing their peritoneal attachments, and both ureters are identified. The tissues behind the superior hemorrhoidal vessels are divided and the dissection is carried downwards, first posteriorly, then laterally, and finally anteriorly. Retraction of the rectum backward and the bladder upward aids in the anterior dissection. Care must be taken to avoid injury to the small vasa deferentia which arch anteriorly over the rectum at the level of the bladder neck. By staying close to the rectum posteriorly and following the direction of its curve ventrally as it tapers to meet the urethra it is possible to avoid disturbing the levator ani musculature and to visualize the puborectalis sling. Here again, the Faradic stimulator is useful in precisely locating these muscle fibers.

The communication to the urethra, if present, is usually just below the bladder at the level of the prostate gland. It is important to avoid tenting the urethra at this point. As the fistula (bowel) is divided several millimeters from the urethra, the distal (urethral) end is closed with interrupted sutures of fine chromic catgut. The bowel end is closed with heavy silk sutures. which will later be used to pull the bowel through the puborectalis sling and perineal incision. Usually 2 to 3 sutures are needed on the urethral side of the fistula. As the fistula is completely divided, the closed urethral end will retract down beneath the bladder.

The puborectalis sling is now easily identified. A suture of 4–0 silk is placed through each side of the sling and left long. These are later sutured to the serosa of the pulled-through segment of colon at the end of the procedure just prior to closing the abdomen. In this way the bowel is fixed to the levator.

A curved clamp is inserted through the perineal wound, directing it cephaled and ventrally just behind the urethra. Under direct vision from above, it is carefully passed through the previously identified puborectalis sling. Following this, the sling is gently stretched from below with well-lubricated Hegar dilators progressing through size 10 or 11. The bowel is then pulled through (anterior to) the sling and into the perineal wound.

In some cases the mesentery may be too short to permit the rectum to reach the perineum. It may be necessary to divide the superior hemorrhoidal vessels, being careful to preserve adequate arcades for blood supply distally. Rarely, one may have to discard the rectum and rectosigmoid, take down the proximal colostomy, and by dividing the inferior mesenteric vessels, pull through the proximal sigmoid or descending colon.

The perineal part of the procedure is then completed by suturing the full thickness of the bowel wall to the edges of the four skin flaps within the external anal sphincter muscle. The mucocutaneous line should turn upward to avoid prolapse and to have the skin supply sensation to the newly created anal canal.

Comment.—1. The principal objection we have to the abdomino-perineal procedure, as described by many writers before Santulli's revised edition (1969), and that of Swenson and Donnellan (1967), is the serious omission of defining precisely the route to the perineum anterior to the vital pubo-visceral sling. In many descriptions, the site is referred to only as "between the levator ani muscles." In many earlier papers, it is clear that the rectum was, in fact, brought down *posterior* to the sling through the diaphragm portion of the levator, the erroneous concept being held that it was the "external sphincter" that was important for continence (Fig. 114).

Fig. 114.—Operative *mistreatment* of the levator diaphragm. **A** and **B,** the new rectum is wrongly routed to the perineum through the levator diaphragm behind the pubo-rectalis sling. **A′** and **B′,** damage to pubo-rectalis and levator diaphragm **C,** perineal approach to the pubo-rectalis tunnel damages important fibers. **C′,** the tunnel is found with least damage if approached from the cranial aspect. (*C* and *B* and *A′* and *B′* reproduced with permission from Australian Paediat. J. 1:107, 1965.)

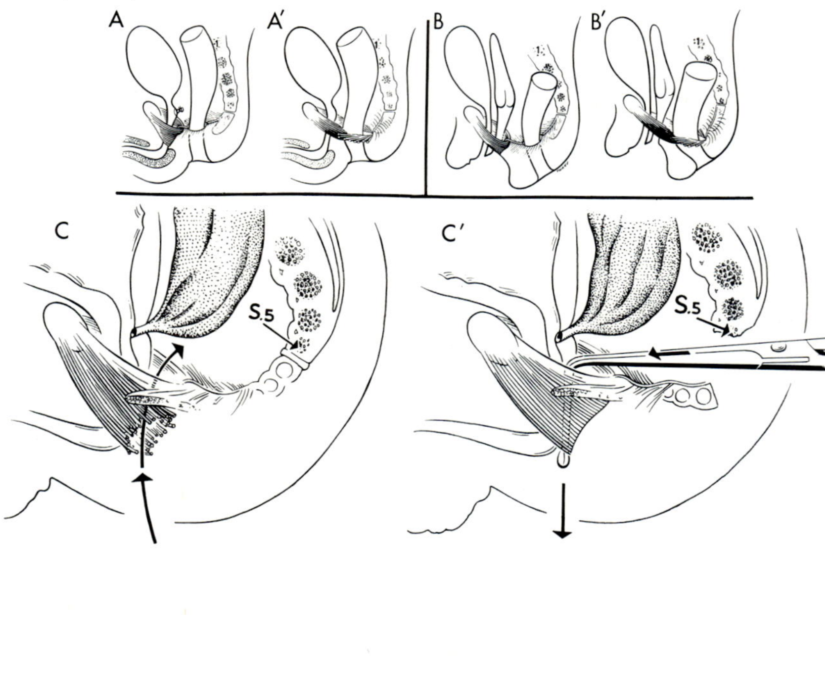

Protagonists of the abdominal route maintain that a good view can be had of the fistula and therefore of the plane of the pubo-rectalis muscle. However, we have found that the problem is not visualization of the fistula, but that from above, it is impossible to see the muscle in its site intimately surrounding the urethra or vagina. Even with a catheter or metal sound in the urethra there is, in our experience, a certain vagueness about the precise midline point hard up against the urethra, as it is obscured in the angle of access to it. As has Kiesewetter (1964), we have re-explored patients incontinent after an abdomino-perineal rectoplasty confidently performed by surgeons with a familiarity with the pubo-rectalis and have found the rectum lying either behind the sling or more eccentrically sited through a torn lateral or posterior edge of the muscle.

Nixon (1961), in describing his technique of abdomino-perineal rectoplasty, correctly stresses the position and importance of the pubo-rectalis and states, "The track is then made by blunt dissection in the hollow of the sacrum in the midline so as to avoid damage to the pelvic plexuses. The instrument is then brought forward so as to dissect through the levator floor just behind the urethra. A sound in the urethra assists in finding the right place."

Swenson and Donnellan (1967) also strongly criticize the original Rhoads operation in an article specifically stressing the vital role of the pubo-rectalis in the repair. In their technique, the muscle is defined principally from below, joined then by the abdominal operator.

Rehbein (1967) has also given a new description of his earlier procedure (to be described later) because of the danger of missing the pubo-rectalis. He now attempts to palpate the levator with a finger above and below to define the plane. Figure 115 depicts the maneuver. Again, however, we cannot feel convinced; compare Rehbein's diagrams with our dissections, and, in fact, there is no convenient hole or deficiency behind the urethra as shown in Rehbein's illustrations for the identification of the anterior border of the pubo-rectalis. The muscle actually fits snugly up against the urethra and fistula (see Fig. 15).

It is our contention that the entrance to the tunnel can never be seen by any approach, even our own sacro-perineal one, nor can it be palpated; only gentle blunt probing with a right-angled clamp can actually open into the minute plane in front of the muscle hard up against the urethra or vagina. It is the virtue of the sacral route that it enables a plane of dissection horizontally on the levator itself and then provides an access in the right direction for the clamp to nudge its way into the tunnel. Kiesewetter and Turner (1963) and Louw (1965) have reported the improved access from the sacral route.

The definition of the pubo-rectalis sling is the principal advantage of the sacro-coccygeal exposure. Apart from this point, which is a

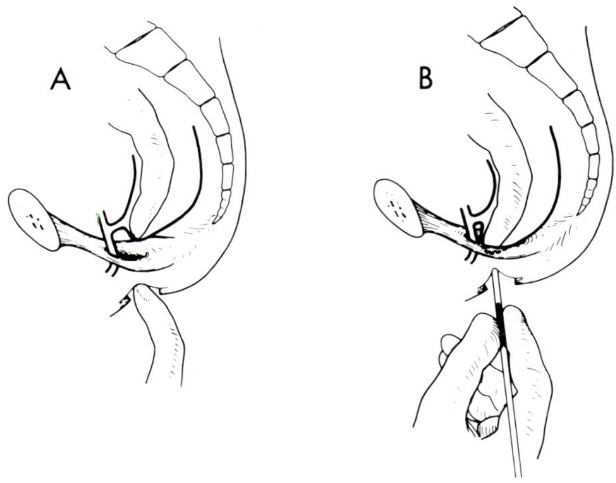

Fig. 115.—Rehbein's abdomino-perineal procedure. The mucosa of the transected blind pouch of rectum is shelled out; the colon is then brought down to the perineum through the denuded sleeve of rectal pouch. The pubo-rectalis sling is tunneled after "bidigital palpation" as indicated in **A** and **B.** (Reproduced with permission from Rehbein, F.: J. Pediat. Surg. 2:99, 1967.)

vital one, we have little disagreement with the other aspects of technique described; indeed, we frequently require an abdominal exposure in addition to the sacro-coccygeal one in order to gain the necessary mobility of bowel. This decision is made preoperatively on the radiographic evidence of the level of the patent bowel relative to the P/C line.

We cannot agree with Trusler and Wilkinson (1962) when they state that although an attempt is made to preserve the pubo-rectalis it is "unlikely that this is possible to any major extent"; however, they state that the functional results are probably better if the rectum is brought through *anteriorly*. In our view, this is the only plane which is acceptable.

2. Comment has been made in other sections that undue stress on the external sphincter is not warranted by its anatomy. This conforms with the observations made in dissections of the rectal malformations (Stephens, 1953). Trusler and Wilkinson (1962) were not impressed by its appearance at operation and stated that it is not technically easy to preserve. Swenson and Donnellan (1967) also believe that the external sphincter has been overemphasized and deliberately place the new anus slightly forward of the normal site to avoid angulated tension on the pubo-rectalis.

3. Excision of an ellipse of skin, or simple vertical incision, in the perineum is more likely to produce stenosis. We prefer not to excise

skin but to turn in at least an anterior flap of skin (and sometimes a posterior flap), as the rectal wall is usually shorter on its anterior than its posterior aspect. It is possible, also, that a skin-lined anal canal may provide some degree of sensation to aid in rectal training (Hiatt and Santulli, 1962; Nixon and Callaghan, 1964; and Kiesewetter, 1966). Turning in of skin flaps also reduces the degree of mucosal ectropion, which is a source of irritating mucus staining.

4. To dilate the tunnel "to admit the surgeon's index finger" we believe overstretches and damages many of the delicate pubo-rectalis fibers; rather, the smallest tunnel possible should be made, and the terminal bowel should be so fashioned as to present a pointed "leader" end that readily follows the pull of the guy sutures along the tunnel. Postoperatively, the tunnel is then gently and progressively dilated for a month or more, a procedure the gradualness of which is made possible by the presence of a colostomy. As far back as 1953, Winkel Smith stressed that "dilatation must be gentle or else the delicate fibres may possibly be ruptured."

5. We do not always suture the urethral side of the fistula (as also Gross, 1953) and do not do a suprapubic cystostomy. A metal sound is better than a catheter in the urethra, to define it during the dissection, and it makes tenting of the urethra less likely when the fistula is being divided. A Hegar dilator is used in the vagina in female repairs.

6. Scott's dissections (Scott and Swenson, 1959) indicate the need to keep the dissection as far posterior as possible on the sacrum, except at the pelvic floor at the site of the pubo-rectalis anteriorly, to avoid damage to the nerve supply to the bladder. His dissections showed that in rectal agenesis, the pelvic plexus and nerves were seen to be grouped in the midline around and below the fistula, so that the fistula should be cleared as close to its wall as possible, or better, as in our technique, approached through the posterior wall of the rectum.

The point that we stress is the relevance of the relation of the rectal pouch to the P/C line, as seen in the invertograms. If the pouch is above the P/C line the nervi erigentes run to the midline below the rectum, and it is imperative that no dissection of pouch or fistula should be done from the sacro-coccygeal route, because such dissection may disrupt the nerves. The dissection posteriorly is confined only to definition of the pubo-rectalis which is below the peritoneal reflection to which the nerves keep close (see Fig. 5). The fistula is approached only from the abdominal exposure. For the same reason we believe the nerves are at a greater risk in endeavoring to locate the pubo-rectalis muscle tunnel from the abdominal route, which perforce must involve a midline dissection through the peritoneal reflection. On the other hand, if the rectal pouch is on or below the P/C line, the nerves are displaced laterally to either side by the rectum.

Dissection of the fistula can thus be safely performed from the sacral route.

7. As it is possible that every centimeter of rectum retained may contribute to rectal sensation and so improve continence, Scott and Swenson (1959), Kiesewetter and Turner (1963) and Kiesewetter (1966) state that only the smallest portion of rectum should be sacrificed. However, we believe that the major source of the sensory receptors is in the pelvic floor muscles, and we do not hesitate to remove the rectum if it is large and hypertrophic.

ABDOMINO-PERINEAL RECTOPLASTY OF SWENSON AND DONNELLAN (1967).—Bearing in mind the foregoing comments we now reproduce in full the operative technique (for recto-urethral fistula) of Swenson and Donnellan*, as representing the best example of the abdomino-perineal approach, with an appreciation of the importance of the pubo-rectalis muscle.

With the legs suspended at 60 degrees by adhesive strapping, the abdomen, genitalia, and perineum are prepared as a single field. Sterile drapes are then applied to isolate the perineum, and a left paramedian muscle-retracting incision is made from just above the umbilicus to the pubis. Better exposure is achieved by angling the incision somewhat medially as it descends. After the peritoneum has been opened, the rectosigmoid is delivered into the wound. In most cases it is very dilated by gas and meconium. It should be aspirated by means of a small trocar which is inserted through a purse-string suture. Unless this is done, the tense distal colon is very likely to perforate during the subsequent manipulations. When the large bowel has been adequately decompressed in this manner, the small bowel is examined and both kidneys are palpated for other possible anomalies.

The sigmoid is drawn medially and its lateral attachments are incised well up along the rectosigmoid. As the sigmoid is freed laterally, the left ureter and spermatic vessels are identified and preserved. The colon is next drawn to the left, and the superior leaf of the rectosigmoid mesentery is incised down to the pouch of Douglas. This incision is carried anterior to the rectum to join the previous lateral peritoneal incision at the junction of the sigmoid colon and rectum. The vas deferens must be identified and preserved at this stage of the operation [Fig. 116, *A*].

It is very important to carry out all manipulations of the bowel with great gentleness, since the intestinal blood supply is always precarious, and peculiarly vulnerable to spasm in newborn infants. This factor may lead to persistent ischemia when the rectum is led down to the perineum.

The rectum, with its blood supply, is freed from the pelvic tissues by sharp dissection. The separation is easy posteriorly in the avascular pre-sacral space, but is more difficult laterally and anteriorly. As the bladder and upper part of the prostate are dissected free, the rectum will be seen to narrow and curve forward to enter the lower substance of the prostate or the urethra, which is identified by the firm Foley catheter within it. The rectourethral fis-

*Reprinted with permission from Swenson, O., and Donnellan, W. L.: S. Clin. North America 47:173, 1967.

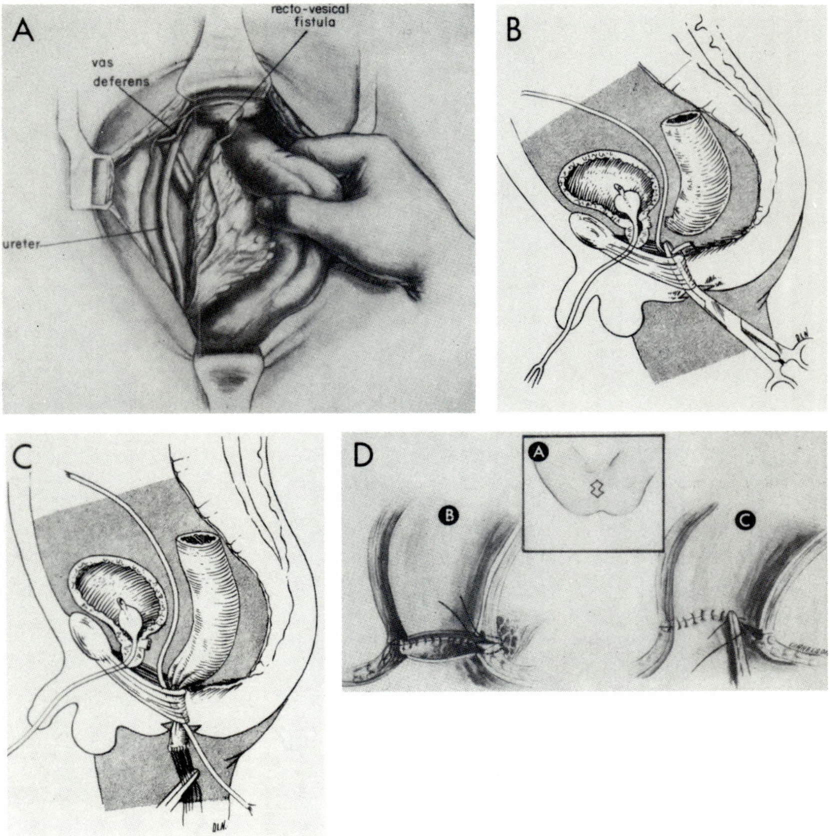

Fig. 116.—Steps in abdomino-perineal operation described by Swenson and Donnellan (1967). **A,** the recto-urethral fistula is detached. **B,** the pubo-rectalis sling is tunneled from the abdominal and perineal aspects. **C,** The rectum is guided to the perineum through the sling and, **D,** sutured to the skin in two layers. (Reproduced with permission from Swenson, O., and Donnellan, W. L.: S. Clin. North America 47:173, 1967.)

tula is cleared on all sides by sharp dissection, and is clamped toward its rectal side in order that it may be drawn upward for better visualization. When its entire circumference is clearly visible, a 4/0 chromic catgut suture is placed and tied through its upper border about 3 mm. from the urethra, and is used to suture the opening on the distal side as the fistula is progressively transected. It is better to leave a slight urethral diverticulum than to run the risk of a urethral stenosis at the fistula.

The rectal fistula is almost invariably the lower end of the narrowed rectum, and so it is discarded when the rectum is opened and sutured to the perineum. For this reason it is only temporarily closed by means of two or three silk sutures, which will be used for traction to deliver the rectum first into the abdomen and later down through the puborectalis sling to the perineum [Fig. 116, *B*].

Great care must be taken to avoid entering the rectum during the above dissections, since the rectal meconium in cases of imperforate anus has been found to be contaminated by bacteria as early as three hours after delivery. Pelvic abscesses and generalized sepsis may result from spillage of meconium during this portion of the operation.

After the fistula has been divided, the puborectalis portion of the levators must be separated from the urethra, and the rectosigmoid mesentry is freed in order to bring the rectum to the perineum without tension. Occasionally one or more of the sigmoid vessels must be cut to lengthen the mesenteric stalk. One surgeon remains above to complete the freeing of the colon, while the responsible operator proceeds to the perineal dissection from below.

In order to provide for a rectal opening approximately 50 per cent greater than appears necessary, so that later scar contraction will not lead to stenosis, a double diamond-shaped incision is made at the site of the proposed anal canal. This incision has two advantages. The irregular shape of the double diamond increases the circumference of the anal margin, and removes the central avascular, poorly healing perineal skin from the site of the stoma. In addition, the margins of this type of incision are elastic and they draw up readily into a good inversion position as healing occurs.

No attempt is made to pass the rectum through the fibers of the external sphincter. As has been discussed, these are often defective, and in any case they play no part in continuous fecal continence. It is usually best to place the anus slightly forward of the normal position, in order to avoid excessive tension on the bowel as it is brought through the puborectalis sling.

Dissection in the perineal fat and transverse perineal muscles is carried upward anteriorly until the urethral catheter can be palpated. Under direct vision the posterior margin of the urethra is freed from surrounding structures. When an 0.5–1 cm length of the vertical portion of the urethra has been exposed, the abdominal operator begins a cautious dissection from above in the plane behind the urethra, and a long medium-pointed curved clamp is advanced from below to meet his dissection. As soon as the two dissections meet, an umbilical tape is passed through the opening, and a larger blunt Pean clamp is drawn progressively through it along this guideline [Fig. 116, *B*]. By cautious spreading of the clamp, the fibers of the puborectalis are gently dilated until an opening large enough to accommodate the bowel is produced. Gentle dissection is necessary so that the muscular fibers and nerve supply of the sling are not torn or otherwise damaged.

As the rectum is drawn through the puborectalis sling [Fig. 116, *C*], its proper orientation is checked from above. The mesentery should lie on its right posterior side and the lower portion of the bowel must not be twisted.

In order to bring the puborectalis to the lowest possible position on the rectum, and to achieve inversion of the perineal skin to form new buttocks folds, 5/0 chromic catgut interrupted sutures are used to unite the dermis of the perineal skin, the edge of the puborectalis sling, and the seromuscular layer of the rectum. If healing proceeds well, this suture brings the contracting puborectalis muscle to the lowest point of the newly formed rectum. After the deep sutures have all been placed and tied, the lower rectum is excised about 2 to 3 mm below them, and the full thickness of the rectal wall is united to the skin with 5/0 silk interrupted sutures which also take in a small amount of the puborectalis muscle. These are tied very loosely over the tip of a hemostat so that the usual reactive oedema will not cause them to cut through [Fig. 116, *D*].

As the perineal portion of the operation proceeds, the abdomen is closed in layers, using interrupted 5/0 silk sutures to the peritoneum and anterior fascia, and a running subcuticular suture of 5/0 plain catgut or interrupted 5/0 silk to the skin. We use a suprapubic cystostomy tube for bladder drainage for the first six post-operative days in order to avoid damage to the urethra by an indwelling catheter.

C. Abdomino-Perineal Rectoplasty Using a Buttock-Reflecting Incision

In 1965 Sauvage and Bill described an alternative approach to define the pubo-rectalis, and the correct plane of dissection. The technique is essentially that of a perineal exposure of the pubo-rectalis from below through the ischio-rectal fossa, the division of the fistula and mobilization of rectum being completed by the abdominal route. The original paper and its illustrations should be consulted, but the principles are as follow:

(a) The pubo-rectalis muscle is identified from the ischio-rectal fossa below the levator diaphragm.
(b) The external sphincter fibers are utilized in addition to pubo-rectalis.
(c) The procedure is a combined abdominal and perineal undertaking.
(d) The anus is skin lined.

The technique is as follows:

(i) A curved incision is made along the lateral aspect of the buttock, extending medially above the sacrum and below to the posterior perineal fold. This large flap is reflected medially. The dissection is carried through the ischio-rectal fossa to reach the back wall of the urethra or vagina and to expose the anterior fibers of the pubo-rectalis sling, which are separated gently from these structures. The "passage" for the rectum is thus established.

(ii) From the abdominal route, the fistula is divided, and the bowel mobilized through the passage in front of the pubo-rectalis.

(iii) Care is taken to define the central portion of the external sphincter, to be utilized in conjunction with the pubo-rectalis.

(iv) A deep skin-lined anal canal is fashioned from anterior, posterior and lateral skin flaps extending up to the level of the deep external sphincter. Such a canal is said to lie within the circular grasp of the superficial sphincter, improve sensory perception to the anus and avoid the constant mucoid discharge of exposed rectal mucosa.

Sauvage and Bill described 4 patients (3 males with recto-urethral fistulae, and 1 female with a high recto-vaginal fistula). The longest follow-up was only 10 months, but the results at that time were gratifying. The long-term results will be awaited with interest. The authors also describe 3 children with low anal anomalies (recto-fourchette fistulae, and 1 male with a fistula at the base of the penis), in whom the same perineal approach has been used successfully.

Comment.—The worrying feature of approaching the pubo-rectalis from below is that the main branches of the pudendal nerve to the pubo-rectalis muscle cross the ischio-rectal fossa to reach the sling. They may be at risk in this approach (see Fig. 7).

D. Submucosal Resection and Abdomino-Perineal Rectoplasty and Abdomino-Sacro-Perineal Rectoplasty [Rehbein]

In order to minimize injury to the nerve and blood supply to the pelvic viscera, Rehbein (1959) described a technique in which pelvic dissection is largely eliminated by bringing the colon through the lower rectum in a submucous plane. The technique is an adaptation of a procedure used in adults with carcinoma of the rectum, inaugurated by Babcock (1947) and Bacon (1949) and in polyposis coli by Ravitch (1948) and Ravitch and Handelsman (1951). It has been presented also by Romualdi (1960 and 1961); Soave (1964) has described a recent modification. Hartl (1960) and Hecker (1961) have also reported good results.

The procedure is performed in the newborn period.

The method is described by Nicolai and Rehbein (1963)* as follows:

After laparotomy the recto-sigmoid junction is freed close to the wall for about 1 cm of length only, the upper rectum is opened, cleaned and cut across. The proximal stump is temporarily closed; then tension sutures are placed around the lumen. Then starting at the edge, the mucous membrane of the rectal pouch is carefully removed. The mucous membrane is held by tension sutures which facilitate mobilisation in the right layer. We found that removal of the mucous membrane was easier in newborns, but was possible also in older infants and children. After complete mobilisation the mucous membrane is cut off at the level of the fistula. Next, the right index finger is introduced into the rectal pouch and the left one into the anal dimple. Bringing both fingers together as close as possible one can easily feel the deepest point of the pouch as well as the middle of the sphincteric muscles. At the perineum an oval excision of skin is made, and with the finger acting as a constant guide, forceps are introduced into the pouch. This artificial channel is carefully widened and the sigmoid colon, which was closed temporarily, is

*Reprinted with permission from Nicolai, I, and Rehbein, F.: Arch. Dis. Childhood 38: 167, 1963.

pulled through the remaining pouch, care being taken to avoid stretching. After re-opening, the sigmoid colon is fixed around the skin excision.

It is very important to ensure that the blood supply is in no way jeopardised and to make sure that there is no tension.

The Figure [117, *A*] demonstrates the technique; the interrupted line in (a) indicates the cut across the upper rectum. The pouch descends distal to the fistula. At (b) the mucous membrane is completely removed and cut off at the level of the fistula; (c) shows the position at the end of the operation with the sigmoid colon pulled through the remaining pouch and fixed around the newly-built anus.

It is not necessary to close the fistula, because the wall of the sigmoid colon fits tightly over it.

Comment.—1. Theoretically, the dissection within the rectum should lead the surgeon to the precise plane of the pubo-rectalis, which immediately surrounds the urethra or vagina. However, as shown in the illustration, the "deepest point of the pouch," being tethered anteriorly by the fistula yields posteriorly and caudally to pressure from within. The pubo-rectalis sling may not escape damage from the obturator with this method of rectoplasty, or it may

Fig. 117.—Rehbein's abdomino-perineal procedure. **A,** steps in his operation as reported in 1963 (*a, b* and *c*). (Nicolai and Rehbein.) See text. Note that the bowel may be behind the pubo-rectalis sling. **B,** modifications reported in 1967. Additional sacral approach performed during the abdomino-perineal procedure designed to locate and tunnel the pubo-rectalis sling with greater precision. This additional maneuver is necessary if the sling cannot be located by "bidigital palpation" as shown in Figure 115. (Rehbein, 1967.) (*A,* reproduced with permission from Nicolai, I, and Rehbein, F.: Arch. Dis. Childhood 38:167, 1963; and *B,* Rehbein, F.: J. Pediat. Surg. 2:99, 1967.)

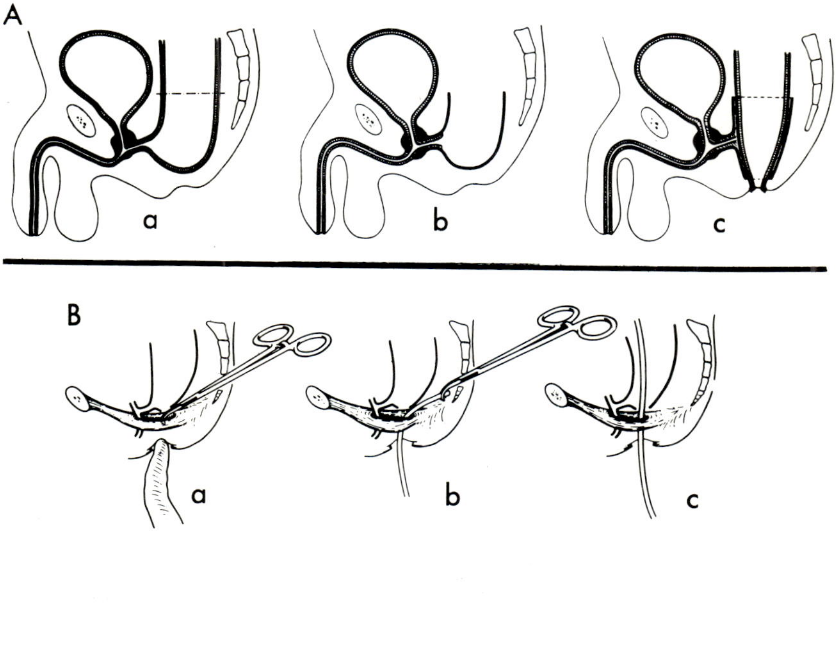

escape altogether as actually shown in Figure 117, *A*, (*c*), lying ineffectual in the angle between fistula and the new rectum. Further, where there is no fistula but a blind rectum, the technique would similarly risk by-passing or damage of the pubo-rectalis sling, because no precise pelvic dissection is performed to define the narrow path of entry to the tunnel.

As described at that time, therefore, the method of finding the tunnel anterior to the pubo-rectalis was open to serious objection.

For this reason, Rehbein (1965 and 1967) revised his method of approach to the muscle, which he now defined by finger palpation above and below the levator (Fig. 117, *B* (*b*). The point has already been discussed and depicted in this chapter, with our comment upon its difficulties.

As Rehbein does not believe it is necessary to define the site of the fistula before operation, he always starts with the abdominal dissection first, being led to the fistula by the submucosal resection of the rectum. When it is certain that the site of the fistula and the plane of the pubo-rectalis is clear, the operation is completed by an abdomino-perineal combination only—termed by Rehbein, "*abdomino-perineal pull-through*." If, however, palpation still leaves doubt, Rehbein then temporarily closes the abdomen, turns the infant over, and the levator is then defined by the sacro-coccygeal route of Stephens, to be shortly described. This combined operation is termed "*abdomino-sacro-perineal pull-through*," differing from the Stephens technique in that the dissection starts abdominally.

2. With respect to the principle of submucosal resection of the terminal rectum, there would seem to be an important advantage in eliminating all pelvic dissection outside the bowel wall, so that bladder control, and perhaps other parasympathetic pathways to the bowel, should not be affected. Further, no muscular part of the rectum is sacrificed, so that afferents from this source for sensation are preserved.

However, mucosal and submucosal afferent pathways are still destroyed, although it is not certain these are important. In one case of the Rehbein procedure investigated by pressure measurements by Nixon and Callaghan (1964), the rectal reflex was lost.

3. We would not agree with Rehbein that preoperative investigations to site the level of anomaly are unnecessary; in all but the lowest anal imperforations, Rehbein is committed to opening the abdomen, yet in intermediate type anomalies, e.g., recto-bulbar fistula and anal agenesis, the lesions can be approached safely from behind and below, without the necessity for the extensive procedure of laparotomy and submucosal resection. The procedure cannot be without morbidity, and in fact 2 of 5 deaths in 30 patients, operated upon by Rehbein as neonates, were from peritonitis and mesenteric-vein thrombosis, respectively, whereas in 3 additional patients the pulled-

through colon retracted, fistulae recurrence requiring reoperation.

4. It still remains to be seen whether fibro-cystic reaction in the denuded rectum prevents adequate rectal function or whether retention of rectal musculature improves the sensation in the terminal bowel.

E. Sacro-Perineal Rectoplasty and Sacro-Abdomino-Perineal Rectoplasty [Stephens]

The essential principles of the Stephens technique may be summarized as follows:

(i) The essential muscle contributing to continence—the puborectalis section of the levator ani—is accurately identified from its posterosuperior aspect, and the narrow plane anterior to the sling defined prior to mobilization of the gut. This definition is achieved via a posterior route through the sacro-coccygeal junction and is the preliminary step to all rectoplasty procedures; from this step onward, the operation may be completed through the same incision or combined with an abdominal exposure.

(ii) In rectal lesions in which the pouch lies on or below the pubococcygeal line (e.g., most recto-urethral fistulae, ano-rectal and anal ageneses without fistulae, recto-vaginal fistulae and the long recto-vestibular fistulae), the division of the fistula and mobilization of the rectum can be completed by the sacro-coccygeal route, thus making abdominal exploration unnecessary, with a consequent saving of morbidity from adhesions, damage to bladder nerve supply, etc.—*sacro-perineal rectoplasty.*

However, when the pouch of the rectum is even fractionally higher in the pelvis than the P/C line, it is an essential part of the procedure to open the abdomen to gain necessary length of bowel and to reach the perineum without tension. This applies to recto-cloacal fistula with long cloacal canal, recto-vesical and unusually high recto-urethral and recto-vaginal fistulae.

When abdominal exploration is added, however, it is always preceded by definition of the pubo-rectalis from the sacral route—*sacro-abdomino-perineal rectoplasty.* No dissection whatever should be made of the fistula or terminal rectum from the sacral aspect when the rectal pouch is above the P/C line because the nervi erigentes to the bladder are particularly vulnerable.

(iii) After incising the bulbous end of the rectum sagittally, the fistula is viewed and identified with a probe within the rectal lumen. This avoids undue dissection in the plane of nerve fibers outside the fistula and avoids cutting the urethra or vagina if traction is applied to the fistula.

(iv) The plane of dissection is in the midline posteriorly behind the rectum, thus minimizing the risks of damage to the nerve supply

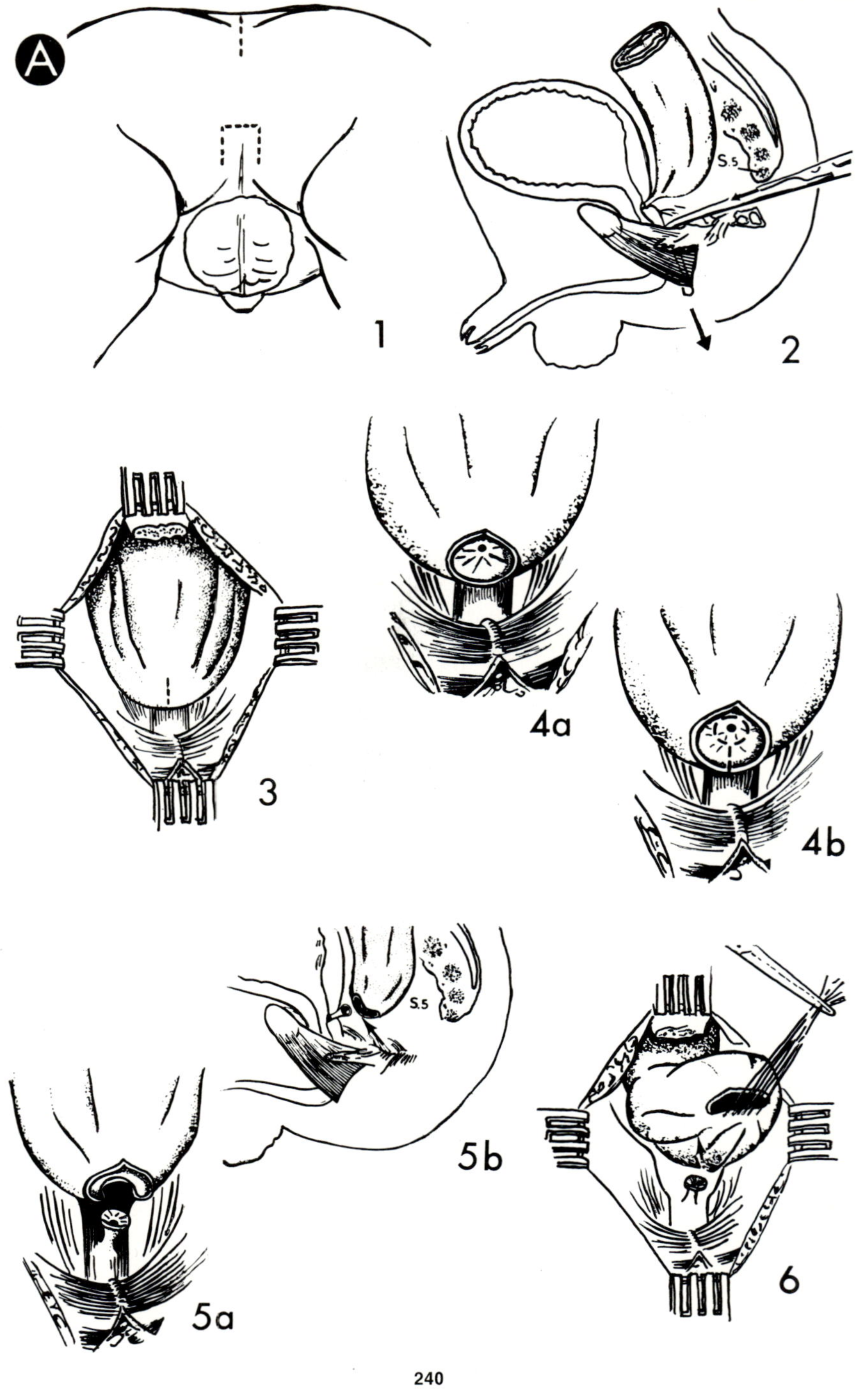
A
1
2
S.5
3
4a
4b
5a
5b
S.5
6

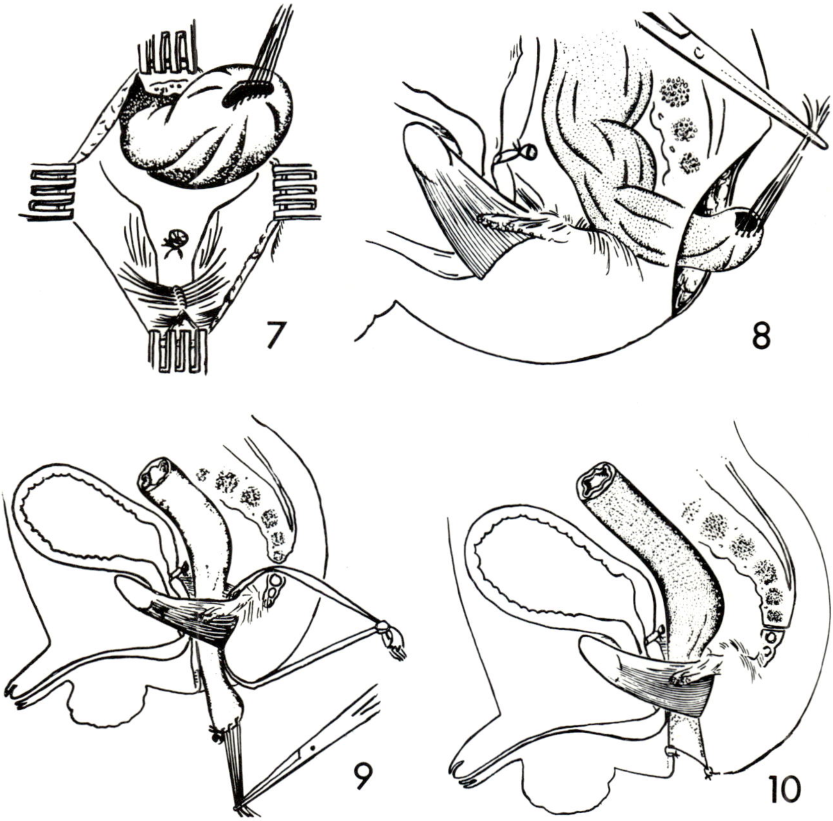

Fig. 118.—A, recto-urethral fistula—rectoplasty by sacro-perineal approach (Stephens). See text. *1,* Sacral and anal incisions. *2,* Tunneling the pubo-rectalis sling. *3,* Rectum exposed and incised. *4a,* Rectal end of the fistula identified within the rectal lumen. *4b,* Incision in rectum extended as a racket around the orifice of the fistula. *5a,* Rectum disconnected from fistula as viewed through the sacro-coccygeal incision. *5b,* Rectum and fistula in lateral view—arrow indicates the mid-line plane in which to start mobilizing rectum. *6,* Traction stitches inserted and arrow again indicates the important midline plane of free dissection close to the bowel wall. Keeping in this plane, the surgeon should dissect laterally and divide tethering tissues under vision as they attach to the rectum. *7,* Ligate fistula and mobilize the rectum. *8,* Lateral view indicates the amount of mobilization required. *9,* Rectum redirected to the anal incision in the perineum through the pubo-rectalis sling. *10,* Rectum sutured to the skin of perineum and also to deeper tissues by buried sutures. (*Important:* The sacro-perineal rectoplasty procedure can be done only on those deformities in which the convex terminal end of the rectum descends to lie comfortably on or caudal to the pubo-coccygeal line. If the convex terminal end is even slightly cranial to this line, the tunnel should be made only through the sacro-coccygeal incision and the rectum and colon should be mobilized through the abdominal incision as described in the text.) (*continued*).

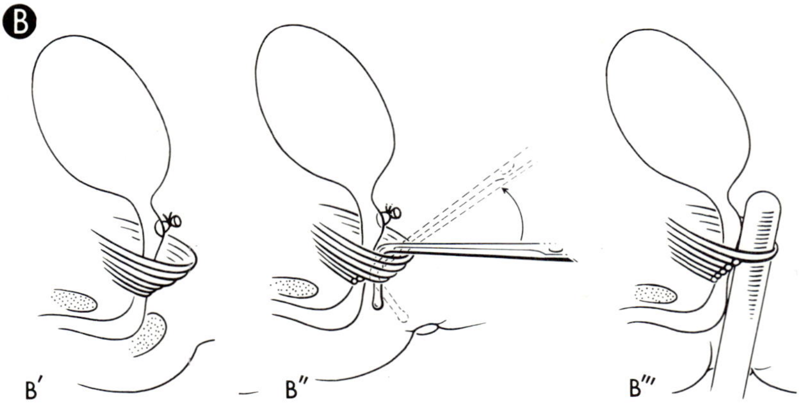

Fig. 118 (cont.). – **B,** Correct and incorrect methods of tunneling and dilatation of the pubo-rectalis sling. *B′*, normal conical disposition of the pubo-rectalis. *B″*, tunneling from the posterior sacro-coccygeal aspect with a right-angled clamp, and dilatation using this clamp, thereby damaging only a minimal number of the shortest fibers. *B‴*, it is incorrect to dilate the muscle with straight dilators which tear too many of the short fibers of the cone.

to the bladder, bowel and pubo-rectalis, and preserving function.

(v) No rectum need be sacrificed, thus perhaps preserving available afferent nerve fibers accompanying the vessels for rectal sensation.

(vi) The technique of tunneling the rectum to the perineum is executed with minimal trauma and preserves the integrity of the muscle.

(vii) A skin flap trap-door incision at the anal site (rather than excision of an ellipse of skin) to provide a partially skin-lined anal canal.

(viii) The pubo-rectalis sling is stretched slowly in an unrushed and graduated fashion for several months through the lumen of the new rectum.

(ix) The colostomy is closed approximately 3 months after the rectoplasty, when a satisfactory anal lumen has been assured.

TECHNIQUE. – 1. Preoperative Preparation. – In bowel preparation for the usual case with a colostomy, the distal bowel requires cleansing, but as the colostomy is maintained after the rectoplasty no restriction of diet is required nor is any oral medication given to reduce the bowel flora. The distal limb of the colostomy is given daily saline washouts on the three final days before operation; 16 hours and again 8 hours before operation 160 ml. of neomycin solution (1 in 200) is instilled into the distal limb. In the less common situation of an older child requiring operation, when no colostomy is present (e.g., anal transplantation by the sacro-perineal route, secondary exploration and rectoplasty in a previously unsuccessful case), full bowel preparation is required—low-residue diet for 3 days, followed by nonresidue diet for 2 days; 4 ml. mineral oil three times a day for 4 days; daily enema followed by saline bowel washout for 5 days, the last washout being at 24 hours before operation; antibiotic retention enema as described above; and oral neomycin 16 hours preoperatively (25 mg. per kg. per dose), as one dose per hour for 4 doses, then one dose per 4 hours for 3 doses.

An intravenous infusion is inserted into the right arm (not the leg) for greater facility when changing from the jackknife supine position to the lithotomy position.

2. The Sacro-Coccygeal Exposure.—The steps of the operation are depicted in Figure 118, *A*.

A urethral sound is passed into the bladder in a male or a Hegar dilator into the vagina in a female and anchored in place with a stitch to penile skin or labia and the child postured over a sandbag into the jackknife position. The legs should be apart to expose the whole perineum.

A midline incision is made in the natal cleft, with its center over the sacro-coccygeal junction and stopping caudally at least 2 cm. from the site of the proposed anus (Fig. 118, *A1*). A transverse incision is made through the cartilage of the sacro-coccygeal junction and extended laterally for 1 cm. on each side. The perineal branch (if present) of the 4th sacral nerve lies medial to the ischial spine on the caudal aspect of the coccygeus and is distributed to the posterior fibers of the pubo-rectalis (see Fig. 6). This nerve is at risk if the cuts lateral to the coccyx are extended more than 1 cm. from the midline. The coccyx is excised or incised distally, and the posterior part of the levator is incised in the midline. The lower sharp margins of the sacrum may be nibbled away. A retractor is placed in the opening separating the soft tissues from the terminal sacral vertebra. The Denis Browne retractor with silk guy sutures attached to the ring is excellent for the purpose. A midline window into the supralevator space is fashioned in the fascia overlying the body of the last sacral vertebra. The access to the levator ani and pelvis is obviously improved in those patients with congential absence of the coccyx and some sacral vertebrae.

Dissection through the enlarged window strictly in the midline exposes the pelvic rectum. It is here that the information derived from preoperative radiological studies is so meaningful. *If the terminal rectal pouch is above the P/C line*, it is imperative that no dissection of the pouch or of the fistula be performed from the back because in these lesions the nervi erigentes run a medial course to the midline below the rectum (see Fig. 5); dissection here is likely to result in disruption of the bladder parasympathetic supply. The dissection proceeds immediately to the definition of the pubo-rectalis, which, when completed, is followed by the abdominal exploration. The division of the fistula then follows that described below, but entirely from the abdominal exposure.

If, on the other hand, the terminal rectal pouch is on or below the P/C line, the rectum and fistula can be cleared safely from the sacral route, because the rectum displaces the pelvic plexuses laterally, as in the normal. The dissection then proceeds as follows:

The fascia over the rectum is incised and stripped off by blunt dissection. The plane of dissection is then carried forwards around the caudal curve of the rectum towards the fistula to the bladder, urethra or vagina on its anteroinferior aspect. In the male, the rectum is now incised sagittally at its bulbous end so as to examine for a fistula or define more clearly from within the lumen the walls of the fistula (Fig. 118, *A3*). This is important, firstly because in some wide fistulae (and even with a sound in the urethra), the posterior wall may tent with traction and be resected with the fistula. Secondly, extension of the incision anteriorly in racket fashion around the orifice of the fistula from within the lumen of the rectum is the safest method of dividing the tract (Fig. 118, *A4*). Thirdly, the plane of separation of the anterior wall of the rectum from the back of the urethra and vesicles or vagina is free in the midline, and this plane is readily found after detachment of the fistula by circumcision from within (Fig. 118, *A5* and 6). The dissection should be kept close to the rectum to avoid damage to the nervi erigentes and pelvic plexuses, which are located anterolateral to the rectum, near the bladder base or cervix uteri. At this stage, the fistula is clamped, transfixed, ligated with catgut and divided, or if wide, as with a vaginal fistula, it may be oversewed after division, although this is not essential (Fig. 118, *A7*). The detached rectum is oversewed and further mobilized by extending the anterior midline plane of cleavage laterally on either side (Fig. 118, *A8*). Traction at this stage on the rectum exposes a lateral line of fascia which anchors the rectum on each side and can be divided under vision.

The tunnel of the pubo-rectalis sling (Fig. 118, *B*) is next defined, although neither the muscle as such nor the levator diaphragm are well visualized. Nevertheless, the plane anterior to the sling can be defined. The passage is made by the long beaks of a right-angled clamp which commence dissection adjacent to the fistula immediately posterior to the urethra or vagina, which is readily identified by the metal obturator in the lumen, the dissection being exactly at the midsagittal line (Fig. 118, *A2*). It is important not to stray laterally because muscle fibers may be torn. The clamp gently opens up a tunnel directed caudally, parallel to and contiguous with the urethra or vagina after a passage of approximately 2–3 cm. as far as the perineal body in the male and the vestibule in the female. The tips of the clamp are then turned posteriorly in the perineum to the site of the new anus.

A trap-door incision 1 cm. square and hinged anteriorly is then fashioned at the site of the proposed anus, previously chosen at the point where pinprick indicates maximal concentration of external sphincter fibers. If these fibers can be identified, the right-angled clamp is passed from above through the center of the fibers to the perineal incision, and a piece of tape is engaged in the jaws of the clamp in the perineum. No dissection deep in the perineal incision should be performed, especially laterally, because the most distal fibers of the sling may readily be nibbled away and the pudendal nerve supply to the pubo-rectalis enters across the ischio-rectal space. The tape is withdrawn gently through the pubo-rectalis sling and out through the posterior incision, and both ends are loosely tied. The tape serves as a guide to the narrow tunnel, up which curved artery forceps can be drawn, released and opened to stretch the lowermost fibers surrounding the tunnel. It serves subsequently as the guide from above to feed the traction sutures and the mobilized rectum down the narrow tunnel (Fig. 118, *A9*). The rectum having been shown by x-ray to reach the P/C line and having been mobilized through the posterior incision, as described above, must now be tested for length. It is drawn through the sacro-coccygeal incision, and an estimate is made of the length of mobilized rectal wall. The length of the tunnel from anus to fistula is then measured (Fig. 118, *A8*). Mobilization may be adequate, or a minor or major discrepancy may exist. Any extra mobilization can be obtained safely by the technique described, although mobilization at this stage may require blunt dissection with the little finger along the sides of the rectum.

When sufficient length of rectum has been achieved from the posterior route, thread sutures are inserted into the pointed "leader" end of the rectum (Fig. 118, *A6*). Using the tape as a guide, forceps are passed up from below through the levator sling and the thread sutures grasped and pulled back to the perineum. The slanted edge of the rectum is then led and "squeezed" very slowly and gently down through the sling by seesaw traction on the sutures (Fig. 118, *A9*). In performing this maneuver the rectum must not be spirally twisted. No attempt is made to enlarge the tunnel beyond that required to accommodate the collapsed rectum and its blood supply, and, above all, attempts at forceful digital thrusts must be resisted. The rectum is led into the perineal incision, and the anterior flap of skin is let into the anterior rectal wall and sutured with 3–0 chromic catgut. A row of 4–0 chromic catgut sutures is then inserted between the lateral and posterior walls of the rectum and the perineal connective tissue (Fig. 118, *A10*). The rectum-skin anastomosis is maintained by a single layer of interrupted fine silk sutures. The tape is withdrawn, the posterior part of the levator diaphragm is sutured, and the poster-

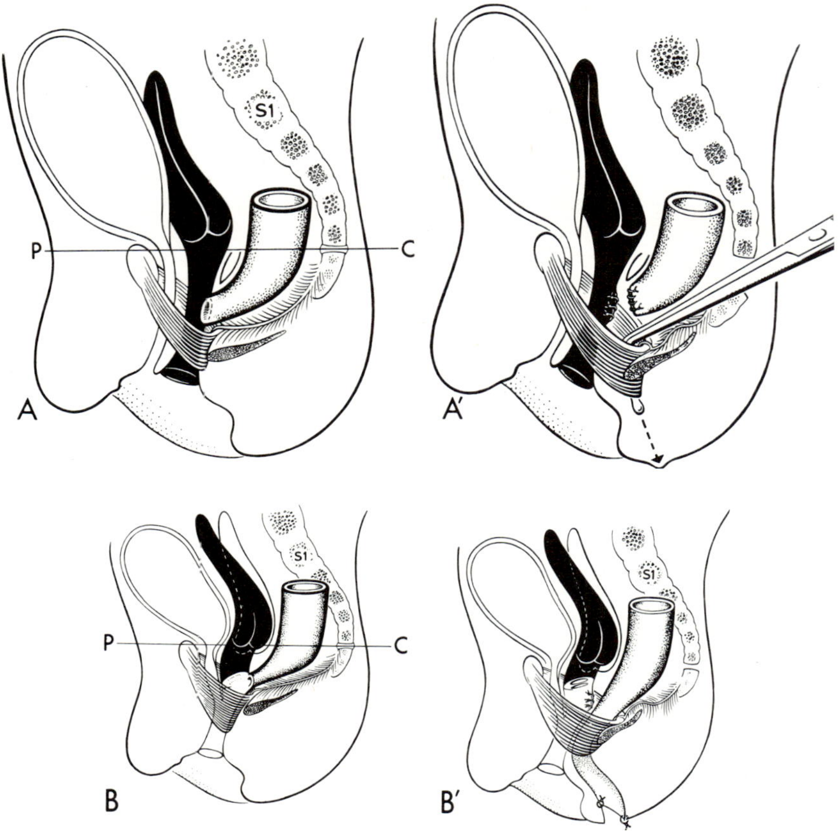

Fig. 119.—The pre- and postoperative location of the pubo-rectalis sling in relation to the anal canal. **A** and **A′,** recto-vaginal fistula. **B** and **B′,** recto-cloacal fistula. (*A′* reproduced with permission from Australian Paediat. J. 1:107, 1965.)

ior incision is drained with corrugated rubber dam and closed in layers with fine, plain catgut, with silk for the skin. If the coccyx has been retained, it is resutured by its perichondrium to the sacrum.

When it is prejudged that there would be insufficient rectum for a safe anastomosis by the sacro-coccygeal route alone or when on x-ray the sigmoid colon exhibits evidence of massive enlargement, an abdominal approach is also required. In this event, the proximal end and the long coil of tape adjoining it is packed into the supralevator space, and the other end is left protruding from the perineal incision. The sacro-coccygeal incision is then closed with a small corrugated drain in place. The child is then turned into the lithotomy position.

3. The Abdominal Procedure.—Through a left paramedian incision the bladder is drawn upwards and anteriorly by stay sutures, and the pelvic peritoneum in the recto-vesical pouch incised along either side of and transversely across the rectum, close to the rectal wall and fistula. The dissection behind the bladder is kept to a minimum, and the rectum is then freed from the pelvis with minimal division of blood vessels.

When the abdominal exploration has been undertaken for a rectal pouch above the P/C line, the pouch and fistula must now be dissected free. The technique is the same as that described for the sacral exposure, avoiding dissection below the rectum wherein the pelvic plexuses lie and keeping close to the wall of the fistula. After the division of the fistula is completed, the rectal stump is delivered out of the pelvis. At this stage, the bulky coil of tape previously fed into the supralevator space from the sacro-coccygeal incision is grasped and drawn upwards through the abdominal incision and held as the guide to the pubo-rectalis tunnel.

The rectum and sigmoid colon are then fully mobilized on their vascular pedicle, and it will be necessary to divide the inferior mesenteric artery, either between the sigmoid branches or at its origin with the aorta, in order to obtain greater mobility and the extra length required. Occasionally, the distal part of the sigmoid is abnormally large and thickened, forming a large terminal reservoir. This focal enlargement should be excised. Usually, however, the terminal colon and rectum are of near normal dimensions, and then all can be saved. The end of the bowel may taper to the fistula or else is tailored on the bias to negotiate the pubo-rectal sling with greater facility.

Long traction sutures are inserted into the tapered end of the bowel and threaded through the levator sling to the perineum, along the path of the tape. The bowel is then led through the tunnel to the perineum. The operation is then completed as described above.

It is important to palpate the kidneys and to inspect the ureters while the abdomen is open for further evidence of associated urinary anomalies. Also, as Nixon (1961) says, "It is also important in the case of a female child to see that the form of the genital tract is entered in the notes. For sooner or later, the question of child-bearing will be raised and it is embarrassing to find that the abdomen has been opened more than once and yet the information cannot be given."

The abdomen is then closed in layers and the tape withdrawn. A Foley catheter is left in the bladder.

4. Closure of Colostomy.—The colostomy is closed approximately 3 months after the rectoplasty, when it is certain that the pubo-rectalis has been gently dilated, and the anal canal has an adequate lumen.

F. Sacro-Abdomino-Perineal Rectoplasty (Combined Sacro-Perineal Approach with Rehbein Procedure [Kiesewetter])

In previous communications (1963 and 1964), Kiesewetter and his colleagues have supported the sacro-coccygeal approach in offering a more certain route to the plane of the pubo-rectalis. Being impressed also with the protection to the pelvic nerves afforded by the Rehbein procedure of submucosal resection, Kiesewetter has combined the two procedures. The procedure and diagrams are reproduced in full (Kiesewetter, 1967)*:

Neonatal Care.—In those patients who will require an abdominoperineal pull-through to correct their abnormality, a colostomy should be instituted as soon as the diagnosis is made in the newborn period. The most effective colostomy in our hands has been the divided left transverse colostomy with the distal stoma higher than the proximal. Such a divided colostomy lessens the chance of fecal material from the proximal bowel entering the distal bowel. When the abdomen is open, a catheter should be placed in the distal limb of the colostomy and the meconium irrigated out to prevent inspissation and reduce the chance of urinary tract infection in those patients with a fistula. Layer by layer arterial silk sutures are placed joining the peritoneum, fascia and skin to the divided segments of bowel. A skin bridge of at least 2 inches between the stomas should be created.

Appropriate urinary studies should be undertaken to rule out any major urinary tract anomalies. A distal colostomy loop barium study should be done for the purpose of estimating the distance from the blind bowel to the skin and defining its relationship to the pubococcygeal line. At the same time, indigo carmine can be given with the barium to ascertain or confirm the presence of a rectourinary fistula.

Sacral Portion of Definitive Procedure.—The time of election for definitive therapy is 6 to 12 months of age. Mechanical cleansing of the distal loop of the colostomy is the only bowel preparation employed. A large Levine tube is put down the distal colostomy to help in identifying the end of the blind pouch through the subsequent sacral incision.

The patient is placed in the face-down position after having had a metal urethral sound inserted. The buttocks are strapped apart. The incision is made from the tip of the coccyx to 1–2 cm from the projected anal opening. The coccyx is left untouched, and a midline dissection is carried out with central division of the levator sling if the puborectalis muscle is below the coccyx. The level of the puborectalis will be determined by the position of the blind rectum in the distal loop barium study. It will lie just beyond the lowermost portion of that structure. If the descent of the bowel has proceeded beyond the coccyx, the pubococcygeal portion of the levator sling will have to be divided in the midline to look down from above on the blind bowel and the puborectalis muscle. If the blind bowel is at or above the tip of the coccyx, the puborectalis sling will be found at the tip of the coccyx, by dissection in the

*Reprinted with permission from Kiesewetter, W. B.: J. Pediat. Surg. 2:106, 1967.

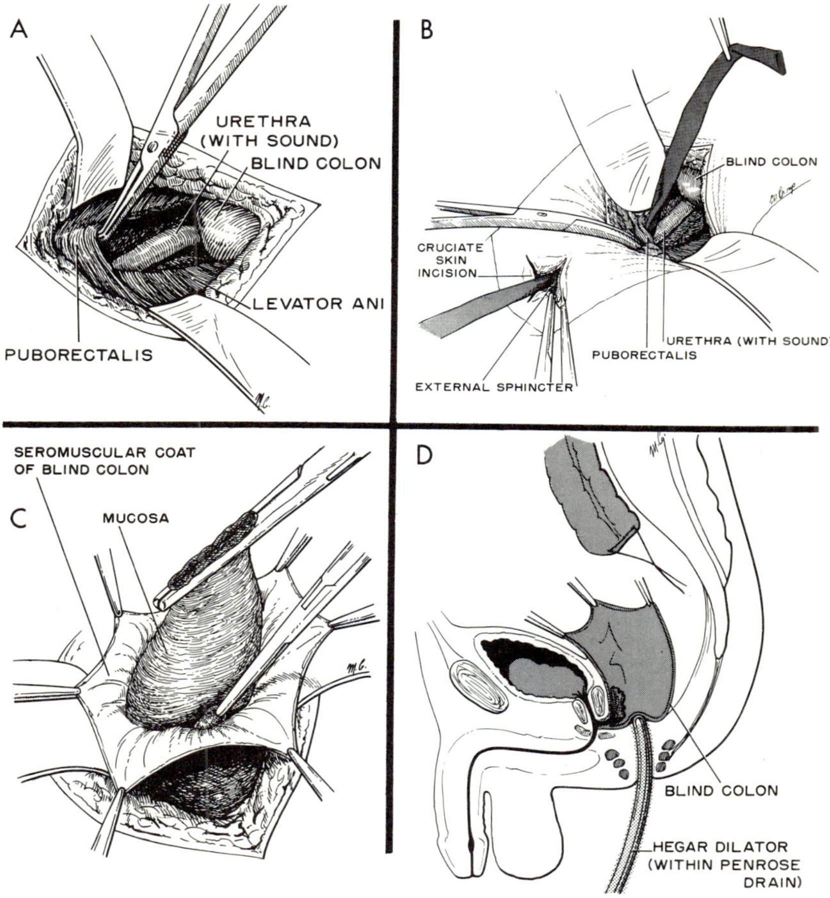

Fig. 120. – Steps of the operations described by Kiesewetter (1967). This operation combines the sacro-perineal delineation of the pubo-rectalis sling and tunnel (Stephens) with the Rehbein procedure. **A** and **B,** hemostat and Penrose drain depict the pubo-rectalis muscle and tunnel through the sacro-coccygeal incision. **C,** mucosa of rectal pouch is denuded through the abdominal approach. **D,** the dilator is passed upwards along the Penrose drain to indent the sero-muscular sleeve of the rectal pouch and so indicate the site through which the colon is to be led through the perineum. (Reproduced with permission from Kiesewetter, W. B.: J. Pediat. Surg. 2:106, 1967.)

midline from below. These relationships can readily be seen in Figure [120, *A*]. The puborectalis is gently dilated to make a canal about 2–4 cm in diameter.

A cruciate skin incision is made over the external sphincter [Fig. 120, *B*]. The skin is separated from the muscle and preserved in toto. An opening is made in the middle of the muscle and it is gradually dilated with Hegar dilators until large enough to accept the prospective pull-through segment (usually 2–4 cm in diameter). The previously made puborectalis tunnel and external sphincter opening are joined and dilated with Hegar dilators in such fashion as not to tear the muscles. A ½ inch empty Penrose drain is placed in the tunnel up to the level of the blind pouch [Fig. 120, *B*]. We emphasize that an empty Penrose drain should be utilized so that a Hegar dilator can be inserted through it at a later stage in the procedure.

The posterior incision is closed so as to carefully rejoin any pubococcygeal and anococcygeal fibers that may have been divided in the course of the dissection.

Abdominal Portion of Procedure.—With the child in the supine position, a left paramedian or left lower quadrant hockey stick incision is made. No pelvic dissection is carried on outside of the bowel. A small amount of saline is injected beneath the seromuscular coat of the bowel just above the peritoneal reflection so as to leave a distal pouch of approximately 8–10 cm. The seromuscular coat is incised vertically through the saline injection and a 2–4 cm wide band of mucous membrane is dissected free from the seromuscular coat in circumferential fashion. It is preferable to leave the bowel intact in the course of this dissection, for it makes it easier to separate the seromuscular and mucosal coats. These 2 layers are then separately divided, the mucosa is cored out in its entirety as shown in Figure [120, *C*]. This removal of mucosa should include its attachment to the urinary tract or high vagina if a rectourinary or high rectovaginal fistula is present. The fistula should be divided and oversewn with fine catgut.

The projected pull-through segment of rectosigmoid is then prepared so as to provide adequate length to reach the skin without tension. This should be done by dividing vascular attachments centrally in the mesentery and preserving the marginal arcades.

A Hegar dilator is inserted through the hollow portion of the perineal Penrose drain until it is felt at the bottom of the seromuscular blind pouch [Fig. 120, *D*]. A blind pouch incision is made on the Hegar dilator and the incision enlarged until it is sufficient to accommodate the prospective pull-through segment. The Penrose drain itself is used only as a guide for the insertion of grasping forceps which can be placed on the drain from the outside and drawn up into the seromuscular cuff. We have used 2 Allis clamps for this purpose. It is preferable not to sew the pull-through segment of bowel to the Penrose drain, because in the pull-through the stitches may tear out and the localization of the puborectalis tunnel lost. Grasping the rectosigmoid segment with the Allis clamps, this bowel is brought onto the perineum without tearing the puborectalis tunnel or the external sphincter circle. If the external sphincter opening is too small, it is desirable to enlarge it by cleanly dividing the muscle in its anterior portion.

The bowel should be under no tension prior to interdigitation of the pull-through with the quadrant skin flaps. Cutting out V-portions in the full thickness of the bowel facilitates placing the skin tips as far up in the reconstructed anal canal as possible. The only stitches used in the perineum are for close approximation of the interdigitated mucocutaneous junction.

The seromuscular sleeve should be drained through a stab wound in the abdominal wall. The sleeve itself should be attached loosely to the bowel with a few stitches. Reperitonealization of the abdominal cavity should be carried out before closure of the abdominal wound in layers.

Postoperative Care.—The seromuscular sleeve drain should be removed in 3 to 5 days. Gentle dilatation with Hegar dilators should not be started until at least 14 days postoperatively.

It is desirable to close the colostomy as soon as an adequate anorectal channel has been established. The fecal stream is the best dilator. Such colostomy closure can generally be accomplished by the end of the third postoperative week. Antibiotics are not used pre- or postoperatively without specific indication.

Comment.—With the initial definition of the pubo-rectalis achieved by the posterior route, we agree that this combination of procedures is a most valuable and important contribution. Our comments, therefore, are only those already made about the Rehbein procedure above, in particular, the procedure always requires the additional abdominal exploration. We prefer, in rectal deformities at or below the P/C line (and this is the majority), to perform the entire procedure from the posterior route, without necessitating abdominal exposure. On the other hand, the Kiesewetter-Rehbein procedure gives a direct and safe approach to the fistula, for the dissection of the terminal rectum at the fistula is the most difficult part of the Stephens sacro-coccygeal approach; in fact, it was this difficulty that led Kiesewetter to look for an alternative.

Perhaps the best compromise is to advocate the sacro-coccygeal route alone for lesions at or below the P/C line, but for higher deformities the Kiesewetter-Rehbein procedure of submucosal resection could be added.

It is emphasized that the sacro-perineal operation is meticulous, dependent for success on absolute criteria obtained through thorough preoperative investigations and perhaps more difficult than the combined abdomino-perineal procedures, especially for the occasional investigator and operator. Hence, many surgeons will prefer a combined operation such as that described by Swenson and Donnellan (above) or that of the Kiesewetter-Rehbein refinement.

Functional Considerations in Rectoplasty

In any technique of rectoplasty, the principal determinant of continence is the integrity of the pubo-rectalis muscle and its nerve supply. The foregoing sections outline fully the means by which damage to these structures can be avoided (see Figs. 4–7).

In addition, however, some discussion is required on the contribution to continence of afferent sensory reception from the rectum and the anal canal and on the technique of construction of the anal anastomosis.

(1) The Rectal and Para-Rectal Afferents.—(See Chapter 2.) The parasympathetic and sympathetic nerve trunks and ganglia disposed around the terminal rectum and bladder base are at risk in a recto-

plasty operation, and it is inevitable that the main branches to the rectum, being extremely short, must be divided when the rectum is used as the new anal canal in pull-through procedures. The techniques described are designed to protect them as much as possible, for severance of the nervi erigentes leads to bladder disturbance. The question here, however, is whether their integrity is essential to fecal continence and whether afferent sensation from the distending rectum in some way facilitates control by the available sphincters. In the same way, if rectal sensation is important, then a necessary part of the operative technique would be to preserve as much of the rectum as possible. In all the rectal deformities, both the internal and external sphincters are rudimentary, so that any relation between the rectal afferents and continence must be one between these afferents and the pubo-rectalis.

Bryndorf and Madsen (1959) and Kiesewetter and Nixon (1967) found that some postoperative patients possessed satisfactory pubo-rectalis contraction on rectal examination and yet remain incontinent; the former authors suggest that trauma to the rectal innervation might account for such bad results.

Two questions need answering: Are there afferents from the rectum itself, and, if so, do they play a part in the nerve pathways and arcs that control the pubo-rectalis muscle?

In the normal adult, there is agreed evidence that distention of the distal 5–7 cm. of rectum initiates a relaxation of the internal sphincter (Gaston, 1948; Gaston and Walls, 1958; Duthie and Bennett, 1963; Duthie and Watts, 1965; Schnaufer *et al.*, 1967; and Scharli and Kiesewetter, 1969), although this stretch reflex passes off rapidly and there is no threat to continence while the intraluminal pressure remains low (Edwards and Phillips, 1965). There is also a contraction of the external sphincter. Similarly, Kiesewetter and Nixon (1967) in 2 normal infants found (by electromyography) changes in the external sphincter to rectal distention. On the other hand, Harris and Pope (1964) could find no changes in anal sphincteric pressure to varying degrees of rectal ampullary pressure. Further, Duthie and Bennett (1963) found no sign of sensory receptors in the rectal mucosa (freely present below the anal valves), and the rectal mucosa did not respond to the tactile stimuli applied. While recognizing the fact of a defecation reflex, it is by no means certain that this reflex necessarily arises in the rectal mucosa, and no information is available as to its effect on the pubo-rectalis as distinct from the effect on the internal and external sphincters.

In the rectal and anal deformities discussed in this book, little information is available on the sensory arcs present. Kiesewetter and Nixon (1967) found no sensation to touch in the rectum in 3 patients following abdomino-perineal resection, except in the distal 1–2 cm. above the muco-cutaneous junction and over the pubo-rectalis zone, but normal sensation was present for 4–5 cm. in 2 patients after rectoplasties from the sacro-coccygeal route. Nixon and Callaghan (1964), in 10 patients with colostomy before rectoplasty, found that balloon distention of the rectum produced electromyographic changes in the external sphincter zone but that in 6 of 12 patients after rectoplasty the response could not be recorded. Similar results were recorded by Schnaufer *et al.* (1967). Again, no information is available on the response of the pubo-rectalis, and the response of the "external sphincter zone" may have included the pubo-rectalis in these studies.

From these investigations, surgeons have concluded that operation destroys a useful reflex derived from the rectal wall and that, in particular, it is important to preserve every centimeter of rectum to facilitate afferent sensation.

However, we interpret the available facts differently. We believe that the receptors of fine appreciation of distention lie in the pelvic floor muscles and, in particular, the sleeve-and-sling combination of pubo-coccygeus and pubo-rectalis around the anal canal. Balloon distention of the rectum in normal subjects, with its reaction on the external and internal sphincters, may only represent pressure changes transmitted to the surrounding muscles and not necessarily stretch of receptors in the rectal wall. Indeed, in the rectal deformities with no internal sphincter and rudimentary external sphincter and with some rectum removed, a high degree of continence can be achieved by the pubo-rectalis alone. Rather than linking rectal wall afferents with the pubo-rectalis, it seems more likely that the muscle is its own sensor; the bad results after rectoplasty are perhaps due not to damage to the rectal afferents either in the rectal wall or in the pelvic plexuses but to damage to the sensory apparatus of the muscle itself. It was interesting to note that in 3 older patients of Kiesewetter and Nixon (1967), apart from the zone just above the muco-cutaneous junction, the only site receptive to touch was overlying the pubo-rectalis. That the pelvic floor muscles themselves may be the site at which distention is felt, in part at least, is suggested in the papers by Golligher and Hughes (1951), Parks *et al.* (1962), Porter (1962), Edwards and Phillips (1965) and Kiesewetter and Nixon (1967).

The facts available do not lead to any certain conclusions, but it is our view, that while we do not advocate indiscriminate removal of the distal rectal pouch the loss of some rectum is not of vital concern. In fact, if the rectum is bulbous and hypertrophic, as it may be in some children, it is more important to remove it—such blind segments may act discordantly, as in those of the proximal pouch in ileal atresia, and, furthermore, the large bulk of bowel may overstretch the pubo-rectalis tunnel at the time of operation. More important than the rectum is the integrity of the muscles and their nerve supply.

(2) Afferents from the Anal Canal.—Although no sensory receptors can be demonstrated histologically in the rectum, there is no doubt about the abundant source of receptors in the normal anal canal. Duthie and Gairns (1960) demonstrated a wide variety of receptors in the canal at and distal to the valves, in the pecten, especially in the hair-bearing skin, and above the valves in some for a distance of 0.5–1.5 cm. These receptors have central connections to the brain so that sensation can be consciously recorded, a phenomenon not possible from the rectum. Nixon and Callaghan (1964), Kiesewetter and Nixon (1967) and Schnaufer *et al.* (1967) recorded normal sensation in the anus after operation for low anal anomalies and in patients in whom sphincteric control was normal. Many workers (Hiatt and Santulli, 1962; Gans and Friedman, 1963; Kiesewetter and Nixon, 1967) believe it is important to line the new anal canal with skin to provide a sensitive area from which these reflexes can be developed. However, it is difficult to see how the presence of tactile sensibility in such an anus can help continence by the pubo-rectalis, for by the time feces or flatus have reached the anal canal it is already too late. Perhaps reflex contraction of the pubo-rectalis induced thereby may stop continued fecal flow, but it could not stop the initial bolus of feces which has already passed the pubo-rectalis, there being no effective external sphincter in rectal anomalies to act as a last line of defense. The fact that patients can be fully continent after rectoplasty, without a skin-lined anal canal, is further evidence that the reflex control is derived from and exerted through the sleeve-and-sling muscles surrounding the rectum. Such patients, however, do have some mucus staining, but this is derived from the mucosa-lined canal itself; lining the canal with skin may diminish this staining and soiling, by removing the mucosa.

(3) The Technique of the Bowel-Skin Anastomosis.—We also advocate a skin-lined anal canal provided by laying in skin-flaps but not primarily because of the possibility that it contributes to the reflex control of continence. The advantages are as follow:

(i) It enlarges the anal orifice.
(ii) The long anastomotic line inhibits stricture.
(iii) In females, the anterior hinged wall ensures a wider skin bridge between vagina and anus.
(iv) If the length of mobilized bowel is insufficient anteriorly, the gusset fills the deficiency.
(v) It diminishes the degree of mucus straining from anal ectropion.
(vi) Sensation from such a canal may possibly contribute to the reflex control of continence, but this is doubtful in view of the comments above.

The prevention of anal mucosal ectropion is an important advantage of skin-lining, for the mucus staining may require special toilet attention and is cosmetically displeasing. The explanation of the staining is the absence of an effective external sphincter whose normal function is to close the anal verge. Although we have shown the inadequacy of the external muscle as a sphincter, it seems logical to locate the bowel within its mass of fibers if possible and to use what is there, but the solution probably rests mainly on the use of skin lining. In our technique, we use an anterior skin flap, and occasionally a posterior one, but a minor degree of mucosal ectropion is common.

Hiatt and Santulli (1962) use a two-stage procedure. After defining the exact site of the external sphincter by faradic stimulation, a cruciate skin incision is made to provide four flaps. The rectum is pulled through beyond the anus, and the skin flaps are "tucked up" into the wound beside the bowel and sutured to the serosa of the bowel and to the levator ani attachments. The cuff of exposed bowel is left for 1–6 months, and when cicatrization and healing is complete the cuff is trimmed to the cutaneous attachments within the anal canal.

Kiesewetter (1967) uses a cruciate skin incision to provide four quadrants of skin which are interdigitated with V-cutouts of the terminal bowel wall.

Swenson and Donnellan (1967) describe a neat procedure which seems to offer real advantages, and we await with interest the late follow-up survey. (The technique is described earlier in this chapter.)

Operative Technique for Rectal Atresia

Nixon (1961) describes a simple technique of a nonsutured anastomosis which appears to be satisfactory.*

> The rectum is mobilised by an abdominal approach. In this condition it is not attached to the urethra (or vagina in the female). A large bougie is passed up the blind anal pouch and the apex of the pouch can be felt from within the abdomen as it comes through the levator floor. A cruciate incision is made in the apex of the pouch. Four catgut sutures are inserted – one in each corner of the incised pouch – each then takes a bite of the rectal wall about 1½ inches from its end leaving the sutures loose. The rectum is then drawn through to the perineum and the internal sutures can be tied. The excess rectum is loosely sutured to the perineal skin. The rectum adheres to the upper end of the anal pouch. In practice the excess bowel shrinks and sloughs off and its excision is not required. Dilatation of the non-suture anastomosis should be carried out to avoid stenosis from the tenth day onwards.

---

*Reprinted with permission from Nixon, H. H.: *Imperforate Anus, British Surgical Practice* (Surgical Progress Volume, 1961) (London: Butterworth & Co., Ltd., 1961).

However, we would agree with Louw (1965) that it is preferable to define the pubo-rectalis initially from the sacro-coccygeal route to be quite certain that the rectum is drawn through in the correct plane.

Postoperative Care

IMMEDIATE.—Intravenous infusion and nasogastric aspiration are continued until adequate bowel sounds are detected, and until the volume of aspirate is suitably reduced. Urethral catheter drainage is discontinued after 48 hours provided the fistula was tied off, but longer otherwise, and while the catheter is in situ infection is prevented by two daily washouts with 0.2% neomycin solution. In the presence of a colostomy, normal diet may be resumed once intravenous infusion has ceased. Antibiotics are prescribed. The nursing staff is instructed to avoid taking rectal temperatures. The buttock is left exposed.

PROLONGED AFTERCARE.—Success or failure may often depend upon the ability of the surgeon to supervise the aftercare management over the next few months. Inadequate follow-up may result in severe degrees of constipation and secondary megacolon, which seriously interfere with bowel training and result in almost certain incontinence.

(1) Dilatation of the Pubo-rectalis Sling.—On the 14th postoperative day, the pubo-rectalis sling should be gently dilated through the new anal canal daily with urethral sounds or Hegar dilators. The dilatation must be slow and gentle so that the tunnel is gradually enlarged. Before hospital discharge, 12–14-size dilators will usually be accommodated, and the child is discharged for the mother to continue daily digital dilatation. At approximately 2–3 weeks after operation, she is instructed in the method of dilatation, first with the little finger and progressively to work through the 3d to the index fingers during the next 2 months. Once the dilatation has achieved sufficient size and suppleness of the sling, no further dilatations are necessary. The surgeon should check the anal lumen and the mother's technique from time to time during this period.

(2) Prevention of Constipation.—Several factors predispose to constipation—any tendency to anal stenosis, inadequate dilatation of the pubo-rectalis tunnel and lack of neural reflexes to the rectum. From the time of closure of the colostomy, we place these infants on a regular daily dose of aperient and instruct the parents to examine the stool. The stools should be soft and regular. Should the stools become hard, the child is in danger of developing rectal inertia and secondary megacolon, which necessitates a regimen of bowel washouts. An established secondary megacolon is a complication, and its treatment is described in Chapter 14.

(3) Bowel Training.—The baby should be "sat out" regularly to develop the habit of daily defecation, and training proceeds as in a normal child. There may be frequent accidents during the toddler period, but rectal control may be expected to occur soon after the age of normal children if a strong pubo-rectalis action can be detected on rectal examination. Parental encouragement is required over the early years when soiling seems to imply failure. The preadolescent child is frequently quite unconcerned about anal dirtiness, and the parents are prone to make accusations of laziness. Small degrees of soiling may dramatically improve when the child begins to take an interest in cleanliness and learns to evacuate completely.

(4) "Toilet Tricks."—Despite the use of a skin flap in rectal repairs, and in most anal repairs, there is usually some degree of exposed mucosa at the anus, below the level of the levator muscle. Even with perfect control of the fecal stream, a little feces or mucus may remain in this exposed sleeve of mucosa after defecation and make a stain on the pants. The child must be taught to evacuate completely at the time, and to clean the whole sleeve at the end of defecation. This is not difficult because the anal verge is not tightly closed. Furthermore, it is useful to carry tissues and, according to need, dry the mucus from the sleeve. Such "tricks" may almost eliminate itchy perineal skin and stains on pants.

CHAPTER 10

Operative Management of Anal Deformities
(Translevator and Intermediate Lesions)

THE PRESENT chapter is confined to the operative techniques and postoperative care applicable to the anal anomalies. The rationale of choice of procedure in each specific anal deformity has been discussed in Chapters 3 and 4, which should be referred to in conjunction with this chapter.

As in high rectal deformities, the chief effective sphincter available for subsequent fecal control is the pubo-rectalis section of the levator ani muscle. In anal deformities, the internal sphincter is often absent or rudimentary. The deep external sphincter is sometimes effectively developed, but the remainder of the external anal sphincter rarely provides a useful contribution to control. However, in the low anal deformities, the surgical problem is considerably easier as the rectum is embraced by the pubo-rectalis sling, and operation is confined to establishing a satisfactory anal orifice where it lies, or at the anterior location of the fistula or after transplanting it backwards to its normal site.

Management Before Newborn Anoplasty

1. Preliminary Investigations.—Reference should be made to Chapter 8, Diagnosis and Investigations, and to the individual lesions discussed in Chapters 3 and 4 for details in obtaining the maximal information about the internal anatomy of the pelvis and other deformities.

These are summarized as follow:

(a) Careful inspection of the perineum, especially in females, by clinical examination, probe or scope for all orifices or for a tract containing meconium or gas. In the presence of a "covered vulva," the midline fusion may need to be divided before adequate inspection is possible (see Fig. 105).

(b) Examination for other anomalies, especially the passage of a nasogastric tube to exclude tracheo-esophageal fistula.

(c) An anteroposterior radiograph to indicate the presence of vertebral, especially sacral, defects.

(d) Invertography is essential for defining the noncommunicating anomalies. In the communicating lesions with a demonstrable perineal fistula, although it is not essential for diagnosis and is open to errors of interpretation, invertography is still worthwhile to define the lowest level of the rectum.

(e) Similarly, a small amount of radiopaque dye injected into the fistula, into a stenotic orifice, or by percutaneous injection of the rectum, may add further useful information, especially in regard to length of the fistula or the stenosis or the depth of the rectum from the perineum.

(f) Clinical assessment of the sacral nerve supply—a "dropped" paralytic perineum, expressible bladder and perineal anesthesia, in the presence of severe sacral agenesis or myelomeningocele indicates involvement of rectal sphincters. Such paralysis does not necessarily preclude the performance of anoplasty. Anoplasty establishes an opening for the bowel, and, if total incontinence ensues because of the neurogenic state, a decision to perform colostomy can be made much later after thorough trials of treatment.

2. Preoperative Preparation.—The usual steps prior to any neonatal operation are instituted and are summarized without discussion.

(a) Recording of weight
(b) Isolette nursing at controlled temperature, humidity and oxygen concentration
(c) Nasogastric catheter and aspiration
(d) Vitamin K
(e) Antibiotics
(f) An intravenous infusion may be required occasionally

Anoplasty

The term "anoplasty" is a confusing one and should be reserved for techniques which enlarge or define the anal orifice and which do not involve mobilization of rectum. However, so many variants of perineal procedure have been described, varying in degree from a simple "cutback" of a fistula, through transplantation of an anus, to radical rectoplasty via the perineum or sacro-perineal route, that we now use the term for any procedure in the perineum involving reconstruction of the anal canal for anal anomalies.

A. Anal "Cutback" Procedure

In this simple procedure, no dissection is made into the sphincters. We favor this operation for *ano-cutaneous fistulae, covered anus*

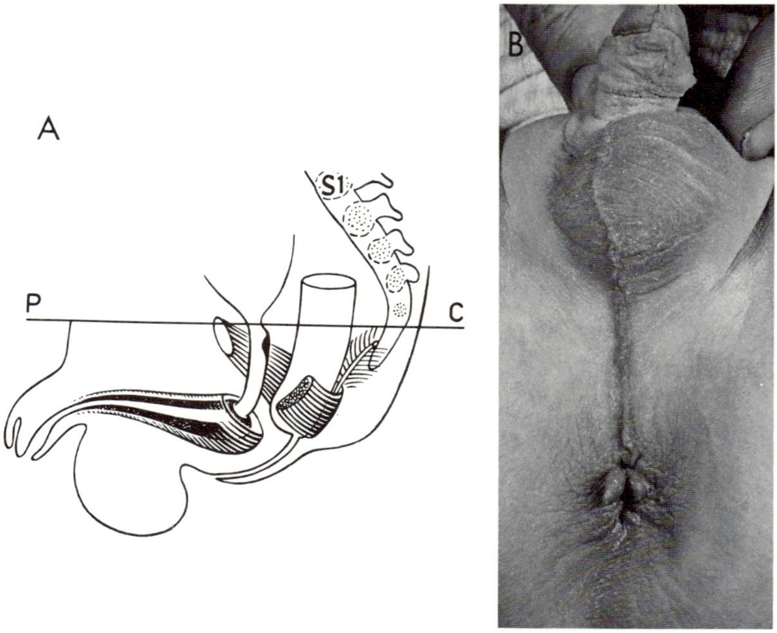

Fig. 121. – Covered anus – ano-cutaneous fistula – male. **A,** subcutaneous tract leads back towards the anal dimple and to the patent rectum. Note that no significant muscle is destroyed by laying open the tract. **B,** postoperative appearances after the laying open of the tract. Skin tags are present, but anus is normal in size and suppleness. Compare preoperative appearance in Figure 44,*A*.

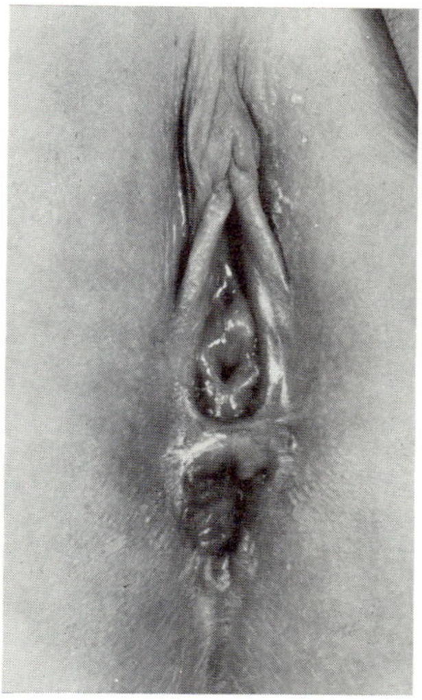

Fig. 122. – Covered anus – ano-cutaneous fistula – female. Appearance after cutback procedure. Note gaping anus, skin bridge between anus and vestibule. Compare preoperative appearances in Figure 106,*B*.

complete and covered anal stenosis, imperforate anal membrane and *anal membrane stenosis*, in either sex, and in the female for *ano-vulvar* and *ano-vestibular fistulae*. It is advised in most of the British literature, e.g., Stephens (1953), Partridge and Gough (1961) and Nixon (1961) and also favored by Sommerschild *et al.* (1964) and by Louw (1965).

The reader is referred to Chapter 11 for a discussion of the value of rectal biopsy at the time of the "cutback."

ANO-CUTANEOUS FISTULA.—*Male.*—A small lachrymal probe is passed along the fistulous tract, which is usually very fine. The tract is laid open by a scissors cut from before backward strictly in the midline. The posterior part of the tract dips into the anal pit, and here the tissues are thicker. At this point, the laid-open tract meets the terminal bowel, and a gush of meconium ensues. The cut is made sufficiently far back to permit the introduction of size 22 urethral sounds. No sutures of anal mucosa to skin are necessary, unless to arrest bleeding. Healing is rapid along the narrow raw area be-

Fig. 123.—Covered anus—ano-vulvar fistula. **A,** posterior border of vestibule overhangs the orifice of the fistula. Small polyp lying beside the orifice; arrow indicates the site of the orifice. **B,** cutback procedure—one blade of scissors in the orifice and one on the skin. A short midline cut is made through the thin skin to enlarge the orifice sufficiently to dilate with the tip of the 5th finger. Dotted line indicates the line of the cut. **C,** appearance after cutback procedure—anus separated from the vestibule by the fourchette (*arrow*). The anus is continent, and feces are directed away from the vestibule. The untidy skin tags may require removal later.

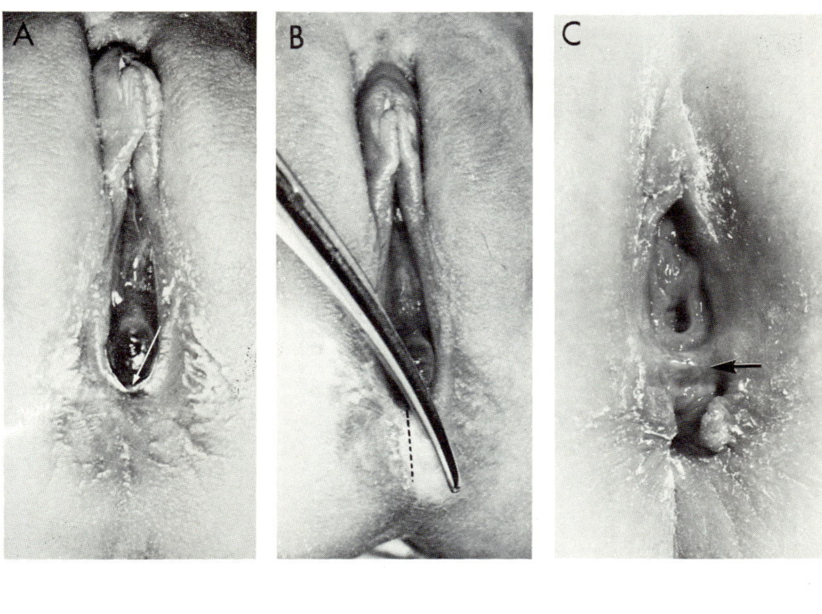

tween epithelium of skin and epithelium of bowel, and scar formation is unusual (Fig. 121).

Female.—The procedure is identical, but the tract is much shorter and wider in caliber, accommodating an ordinary probe or sound (Fig. 122).

ANO-VULVAR FISTULA.—The fistula is longer and more closely resembles that of the male ano-cutaneous fistula, and the same procedure applies. The cut commences on the posterior edge of the fistula, which will be the dry skin on the posterior border of the fourchette (Figs. 123 and 124).

COVERED ANUS COMPLETE AND COVERED ANAL STENOSIS.—Many patients with stenosis require only dilatation (Figs. 125 and 126), but a posterior hypertrophied band of fused genital folds is better incised by "cutback" to hasten the dilatation. Sometimes, the posterior fusion is a rectangular plaque or shield, and this can be undercut and turned in as a small skin flap. Untidy skin tags may require trimming at a later period, but it is surprising how ridges and tags even out spontaneously. No sutures are necessary, apart from those required for hemostasis.

IMPERFORATE ANAL MEMBRANE AND ANAL MEMBRANE STENOSIS.—Cruciate or multiple radial incisions of the membrane are required,

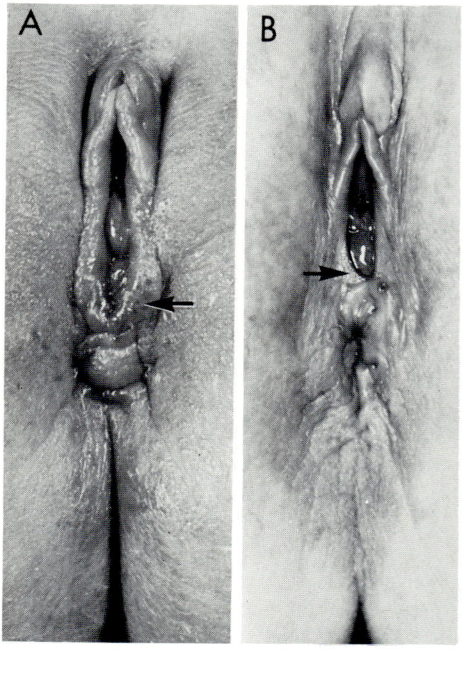

Fig. 124.—Covered anus—ano-vulvar fistula. **A,** anal fistula (*arrow*) covered by fused genital folds. **B,** after cutback procedure, fourchette and rudimentary perineum are exposed (*arrow*), but anus is quite separate from vestibule.

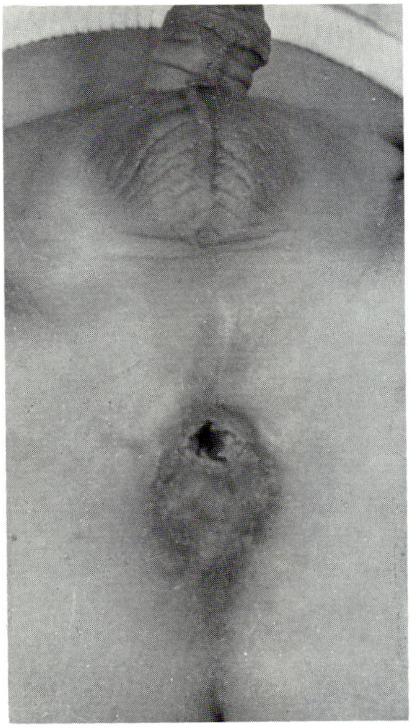

Fig. 125. — Anal stenosis of covered anus type. Anal orifice dilated at and soon after birth; anus patulous but continent. Note heaped-up skin behind anus.

Fig. 126. — Anal stenosis — covered anus type. **A,** arrow marks site of stenosed anus with heaped-up folds posterior to it. **B,** anus (*arrow*) 15 years later after anal dilatation only. Note spontaneous regression of post anal tubercles.

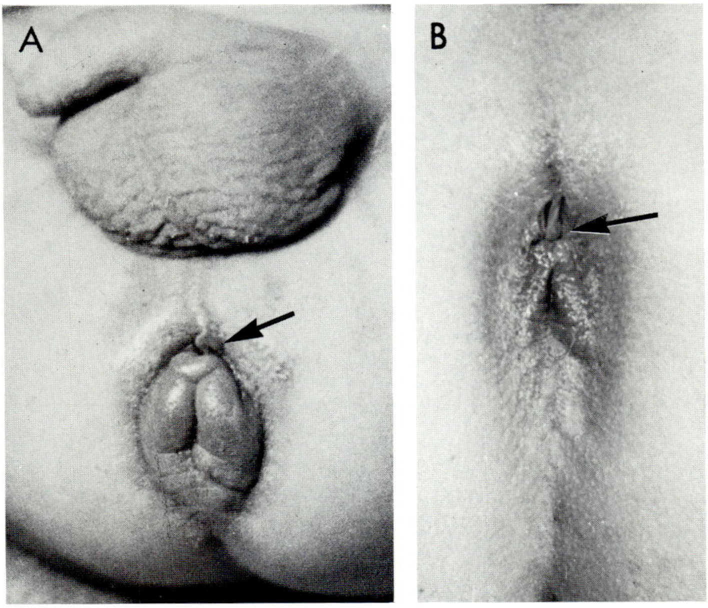

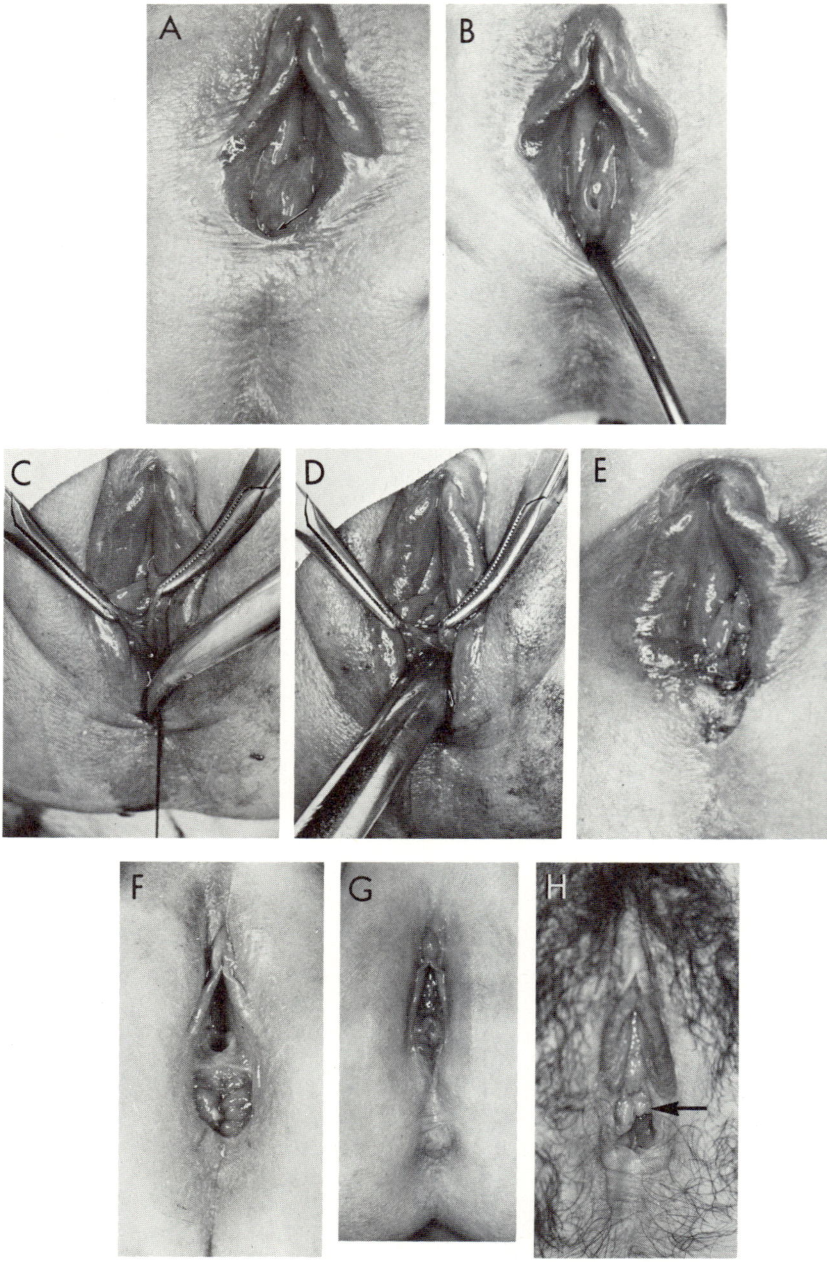

Fig. 127.—Ano-vestibular fistula. **A–E,** cutback procedure. **A,** stenosed orifice of fistula hidden by overhanging border of vestibule (*arrow*). **B,** small sound in

followed by digital dilatation during the subsequent period of infancy. The membrane should not be excised.

ANO-VESTIBULAR FISTULA. – We prefer a cutback procedure for the majority of these patients, even if subsequently a transplantation of the anus backward is desired for cosmetic or psychological reasons. In this deformity, however, only the resistant posterior rim of the orifice is incised, followed by dilatations (Fig. 127). Dilatation alone splits the anterior part of the orifice and the vaginal septum, making one common orifice out of two discrete orifices. This creates soiling and vulvitis and is a complication which is readily avoided.

Sommerschild *et al.* (1964) describe a modification of the cutback procedure. Believing that the external sphincter is divided by the cutback they attributed some cases of incompetence to this occurrence. They recommended a two-stage procedure to ensure anchorage of the anterior portion of the external sphincter before division. In the first stage, "a linen ligature is placed around the anterior portion of the sphincter. The fibrosis which develops during the course of 2–3 weeks fixes the muscle fibers when they are divided at the second session. This ensures that the sphincter will be competent, as was found to be true in our 6 patients so treated."

We do not believe that continence is dependent on the external sphincter.

B. ANAL TRANSPLANT PROCEDURES

As an alternative to "cutback," many American authors dissect and mobilize the bowel freely and establish it amidst the voluntary external sphincter fibers. Judging by the various descriptions, the dissection is apparently quite deep, as indicated by the advice to have a urethral catheter in situ as a guide (Potts *et al.* (1954), Rhoads and Koop (1955), Trusler and Wilkinson (1962) and Santulli (1963).

Santulli's description (1963) of operation for a male "recto-perineal fistula" (ano-cutaneous fistula, our classification) is typical of

---

orifice, which passes cranially. **C,** division of the posterior rim of the orifice and posterior border of vestibule with scissors. Note the thinness of vaginal septum between tips of hemostats. **D,** large sound then readily introduced into the rectum. **E,** shelving incision leading to the enlarged and exposed orifice. **F–H,** appearances after cutback procedure. **F,** ano-vestibular fistula. Patulous anus, but continent anal canal. **G,** ano-vestibular fistula. Orifice of fistula enlarged by midline cut, continent anus. Note the tuft of skin overlying the normal site of anus. **H,** ano-vestibular fistula – patient aged 16 years. Anus patulous but continent, clean and tucked up within the vestibule; arrow marks the vaginal orifice. (For original appearance of vulva, see Fig. 63,*A*.

this approach. Two separate incisions are utilized, one encircling the fistula, the other overlying the external sphincter. The fistula and rectum are mobilized freely from the levator through the anterior incision. The bowel is brought back to the posterior incision within the external sphincter muscle. In some cases, if the fistula is close to the anterior commissure of the sphincter, the muscle fibers are divided and then reconstituted. A urethral catheter is inserted "in order to help identify the urethra and avoid injury to it during mobilisation of the anterior rectal wall."

Similarly, in ano-cutaneous fistula in the female, Santulli (1963) transplants the rectum backwards, utilizing two separate incisions, ensuring that there is a wide bridge of normal skin between the anterior incision near the vulva and the new anus.

Santulli disagrees with those authors (Gross, 1953; Kiesewetter, 1956; and Swenson, 1958) who advocate splitting the external sphincter into lateral halves and deliberately making the anal orifice larger than normal. If more exposure is needed, Santulli divides the posterior commissural fibers but repairs them at the end of the procedure.

We cannot see the necessity for the extensive mobilization of the anus and rectum indicated by these operative descriptions. The anal mucosa is very close to the perineal skin, and the orifice functions adequately where it lies, once an adequate opening has been established by the cutback. We believe that the technique described by Santulli and others is based upon an undue emphasis on the value of the external sphincter and on the erroneous idea that the covered anal canal (and not just the fistula) is sited anterior to the external sphincter. Further, the extensive mobilization would seem potentially dangerous, for, even in low anal anomalies, the levator is still the chief muscle of continence, and its fibers are vulnerable in the dissection.

TRANSPLANTATION FOR RECTO-VAGINAL AND ANO-VESTIBULAR FISTULAE.—As discussed in Chapter 4, we have shown that the rectum in recto-vaginal fistulae at any level lies cranial to the levator ani, and we manage them as in other rectal deformities, by sacro-perineal or sacro-abdomino-perineal exposure. Fistulae low in the vagina can be approached safely by the sacro-perineal route alone, but high fistulae may require abdominal mobilization. Both types are preceded by colostomy, and the technique is described fully in the preceding chapter.

As regards ano-vestibular fistulae, it is our experience that most require only enlargement of the orifice and do not require transplantation at any time of life. We reserve transplantation for selected patients in whom, after several years, there persists some degree of

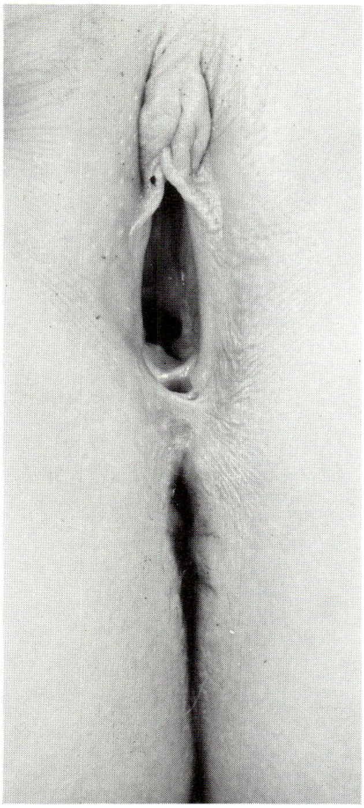

Fig. 128. – Postoperative appearance of anus after transplantation from previous site in the vestibule. Transplantation became necessary because of vulval contamination. The transplantation was performed via a sacro-perineal approach.

genital soiling. Previously, we have used a technique for such transplantation through two separate incisions in the perineum, one encircling the fistula and the other at the anal site; the rectum has been freed and moved back precisely in the manner described by Nixon (1961), below. However, as this dissection requires mobilization of the rectum from below the levator sling, it is not easy to secure the necessary length of rectum without endangering the pubo-rectalis muscle; recurrence of fistula has followed such an operation. Consequently, we now perform the transplant through the sacro-perineal approach (Fig. 128), through which adequate length of bowel can be assured without danger to the pubo-visceral sling. No dissection is required below the levator, except for the disconnection of the fistula from the vestibular wall. This circumcision of the orifice is performed immediately prior to turning the child into the jackknife position for the sacro-coccygeal part of the operation.

This approach to low recto-vaginal fistulae and ano-vestibular fistulae is at variance with that of most other surgeons, in both technique and indications for transplantation. In the view of most surgeons, all are transplanted, and an enlarged orifice of an ano-vestibular fistula is considered not acceptable in its forward site. The entire operation is performed through the perineal incisions. While not agreeing with these views, we include a description of different techniques by several surgeons.

Historically, anal transplantation was a development from the numerous modifications of perineal exploration. Two separate transverse incisions are utilized by a great many surgeons, e.g., Stone (1936), David (1937), Murdock (1941), Hanley *et al.* (1954), Potts *et al.* (1954), Davis (1959), Nixon (1961), Oeconomopoulos (1961), Snyder (1961), Santulli (1963) and Sitkovskii (1966). Most modern procedures are based on Stone's operation (1936).

SANTULLI'S OPERATION (1963).—This procedure is used for recto-vaginal and ano-vestibular fistulae.*

A special table with leg holders and shoulder braces is used, or the infant's legs may be folded over the abdomen and held in place with long strips of adhesive tape. . . .

The external anal sphincter muscle is precisely located with the help of an electrical muscle stimulator and a 1.5 cm vertical skin incision is made within the muscle. The deeper tissues are spread and the muscle is gently dilated with a curved clamp to the size of a number 10 Hegar dilator. Another incision is made encircling the fistula and the lower part of this incision extended laterally on either side. The rectum is freed posteriorly and laterally well up into the hollow of the sacrum. The anterior rectal wall is carefully separated from the posterior vaginal wall. The dissection is frequently carried up to the anterior peritoneal reflection in order to obtain sufficient length for the new position of the rectum. The fistula is brought down beneath the perineum and pulled through the incision within the sphincter muscle. The deeper tissues are approximated anterior to the rectum with a few sutures of chromic catgut. The vaginal defect, if any, is closed with absorbable sutures and the transverse skin extensions of this incision are approximated with fine interrupted nonabsorbable sutures. The anus is constructed by sewing the full thickness of bowel wall to the skin with interrupted nonabsorbable sutures. The mucocutaneous line should turn upward in order to prevent prolapse and to have the skin supply sensation to the newly created anus. However, it is of the utmost importance to avoid any tension on the suture line. At the completion of the procedure, the anal canal should be as large as a number 10 Hegar dilator (32 French catheter).

Comment.—Our principal objection is to the perineal dissection of the rectum "posteriorly and laterally well up into the hollow of the sacrum." We feel such an extensive dissection must be within the levator and could gravely endanger the pubo-rectalis and its lateral inferior nerve supply. Yet without such mobilization, adequate rectal length will not be obtained.

*Reprinted with permission from Mustard, W. T., *et al.* (eds.): *Pediatric Surgery* (2d ed.; Chicago: Year Book Medical Publishers, Inc., 1969).

NIXON'S OPERATION (1961*).—This procedure is used for low recto-vaginal and ano-vestibular fistula, referred to by Nixon as "ectopic anus."

The technique is similar to that described by Santulli above, but without the extensive dissection of the rectum above the levator ani. Nixon performs the operation when the child is about 4 years of age.

1. The ectopic anus should be mobilised from an incision along the posterior border of the vulva and its orifice circumcised. A separate incision should be made at the normal anal site. The midline incision often shown running back from ectopic to normal site gives excellent exposure, but it heals with contracture forwards and upwards so that the anus may return very nearly to the original position. The bridge of intact skin should be preserved between ectopic and normal anal sites.

2. Denis Browne suggested the insertion of a wide rubber tube into the bowel and temporary suture of this to the bowel end before further mobilisation. It forms a very convenient guide in dissection and tractor in transplantation.

3. Mobilisation of the bowel should extend only up to the levator floor. Higher dissection, to minimize the risk of tension, is unwise. The blood supply along the wall of the mobilised bowel is inadequate and breakdown likely. Retraction above the levator can cause a severe disabling fibrosis of the pelvic floor. The aim should rather be to bring skin up to meet the bowel and deepen the natal cleft. Partial breakdown after this limited mobilisation may necessitate dilatations under anaesthesia but does not seem to jeopardize the final result.

4. Care is needed in dissection to avoid cutting into the bowel wall or fistula may follow. Buttonholing of the posterior vaginal wall (the only difficult phase of separation) does not matter. Such holes may be left to heal spontaneously.

5. After mobilisation an ellipse of skin is excised at the normal anal site so as to avoid a tight inelastic ring of skin-mucosal junction. Blunt dissection is carried up through the strap of muscle representing the external sphincter and then forwards superficial to the pelvic floor tunnelling to the anterior dissection. The rubber tube is seized and used to draw the bowel back and out at the new anal site.

6. Suturing should be in two layers. Several catgut sutures should be placed from the bowel to the pelvic floor to take some of the tension inevitable in defaecation, before the skin is sutured to the end of the bowel.

7. A perineal body is formed by one or two deep catgut sutures joining the deep tissues from either side in front of the displaced bowel. This presumably unites the anterior ends of what external sphincter is present as well as building up a more normal appearance. The excellent continence achieved without transplantation, however, suggests that this sphincter is less important than the levator and, in particular, the puborectalis sling.

8. The opening left in the posterior vaginal wall at the original anal site is

*Reprinted with permission from Nixon, H. H.: *Imperforate Anus, British Surgical* Practice (Surgical Progress Volume, 1961) (London: Butterworth & Co., Ltd., 1961).

loosely closed about a suction drain. Gentle hydrostatic suction for 3–4 days prevents the collection of a haematoma—a potential cause of infection and hence fistula formation.

9. Colostomy is not necessary with this technique. In any event it would not prevent breakdown or fistula formation if the safeguards mentioned were not adhered to.

10. It appears that the cases requiring transplantation are mainly the vestibular type.

Louw (1965) describes an almost identical procedure for both lesions, which he performs when the patient is about 4 years of age; he treats the lesions at birth by a simple "cutback."

SWENSON AND DONNELLAN'S OPERATION (1967).—This procedure is used for low recto-vaginal and ano-vestibular fistulae.*

These surgeons also use a perineal approach and perform operation in the neonatal period without colostomy. They admit to the difficulty of the operation in the infant.

The technique begins with a circumferential incision around the opening of the rectovaginal fistula. A number of 6–0 sutures are then placed about the delicate edges of the fistula so that reasonable traction can be accomplished without tearing the tissue. The dissection should be carried along the upper margin of the fistula down to the junction of the vagina with the colonic wall. The most difficult part of the operation is to separate the fistula from the posterior vaginal wall without tearing either structure. By careful dissection with slightly blunt, plastic-type scissors it is possible to develop an adequate plane. At this stage of the operation the levator is densely adherent to the fistula and colon, and it must be dissected away sharply on the lateral and posterior sides. A common mistake is to remove a portion of the levators with the colon during this dissection. It is prudent to check the accuracy of the dissection by placing a clamp inside the lumen of the bowel from time to time, in order to demonstrate the thickness of the colonic wall which is being preserved. The dissection becomes progressively easier as the separation of the vaginal and colonic walls proceeds.

The bowel must be freed extensively so that it can be brought back behind a perineal body about 1 cm in diameter. The site for the anal opening is then selected and a double diamond incision is fashioned which increases the skin circumference and removes the poorly vascularized central perineal skin. This incision should be at least 1 cm posterior to the rectovaginal fistula so that a band of skin of that width is left intact between the new anal opening and the dissection of the area around the rectovaginal fistula. The next step is to undermine the skin so that the puborectalis sling and the levator can be gently stretched posteriorly to permit the colon to be brought out through the new perineal opening. Unless this is performed very diligently, the levator sling will be so unyielding that it will tend to pull the bowel forward again and promote recurrence of the rectovaginal fistula. After the puborectalis and levator sling have been sufficiently stretched, the perineal body is reconstruct-

*Reprinted with permission from Swenson, O., and Donnellan, W. L.: S. Clin. North America 47:173, 1967.

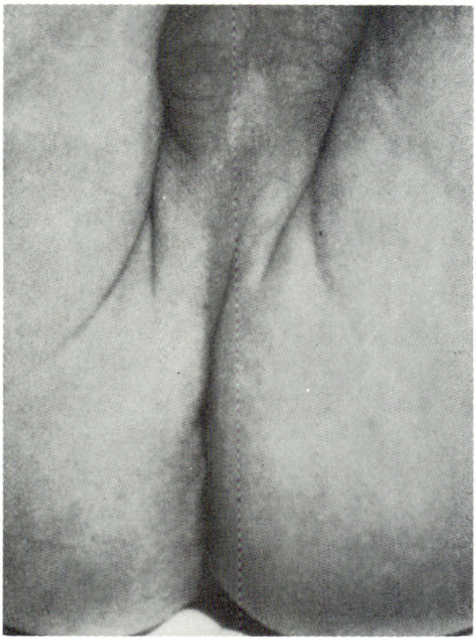

Fig. 129.—Appearance of anus after technique of anoplasty as described by Swenson and Donnellan (1967). Anal mucosa hidden by new buttocks folds created by the operation in both males and females. (Reproduced with permission from Swenson, O., and Donnellan, W. L.: S. Clin. North America 47:173, 1967.)

ed through the vagina with a series of 4/0 chromic catgut sutures. It is not necessary to bring the edges of the vaginal fistula too carefully into approximation, but if the fistula is not entirely vaginal the skin edges should be carefully approximated with silk sutures.

Construction of the new anal opening is then undertaken. In order to maintain the levator sling adjacent to the skin, a series of 5/0 chromic catgut sutures are placed which unite the subcutaneous tissue, the edge of the levator, and the muscular wall of the colon. These sutures are placed all around the bowel and are then tied and cut successively. The object of this row of sutures is to hold the levator and the skin edge close together. As the levator contracts it will pull the skin up into a deep inner gluteal fold, which is advantageous to the patient, because it will prevent the distressing mucus discharge which occurs when the rectal mucosa is allowed to protrude [Fig. 129].

A row of interrupted 5/0 silk sutures is placed between the skin, the edge of the levator, and the full thickness of the rectal wall. As in the perineal portion of the abdominoperineal operation, it is important to leave space for tissue swelling to occur. This can be accomplished by placing a small curved clamp under each suture before it is tied, in order to assure that the knot is not being drawn down too tightly.

Other Modifications.—Minor modifications at the anal anastomosis were suggested by David (1937), and Murdock (1941) in an effort to prevent the bowel moving back to its previous site and also to reduce the area of wet mucosal ectropion. David turned in two lateral skin flaps, and Murdock turned in a U-flap of skin. Sitkovskii (1966) describes a further modification of buckling the rectal wall itself to aid continence. Like other authors, Sitkovskii stresses the use of the external sphincter.

C. Proctoplasty for Recto-Bulbar Fistula and Anal Agenesis (No Fistula)

In these two lesions, we use the term "proctoplasty" to stress (1) the necessity for adequate mobilization of the rectum, (2) that the agenesis of the anus makes the word "anoplasty" seem inappropriate and (3) to indicate some similarity to rectoplasty, in that the procedure is deferred to a later elective time after preliminary neonatal colostomy.

Stephens (1963) described the perineal route to these lesions (after colostomy), with success in those patients exhibiting a very thin perineum (Fig. 130, *B*), but further experience with those in whom the perineum is thick has led us to abandon this route. As in the perineal transplant procedure described above, it was found difficult safely to mobilize sufficient rectal length from below, and this, plus the size of the bulbar fistula, resulted in recurrence of fistula.

Our standard sacro-perineal operation again seemed the logical one to give safe access above the pubo-visceral sling. The lesions are rare, but we have had opportunity to perform three such proctoplasties by this route; the access is adequate to divide the fistula, mobilize the gut and define the pubo-visceral tunnel, and no fistulae have

Fig. 130.—Recto-bulbar fistula. Appearance of anus after perineal anoplasty. **A,** anus widely open and patulous as far cranially as lower margin of pubo-rectalis, which operates quite efficiently, controlling flatus and firm feces in patient C. J., with deep perineum. **B** (see Fig. 33,*C*) with shallow perineum, showing closed shallow anus, also with good control. (Chordee corrected, but hypospadias repair not yet completed.)

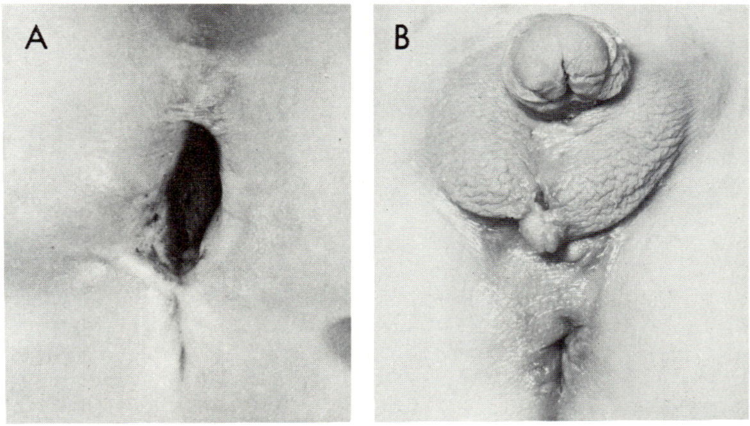

resulted. The technique is identical with that for recto-urethral fistulae.

OTHER AUTHORS.—Recto-bulbar fistula is a lesion rarely referred to in the literature, so that other operative descriptions are rare. In 1928, Barney performed a successful perineal operation for this fistula. Louw (1965) agrees with us in performing neonatal colostomy, but his definitive procedure is a perineal anoplasty.

For the blind lesion of anal agenesis Louw (1965) approaches the bowel through the perineum only, and he does this in the neonatal period. Santulli (1963) similarly uses a perineal approach, although he now precedes this by colostomy (1965).

Postoperative Care

The postoperative care in anal operations is identical with that described after rectoplasty and is only included here in summary form; care is no less important in the anal group, in which severe constipation may develop rapidly.

1. Perineal cleansing of the anus with saline in the first week postoperatively.
2. Anal dilatation after the first 2 weeks and regularly thereafter for several months, as determined from week to week.
3. Prevention of constipation.
4. Commencement of toilet training and use of "toilet tricks."

Follow-up Investigations

Following initial perineal operation, the search for other anomalies, especially urinary, is continued, and bladder control is noted. The special investigations of the ensuing months are outlined in Chapter 8.

CHAPTER 11

Associated Anomalies

(Other Than Genito-Urinary)

ONE OF THE DISTRESSING features of anal and rectal malformations is that there is frequently an associated maldevelopment of other viscera or of the limbs. Unfortunately, many of these associated anomalies are serious, often life threatening, and are related to long-term problems in the urinary, alimentary, cardiac, cerebral and musculo-skeletal systems. The over-all mortality rate is influenced more by these associations than by any other factor.

The fact that there are such widespread developmental errors implies a common influence upon the embryo at a time when many viscera are becoming differentiated from the primitive endoderm and mesoderm. The period of major organ differentiation occurs at the 4–6-mm. stage (4–6 weeks), and it is at this period also that the cloaca is beginning to subdivide. It is not surprising, therefore, that serious multiple anomalies may coexist with rectal deformities.

Over-all Incidence

Excluding the complicated anomaly of "vesico-intestinal fissure," which has been considered as a complex type of rectal deformity, the present series of 246 patients included 149 children with one or more associated anomalies (60.6%).

Many series record the incidence of this association. The figures vary from 20% to over 70% and largely reflect the intensity of investigation to which the infants have been subjected. In many series, only a small number of children had intravenous pyelography performed. The more one investigates, the more anomalies are found. Table 9 is a composite study of the papers of 34 authors, which indicate an over-all incidence of 43.4% with an associated anomaly.

The incidence is much higher in studies of autopsy material, not surprising since death is so often due to an associated anomaly. In the 76 deaths in our series, autopsies were performed on 60 patients,

TABLE 9.—OVER-ALL INCIDENCE OF ASSOCIATED ANOMALIES

	PRESENT SERIES 246 CASES	33 AUTHORS* 3,223 CASES
Associated Anomalies	149 (60.6%)	1,394 (43.4%)

*Crowell and Dulin (1940), Lee (1944), Dmytryk (1945), Norris *et al.* (1949), Mayo and Rice (1950), Arnheim (1951), Bacon and Sherman (1952), Moore and Lawrence (1952), Santulli (1952), Gross (1953), Waite (1954), Palmer (1956), Thompson and Hooks (1956), Parkkulainen (1957), Bradham (1958), Brayton and Norris (1958), Bryndorf and Madsen (1959), Duhamel (1961), Forshall (1960), Scott and Swenson (1960), Shahi and Mishra (1961), Katzen (1962), Lynn and Arcari (1962), McPherson (1962), Swain and Tucker (1962), Swenson and Grana (1962), Trusler and Wilkinson (1962), Kiesewetter *et al.* (1964), Bielowicz (1965), Louw (1965), Shopfner (1965), Berdon *et al.* (1966) and Swenson and Donnellan (1967).

of whom 56 possessed another deformity. In 33 of 34 autopsies in Moore and Lawrence's series (1952), there were associated errors of development.

Incidence in Relation to Sex and Type of Deformity

It is instructive to study the relative incidence of associated anomalies in the various types of anal and rectal deformity. Some guidelines to prognosis may then be deduced.

ANAL AND RECTAL DEFORMITY.—Table 10 indicates relative incidence in the present series compared with three other series.

The occurrence of other anomalies in the rectal group is nearly twice as high as in the anal group. The same tendency was noted by Katzen (1962), Swain and Tucker (1962), Scott and Swenson (1960), Berdon *et al.* (1966) and Swenson and Donnellan (1967). In those series using the Ladd and Gross classifications, a higher incidence is constantly found in types 3 and 4, Norris *et al.* (1949), Brayton and Norris (1952), Moore and Lawrence (1952), Thompson and Hooks (1956) and Duhamel (1960). For the data in Moore and Lawrence's series (1952) see Table 11.

TABLE 10.—INCIDENCE OF ASSOCIATED ANOMALIES IN ANAL AND RECTAL GROUPS

DEFORMITIES	PRESENT SERIES	PARTRIDGE & GOUGH (1961)	LOUW (1965)	SWENSON & DONNELLAN (1967)
Anal	71 of 154 patients (46.1%)	25%	37%	24%
Rectal	78 of 92 patients (84.7%)	62.3%	69%	52%

TABLE 11.—INCIDENCE OF ANOMALIES IN RELATION TO TYPES
(After Moore & Lawrence, 1952)

TYPE	NO. OF CASES	NO. WITH ASSOCIATED ANOMALIES	PER CENT
1	5	3	60
2	20	11	55
3	90	68	76
4	5	4	80
TOTALS	120	86	72

Thus, the prognosis for *rectal deformities* is already biased towards an unfavorable result, not only because of the more difficult technical problems of the rectal repair, but because *over half of them are complicated by a serious associated anomaly.*

The associated deformities in the anal group are not only less common but also more simple to treat and less serious to life.

SEX.—In *anal* anomalies slightly more females have associated aberrations than males, whereas, in the more serious *rectal* anomalies, the males are more frequently affected, thus further militating against success in the male (Table 12).

Mayo and Rice (1950) found that 51.8% of males were affected compared with 36.3% of females. Nineteen (19) of the 24 patients with serious anomalies discussed in the paper by Norris *et al.* (1949) were males, and this same male preponderance of serious anomalies was commented on by Dmytryk (1945), Forshall (1960) and Lynn and Arcari (1962). Berdon *et al.* (1966) found a male preponderance in low anal anomalies, in which one-third had associated anomalies, but none of the females with anal anomalies was so affected in that series.

TABLE 12.—ASSOCIATED ANOMALIES RELATED TO SEX
(Authors' Series)

ANOMALIES	MALES WITH OTHER ANOMALIES	FEMALES WITH OTHER ANOMALIES
Anal	42 of 95 patients (44.2%)	29 of 59 patients (49.2%)
Rectal	56 of 64 patients (87.5%)	22 of 28 patients (78.6%)
TOTALS	98 of 159 patients (61.6%)	51 of 87 patients (58.6%)

RELATION OF TYPES OF ANAL OR RECTAL DEFORMITIES TO THE INCIDENCE OF OTHER MALFORMATIONS.—The incidence of all associated anomalies, including genito-urinary, in the various types of anal or rectal deformities is shown in Table 13 (Melbourne series).

It can be seen that in the common covered anus deformity (in both sexes) of ano-cutaneous fistula less than one third of the patients were affected with an associated problem. Although 92% of recto-bulbar fistulae possessed another anomaly, most of these were relatively minor (9 of 12 anomalies); however, in ano-vestibular fistulae and in the imperforate anal lesions, the spread of anomalies included several serious problems, as in the rectal deformities.

On the other hand, the high incidence of associated anomalies in rectal deformities was spread evenly over all types; many of these problems were serious and often life threatening. Not apparent in Table 13 is the fact that other anomalies were as common in low

TABLE 13.—RELATION OF ASSOCIATED ANOMALIES (INCLUDING GENITO-URINARY) TO TYPE OF ANAL OR RECTAL DEFORMITY

DEFORMITIES	NO. OF PATIENTS	NO. OF PATIENTS WITH ASSOCIATED ANOMALIES
Anal		
Anterior anus	6	3 (50%)
Ano-cutaneous fistula and stenosis	77	24 (31%)
Recto-bulbar fistula	13	12*(92%)
Ano-vestibular fistula	26	15 (58%)
Anal agenesis (no fistula)	11	9 (82%)
Imperforate anal membrane	7	5 (71%)
Anal membrane stenosis	14	3 (21%)
TOTAL	154	71 (46.1%)
Rectal		
Ano-rectal agenesis (no fistula)	18	16 (89%)
Recto-vesical fistula	5	5 (100%)
Recto-urethral fistula	44	38 (79%)
Recto-cloacal fistula	8	7 (88%)
Recto-vaginal fistula (high and low)	8	7 (88%)
Recto-vestibular fistula	7	3 (43%)
Rectal atresia	2	2 (100%)
TOTAL	92	78 (84.7%)

*Includes hypospadias.

vaginal deformities as in other high rectal groups, supporting our contention that low vaginal deformities should be considered in the "high" group and treated similarly. Louw (1965) also found a similar association.

The figures showing the incidence of the various systems involved in each of the subtypes of anal and rectal deformities are too scattered for assessment, but the accumulated figures are shown in Table 14.

These figures are comparable with those reported by Louw (1965). In *anal* deformities, urinary abnormalities occurred in one fifth of the patients, although in approximately half of these the problem was not a serious one. Only 17% possessed a vertebral anomaly, a fact of considerable importance, in that it means that in the large majority of anal deformities the levator muscle is normal, both in development and in its nerve supply.

In *rectal* deformities, however, over one third of the children possessed a urinary abnormality, and usually it was serious. Forty per cent of the rectal malformations were accompanied by a vertebral abnormality. The commonest problem was a variable degree of sacral malformation, affecting the integrity of the levator ani and its nerve supply. Some infants are, therefore, doomed to neurogenic incontinence.

Individual Systems

Very frequently more than one additional anomaly occurs in the same patient. Almost every known congenital malformation has been reported in the comprehensive lists of anomalies prepared by various authors, and, as in our own series, no list will be complete. However, certain associations appear to be more common, and the discussion is confined to these. No attempt is made to discuss the investigation and treatment of lesions having no immediate relation to the anal or rectal deformity (such as cardiac malformations, cleft lip and palate, duodenal atresia, limb deformities, etc.), except insofar as these might affect the timing of intervention.

TABLE 14.–THE SYSTEMS INVOLVED IN THE ASSOCIATED ANOMALIES
(Authors' Series)

		NUMBER OF PATIENTS WITH ANOMALIES				
DEFORMITIES	NO. OF PATIENTS	Genito-Urinary	Verte-bral	Alimen-tary	Cardiac	Other
Anal	154	33(21%)	26(17%)	11(7%)	14(9%)	34(22%)
Rectal	92	34(37%)	37(40%)	14(15%)	8(9%)	18(20%)
TOTALS	246	67(27%)	63(26%)	25(10%)	22(9%)	52(21%)

A. Vertebral

Associated vertebral anomalies are common, especially in rectal deformities. They occurred in 63 of 246 patients (26%) in this series, in 17% of anal deformities and in 40% of rectal deformities. These figures are comparable to those of other authors. Williams and Nixon (1957) found 12 abnormal sacrums in 51 patients with imperforate anus and rectum; Parkkulainen (1957), 7 of 51 patients; Stephens (1953), 19 of 48 patients (17 of 27 rectal cases); Kiesewetter *et al.* (1964), 44 of 146 patients; and Louw (1965), 24 of 95 rectal anomalies but only 5 of 103 anal anomalies.

Berdon *et al.* (1966) describe an unusual lumbo-sacral anomaly (8 cases) consisting of a vertical lucent area dividing the lumbar vertebra into two parts and a narrowing of the adjacent disc space. All were in patients with high rectal agenesis, and all had sacral and urinary anomalies.

In a small number (12 of our 63 patients), the vertebral defect was a diffuse one, consisting of multiple hemivertebrae, vertebral arch deformities, absent vertebrae and fused ribs, affecting the cervical, thoracic or lumbar chain (Fig. 131). The majority (51 of 63 patients) had a deformity confined to the sacrum and/or coccyx. Nearly one half of the patients with rectal deformities had an abnormal sacrum, three times the frequency in anal deformities.

The sole significance, yet the vital one, of these sacral abnormalities is their bearing on the integrity of the sacral nerve roots and the associated development of the levator ani. Severe sacral agenesis may be associated with defective innervation to the bladder and to the anal and levator sphincters as well as with structural deficiency of the levator ani. The types of sacral aberration seen were reported in a paper by one of us (Smith, 1959). Until 1950, only 43 cases of congenital anomalies of the sacrum had been reported since the original description by Hohl, in 1852. Freedman (1950) reviewed these 43 cases and summarized the urological, orthopedic and neurological manifestations. Other reports have followed (Del Duca *et al.*, 1951; Peral, 1953; Katz, 1953; Valentine, 1953; Soothill, 1954; Strom-Matheson, 1954; Jaros, 1956; Giordani, 1957; Paris *et al.*, 1957; and Williams and Nixon, 1957).

Most authors have referred to this anomaly as agenesis of the sacrum, a term which denotes suppression of one or more whole sacral vertebrae. In more than one third of the examples in Smith's series (1959), however, only one side of the sacrum was affected, a condition akin to the hemivertebrae seen more commonly higher up the vertebral column.

These two main groups were identified in an original classification by Foix and Hillemond, quoted by Zeligs (1940), in which they recog-

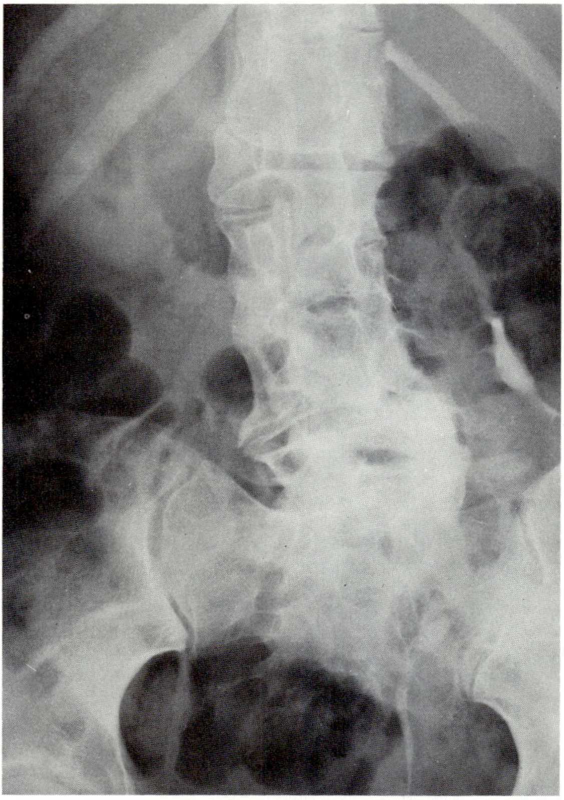

Fig. 131.—Vertebral deformities. Recto-vaginal fistula. Lumbar spine exhibits fused and hemivertebrae.

nized complete and subtotal agenesis, and, in addition, cases of hemiagenesis or hemihypoplasia, terms applied to defects on only one side of the sacrum.

Combinations of both groups make for confusion, as when a sacrum is found exhibiting absence of the 4th and 5th segments (agenesis) combined with defective formation of one lateral mass (hemiagenesis).

It is advisable to exclude from the discussion that condition which has been described as epistasis, a term which connotes a sacrum of four segments in combination with six lumbar vertebrae. Such a short sacrum is better described as an anatomical variant than as a malformation. Epistasis is accompanied by normal innervation of the sacral outflow (Williams and Nixon, 1957).

Epistasis may, nevertheless, be associated with agenesis of the coccyx or one or more of the distal sacral vertebrae, and here the nerve and sacral defects must be equated to the number of vertebrae present in the spinal column rather than to the number absent.

In this study, the sacral anomalies fell into two groups (Fig. 132 and see Figs. 46 and 50).

Agenesis

1. Total—the whole sacrum is absent.
2. Subtotal—the sacrum lacks four, three, two or one of its whole segments.

Hemisacrum

1. Total—in which all sacral segments are present on one side but lack the corresponding half on the other side.
2. Subtotal—in which all sacral segments are present on one side but one or more of the bodies and lateral masses on the opposite side is developmentally defective.

Both lateral and anteroposterior radiographs are necessary to display the abnormalities. A lateral view provides information regarding the number of sacral segments present, but only the anteroposterior view differentiates between the agenesis and hemisacrum groups.

In the young infant, it is not easy to interpret the x-ray film accurately because of minor variations in the rate of appearance of sacral ossific centers, but most anomalies can usually be recognized if the possibility of a sacral defect is kept in mind.

AGENESIS.—In total agenesis the disposition of the iliac bones varies. In 1 patient the iliac bones, being set close together, articu-

Fig. 132.—Associated sacral defects. **A,** recto-urethral fistula—absence of S3, 4 and 5. **B,** recto-urethral fistula—hemisacral defect of S3 and 4 and absence of S5.

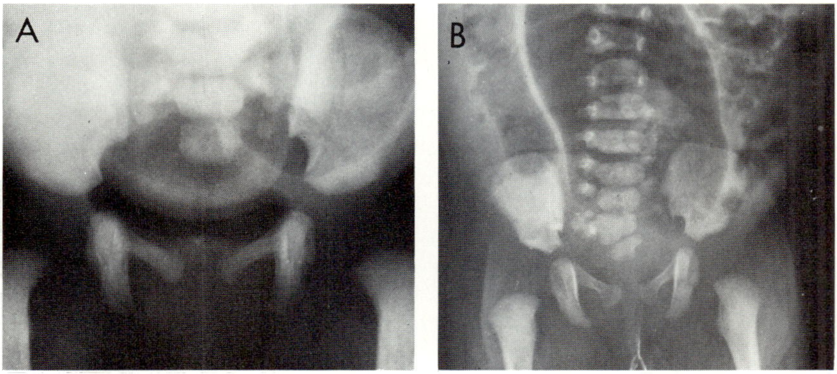

lated – an interiliac articulation. The pelvis is contracted in its dimensions.

In the two other cases of total agenesis, a lumbo-iliac articulation existed. Here the iliac bones were set higher up, articulating with the transverse processes of the lower lumbar vertebrae. In these patients this type of articulation produced a short back and lumbar lordosis.

Both the interiliac and the lumbo-iliac articulations were stable in these patients. The stability is accounted for by the strength of the ligaments of the articulations. Higgs (1924) demonstrated these strong supporting ligamentous structures by dissection of an interiliac articulation of a fetus.

In subtotal agenesis the articulation of the iliac bones was stable, and no obvious postural defect was observed in the surviving children.

HEMISACRUM. – A wide variety of appearances has been seen without any special pattern. They range from lack of development of half a vertebral body and its neural arch to a relatively minor maldevelopment of part of a lateral mass. Scoliosis is a marked feature of total hemisacrum.

Radiographs taken at intervals of 3 – 15 years in 8 patients showed no regeneration in the deficient segments. The ossific centers were absent, not simply delayed in their appearance and development. The corresponding neurological deficit also remained status quo and hence was also part of the original deformity.

B. ALIMENTARY

Alimentary anomalies were less common than those of other systems, 25 of 246 patients (10%) being affected. Of these, 7% of the anal deformities and 15% of the rectal deformities had such an association. The types of deformity are listed in Table 15.

ESOPHAGEAL ATRESIA. – This association with imperforate anus and rectum is the most common alimentary problem. McDonald (1937) noted the association, and cases have been described by O'Hare (1937); Ashley (1941); Freedman (1944); Norris *et al.* (1949), 3 cases; Arnheim (1951); Gross (1953), 18 in 507 patients; Kiesewetter *et al.* (1964), 14 in 146 patients; and Louw (1965), 7 in 95 patients. Blanca Smith (1960) states that the association occurs in about 10% of cases. The esophageal lesion was almost always associated with the rectal deformities, but 7 of our 13 were in anal deformities (1 recto-bulbar fistula, 2 male ano-cutaneous fistulae, 1 female ano-cutaneous fistula, 3 ano-vestibular fistulae; the remaining 6 cases were in 5 males with ano-rectal agenesis (no fistula), recto-urethral fistula or recto-vesical fistula and in 1 female with recto-cloacal fistula).

The frequency of this association suggests the wisdom of the rou-

TABLE 15.—ASSOCIATED ALIMENTARY ANOMALIES
(Authors' Series of 246 Patients)

Anomaly	No. of Patients
Esophageal atresia, with or without fistula	13
Duodenal atresia	4
Annular pancreas	3
Malrotation	2
Volvulus	1
Jejunal atresia	1
Meckel's diverticulum	1
Absent colon	2
Absent appendix and spleen	1
Exomphalos	3
Bile duct stenosis	1
Eventration of diaphragm	1
Total	33

tine insertion immediately after birth of a firm rubber catheter into the esophagus in all patients with imperforate anus and rectum. The severity of the esophageal lesion demands that no more than a colostomy be performed for the bowel lesion in all but the most simple of anal deformities. The management of the esophageal lesion follows the usual lines depending on the general state of the infant; a very fit baby may withstand both colostomy and esophageal anastomosis; a less fit or premature infant may require a staged program of colostomy, aspiration of the upper pouch, gastrostomy and simple division of the fistula, deferring the anastomosis until later.

HIRSCHSPRUNG'S DISEASE.—No case of Hirschsprung's disease occurred in the present series. However, the actual incidence is somewhat of a vexed question, since the publication of the paper by Parkkulainen *et al.* (1959), in which 15 of 25 biopsy specimens in 34 type 3 deformities showed aganglionosis. Yet most other surgeons, on clinical grounds, do not find the association so common. Bacon and Sherman (1952) only found two examples in 111 patients; Stevenson and Herron (1967), 2 patients; and Pellerin (1957), Ragius *et al.* (1957) Riker (1957) and Brayton and Norris (1958) contributed single case reports.

Kiesewetter *et al.* (1965) sent a questionnaire to 32 centers in the United States and Canada and reported the association only when definitive evidence was forthcoming from serial sections of autopsy or resected specimens. These figures are reproduced in Table 16.

This is the most accurate review of incidence so far reported, in which the criteria of diagnosis of Hirschsprung's disease were strictly adhered to.

The importance of Hirschsprung's disease is that it may explain

TABLE 16.—ASSOCIATION OF HIRSCHSPRUNG'S DISEASE AND RECTAL DEFORMITIES
*(After Kiesewetter et al., 1965)**

SURGEON REPORTING	CASES EXAMINED FOR GANGLION CELLS	NO GANGLION CELLS FOUND (CASES)	LENGTH OF AGANGLIONOSIS (CM.) OR SITES	COMMENTS
Trusler (Canada)	30	1	Entire colon	P.M.
		1	Lower sigmoid	Resected specimen
Fisher (Boston)	15	1	10 cm.	Resected specimen
Abel (Houston)	12	1	Entire colon	Ileostomy
Dorman (Dallas)	40	4	2–7.5 cm.	3 Resected specimens 1 Biopsy
Kiesewetter (Pittsburgh)	44	1	6 cm.	Resected specimen
TOTAL	165	10 (3.4%)		

*Reproduction with permission from Kiesewetter, W. B.; Sukarochana, K., and Seiber, W. K.: Surgery 58:877, 1965.

an occasional case of persistent constipation when the anal orifice is adequate and the follow-up supervision has been satisfactory, e.g., see the report of Stevenson and Herron (1967). Pellerin and Saied (1965) reported on the histological findings of the lower rectum and fistulae in ano-cutaneous fistulae and anterior anus in females in whom persistent constipation had ensued. They found that the lower rectum and fistula sometimes contained no ganglion cells, and, at other times, there were abnormalities of distribution and number of ganglion cells, combined with distortion of the muscular layers causing disturbance of function. Magnus and Stephens (1966) in a dissection of an imperforate anal membrane found no ganglion cells in the distal 2 cm. above the membrane and in the posterior wall for a further 3.5 cm. cranially.

Aldridge and Campbell (1968) in a careful study of the number and distribution of ganglion cells in *normal* infants found that there was a zone of absence or diminution in the number of ganglion cells for a varying distance above the anal valves (Fig. 133). This "hypoganglionic" zone was found to extend an average of 4 mm. (maximum 14 mm.) in the myenteric plexus, 7 mm. in the deep submucous plexus (maximum 17 mm.) and 10 mm. in the superficial submucous plexus from and cranial to the anal valves or pectinate line of the anal canal. In the normal rectum, postganglionic dendrites are about 2 cm. long; in rectal deformities in which the internal sphincter is absent, we would not expect to see the first ganglion cells for at least 2 cm. above the end of the two smooth muscle coats of the bowel.

It is not altogether surprising that the most terminal portion of

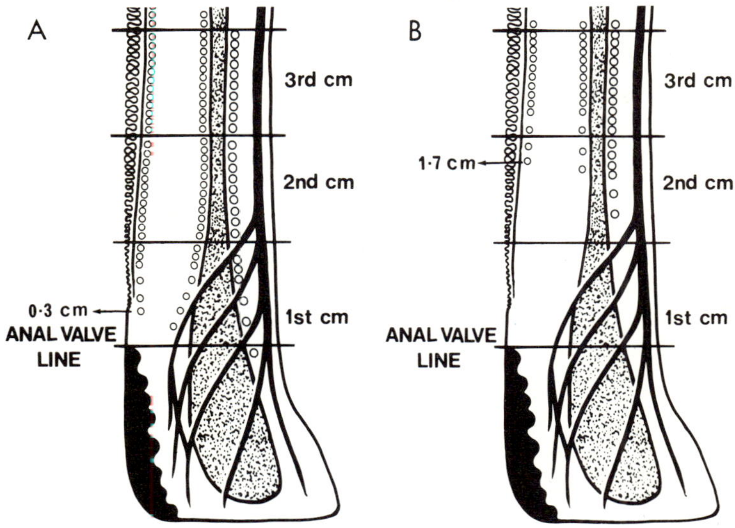

Fig. 133.—Hypoganglionic zone of the rectum in normal infants and children. Ganglia of plexuses of Auerbach and Meissner when searched for in longitudinal sections extend distally in some specimens in normal concentration to within 0.5 cm. of the line of the anal valves and peter out at the valves (**A**). In others, the ganglia extend in normal concentration to a level approximately 2.0 cm. cranial to the valve line and peter out at 1.7 cm. from the valves (**B**). In yet others, the ganglia disappear at levels between those shown in **A** and **B**. The zone distal to the point of disappearance is hypoganglionic, being endowed with sparse ganglion cells and postganglionic nerves. Meissner's plexus is arranged in two layers, one which clings to the muscularis mucosae and one which clings to the circular coat. Aldridge and Campbell (1968) described the two layers of ganglion cells in Meissner's plexus.

bowel, already subject to a process which results in agenesis, might, by the same process, suffer incomplete migration of ganglion cells to its termination (Okamoto and Ueda, 1967).

These findings in the normal infants, and in the anal deformities, suggest that absence of ganglion cells in sections taken of the terminal 1–2 cm. of resected specimens may not be a valid criterion of the presence of Hirschsprung's disease. This might account for the high figure of Hirschsprung's disease reported by Parkkulainen *et al.* (1959) in whose cases most of the aganglionic segments were very short.

On the other hand, it is a fact that some patients with quite simple and low anal anomalies can be stubbornly constipated, and it is a moot point whether the short aganglionic zone should be looked upon as Hirschsprung's disease. Rehbein and Hüther (1957) pointed out that patients with very short aganglionic segments in Hirschsprung's disease may be treated as in idiopathic colonic inertia, and similarly, it is well known how a residual tiny segment of aganglionic internal sphincter left after rectosigmoidectomy may continue to act as an obstructive lesion.

The relevance of the nature of the short aganglionic segment in anal and rectal deformities is in determining whether some terminal gut should be resected. Kiesewetter *et al.* (1965) recommend that a frozen section rectal biopsy should be taken always at the time of an abdomino-perineal rectoplasty to check for Hirschsprung's disease before deciding on the extent of rectal resection. They also recommend subsequent rectal biopsy if constipation persists without adequate explanation, e.g., in anal stenosis. Pellerin and Saied (1965) go further and take a biopsy of the "fistula" at the time of "cutback" in low anomalies; if the rectal wall is normal, then cutback will suffice; if abnormal, they suggest that a Swenson-type rectosigmoidectomy is required. However, it is difficult to be sure what is implied by the term "fistula" in their paper. As Pellerin and Saied describe "rectal wall" in the fistula, it appears that the biopsy is not of perineal skin tract, usually taken as the fistula, but of the anal or rectal canal itself.

Our experience of the postoperative care of rectoplasty and anoplasty for these deformities is that most patients can be freed of the risks of constipation if their follow-up is diligently supervised, and other factors such as a stenotic orifice are avoided. We believe that the association with true Hirschsprung's disease must be very rare indeed and that biopsy of the terminal gut may mislead the surgeon into believing that a more radical procedure is necessary. In the light of our present state of inadequate information of the distribution of the ganglion and postganglionic disorders in these deformities, a conservative approach should be invoked pending more certain work to determine the true ganglion status and the innervation of the smooth muscle.

OTHER ALIMENTARY ANOMALIES.—Apart from duodenal obstructions, other alimentary lesions have occurred only as isolated entities. Duodenal obstructions have occurred in 1–2% of all series. Small bowel obstructions do not provide difficulty in diagnosis because they produce symptoms early and are suggested by the gas patterns in the plain radiograph. Their serious nature demands attention even more urgently than the rectal anomaly. The presence of a small bowel obstruction destroys the possibility of using the inverted film in assessing the level of the rectal or anal imperforation, because obviously gas does not reach the rectum. A colostomy should be performed at the time of the laparotomy for all but the most obvious low anomalies, even though subsequently the colostomy may be found to be unnecessary.

TABLE 17.—INCIDENCE OF OTHER ANOMALIES
(Authors' Series of 246 Cases)

Central Nervous System	
Myelomeningocele	8
Down's syndrome	8
Mental retardation	2
Craniorachischisis	1
Hamartoma of cerebellum	1
Absent corpus callosum	1
Sacro-coccygeal tumor	1
Musculo-skeletal System	
Talipes	9
Arthrogryposis	3
Madelung's deformity	3
Absent metacarpals, digits, etc.	5
Phocomelia	2
Congenital amputation (leg)	1
Accessory thumb	1
Arachnodactyly	1
Congenital hip dislocation	4
Klippel-Feil deformity	3
Other "Systems"	
Prematurity	11
Cleft palate	4
Pectus excavatum	1
Bilateral microtia	1

C. CARDIAC

Associated cardiac malformations occurred with an incidence similar to that of alimentary anomalies, 22 of 246 patients (9%), being equally distributed in anal deformities and rectal deformities. All varieties of congenital heart disease have been seen—atrial and ventricular septal defects, tetralogy of Fallot, truncus arteriosus, transposition of great vessels, infundibular stenosis, coarctation of aorta, etc.

When recognized in the neonatal period, their presence calls for the most minimal anal procedures—operations for anal anomalies may be performed under local anesthesia, and no more than a colostomy should be attempted for other levels of imperforation. Subsequent management of the cardiac anomaly varies. Some anomalies are incompatible with life; some need correction prior to rectal operation, whereas treatment in the majority may be deferred to an elective time after completion of rectoplasty.

D. OTHER SYSTEMS

Almost every system of the body has been reportedly involved in association with anal and rectal deformities. Apart from central nervous system malformations, no one condition predominates. *Prematurity*, although not a "malformation," occurs with higher incidence than in "normal" infants. It occurred in 13 of 93 patients of Brayton and Norris (1958); in 53 high rectal anomalies reported by Forshall (1960), 20 were in premature infants, of whom 14 had some other severe associated anomaly. None of these 14 infants survived the postoperative period, and 3 additional female premature infants without another serious anomaly died. Prematurity must, therefore, rank high as a cause of mortality in assessing the results in any series.

Central nervous system malformations appear frequently in most series—spinal myelomeningocele, Down's syndrome, mental retardation, cerebellar malformations, craniorachischisis, etc.

The incidence of all these other anomalies in this series was 52 in 246 patients (21%), being equally distributed amongst anal and rectal deformities. They are listed in Table 17. Their management can be considered quite apart from the rectal deformity, except in relation to the paralytic conditions (myelomeningocele, etc.).

CHAPTER 12

Genito-Urinary Anomalies and Their Complications

GENITO-URINARY ANOMALIES and complications in the urinary tract after operation contribute a significant degree of morbidity in the over-all management of ano-rectal deformities.

Some of these anomalies present as problems in their own right, without urinary infection; some present as urinary infection, either because of stasis in the abnormal tract or by contamination through a recto-urinary fistula; others present as problems of urinary incontinence.

The nature and timing of the investigations to establish the diagnosis of genito-urinary abnormalities is discussed in Chapter 8.

Incidence of Associated Urinary Abnormalities

Except for rare complicated anomalies (Chapter 13), genito-urinary deformities occurred in 67 of the 246 patients in our series, 21% being associated with anal and 37% with rectal malformations. In anal malformations, apart from the lower incidence, the type of urinary problem was usually not serious. In rectal deformities, the associated urinary problem was usually a serious one, especially in males. Finally, the possibility of neurogenic urinary incontinence is much greater in the rectal deformities, because in 40% there was some degree of sacral agenesis, as against only 17% in anal deformities. In 20 patients (12 sacral agenesis, 8 myelomeningocele) neurogenic incontinence resulted.

The urinary lesions encountered in these 67 patients are shown in Table 18.

Structural Abnormalities without Infection

A coexistent lesion may be obvious on clinical inspection, as in hypospadias, or be revealed by the investigations, for example, pelvi-ureteral obstruction, horseshoe kidneys, polycystic kidneys or degrees of renal hypoplasia or agenesis.

TABLE 18.—GENITO-URINARY ABNORMALITIES IN 67 PATIENTS
(Authors' Series of 246 Patients)

Upper Urinary Tract	
Horseshoe kidneys	4
Polycystic kidneys	2
Hypoplastic or nonfunctioning kidneys	7
Renal agenesis (unilateral)	3
Renal agenesis (bilateral)	1
Hydronephrosis (unspecified)	4
Ureteral reflux—normal ureters	2
—megaureters	17
Megaureters without reflux or obstruction	1
Megaureters with obstruction	2
Duplex systems	5
Lower Urinary Tract	
Hypospadias	15
Urethral diverticula	2
Urethral valves	1
Urethral stricture or septum (congenital)	2
Bifid urethra	1
Penile sinus (not hypospadias)	1
Ectopia vesicae	1
Megacystis with absent abdominal muscles	2
Absent bladder and urethra	1
Absent urethra	1
Urachal fistula	1
Genital Tract	
Absent genitalia	1
Double uterus and tubes (not cloacal deformities)	3
Multiple Anomalies	
Vesico-intestinal fissure	11
Duplication of anus with genito-urinary anomalies	2

The attack upon overt lesions of hypospadias and ectopia vesicae may be undertaken later as elective procedures after the completion of the rectal operation. In *hypospadias* associated with recto-bulbar fistula in a fit child with no special difficulties encountered in the anal repair, it may sometimes be appropriate to perform the first stage of the repair at the time of proctoplasty (See Fig. 33).

Incidental abnormalities of the urinary apparatus (Figs. 134, 135 and 136) require independent assessment. Obstructions (e.g., pelvi-ureteral and lower ureteral) should be relieved; a derelict kidney (e.g., hypoplasia), especially if associated with vesico-ureteral reflux and infection, may need nephrectomy. But intervention for these problems can proceed quite independently of decisions concerning the rectal anomaly.

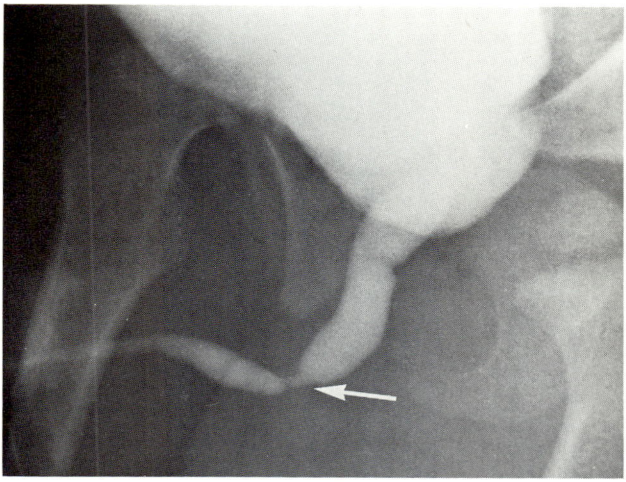

Fig. 134.—Associated urinary anomaly. Patient with recto-urethral fistula. Stricture (*arrow*) of the bulbous urethra shown by micturition cystourethrography.

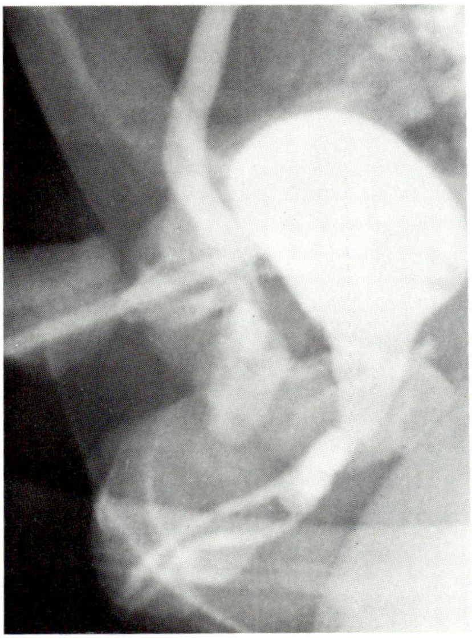

Fig. 135.—Associated urinary anomalies. Patient with covered anus. Double penile urethra joining at the bulb to form a single posterior urethra; also vesico-ureteral reflux.

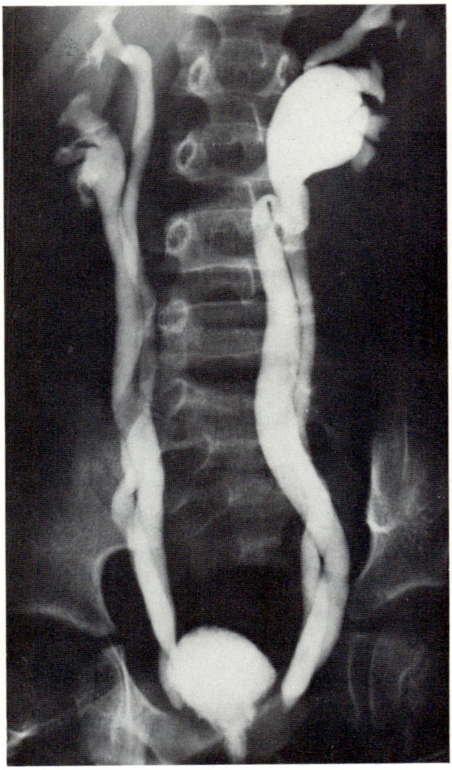

Fig. 136. —Associated urinary anomalies. Patient with ano-vestibular fistula. Bilateral double ureters with reflux and with dilatation of the ureter from the lower renal pelvis.

Urinary Infection

Urinary infection may result from a variety of causes, e.g., from contamination through a fistula, from associated urinary anomalies, from neurogenic stasis or from surgical damage to the urethra.

Mechanisms

(I) Infection Through a Recto-Urinary Fistula.—After establishment of a colostomy in the newborn period, and prior to delayed recto-plasty, fecal organisms may contaminate the urinary tract through the fistula (recto-vesical, recto-urethral and recto-bulbar). This risk has long been recognized and is mentioned in the papers by Bevan (1920) and David (1937), as well as those of subsequent writers. In recto-vesical fistulae, the risk of infection is maximal, whereas, with fistulae into the urethra, some protection to the bladder is afforded by the closed bladder neck. In our own series, there were 5 patients with recto-vesical fistulae, but 4 died from other anomalies within days of birth; the remaining patient died at 2 years from pyelonephritis complicating severe hypoplastic kidneys. Table 19 indicates the incidence of infection in patients with recto-urethral and recto-bulbar fistulae compared with those without urinary communication, but it is important to interpret Table 19 in the light of subsequent discussion concerning relation of infection to associated anomalies and the adequacy of colonic washouts. Of 44 patients with recto-urethral fistulae, 14 are dead, and only one of these survived sufficiently long for adequate follow-up; with 30 surviving patients, this provided 31 for analysis. Similarly, of the 13 patients with recto-bulbar fistulae, 10 were available for analysis: and of 194 patients with no urinary communication, 138 patients were studied.

It can be seen that the risk of infection is considerable in recto-urethral fistulae and much less so in recto-bulbar fistulae.

In the 138 patients without a recto-urinary communication, only 14 developed infection. The principal reason for this low incidence is the small number of associated urinary anomalies in the anal group which comprise the bulk of these 138 patients.

It is apparent from Table 19 that the higher the fistula the greater the infection rate, but it must also be borne in mind that the higher the fistula the more serious is the deformity, and with it come more widespread and serious urinary and other defects. The fistula may provide the route of infection in the first instance, especially if the colon contains decomposing meconium, but stasis in the urinary tract promotes the infection. Furthermore, a fine fistula may be valvular, permitting meconium or infection to enter the urinary tract only under high pressure of bowel obstruction, but not after colostomy when the pressure is low; it may permit small amounts of urine to pass from bladder or urethra into the rectum, but not in the reverse direction and may not be a cause of infection; but a two-way flow may occur if the fistula is wide, creating stasis and infection.

The risk of direct infection is avoided by early disconnection of the fistula, but we believe these risks can be minimized in many patients by other means (see below).

Infection may also occur from the *recurrence* of a recto-urinary

TABLE 19.—Incidence of Urinary Infection in Relation to Recto-Urinary Communication

Recto-Urinary Communication	No. of Patients	Infection	No Infection
Recto-vesical fistulae	5*	1	
Recto-urethral fistulae	31	21	10
Recto-bulbar fistulae	10	2	8
No urinary fistulae	138	14	124

*Four neonatal deaths from other deformities.

fistula after operation. This was a common event in the era of perineal exploration for high deformities. Four patients exhibiting such recurrence of fistula were subsequently seen and treated by us; of 10 recurrent fistulae reported by Partridge and Gough (1961), 7 appeared after perineal reconstruction. Recurrent fistulae (and infection) are much rarer after abdomino-perineal rectoplasty, occurring in only 3 patients of Partridge and Gough (1961), and in no patients in our series of 37 sacro-abdominal repairs.

(II) INFECTION AS A CONSEQUENCE OF STASIS DUE TO ASSOCIATED ANOMALIES.—The commonest incriminating cause of stasis is vesico-ureteral reflux, with or without megaureters, which occurred in 19 of the 64 patients in this series with urinary abnormalities (Fig. 137). Megaureters due to ureteral obstruction, or megaureters without obstruction or reflux, occurred less commonly. Other associations with static pooling of urine were various arrangements of duplex renal systems, bladder and urethral diverticulae, urethral stricture, and megacystis associated with absent abdominal muscles and cryptorchidism (triad syndrome).

Any of these anomalies may result in infection quite apart from the rectal deformity, but, in addition, a rectal fistula may be the initi-

Fig. 137.—Micturition cystourethrogram in recto-urethral fistula (the latter shown by the posterior angulation of the urethra and contrast medium in the terminal rectum) reveals associated bilateral vesico-ureteral reflux.

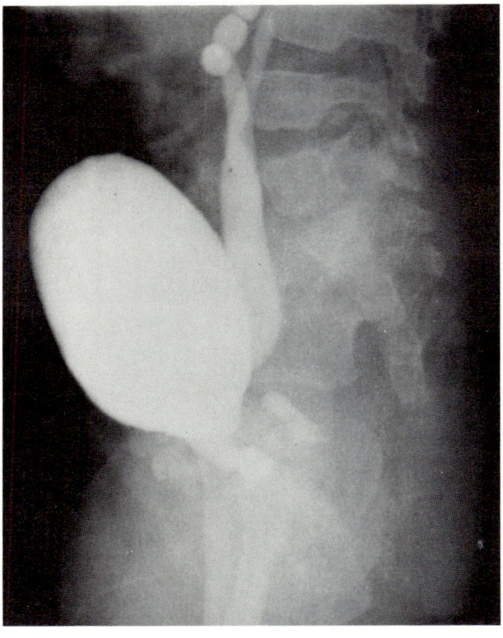

ating cause of infection. The relationships between urinary infection, rectal fistulae and associated anomalies are shown in Table 20 (only patients surviving at least 6 months are considered).

In recto-urethral fistulae, 14 of 15 patients with associated urinary tract anomalies developed infection, whereas only 7 of 16 without anomalies became infected. The anomalies in the 14 infected patients constituted significant causes of infection (megaureters with reflux, some duplex, 10 patients; horseshoe kidney, 1; nonfunctioning kidneys, 2; and only 1 patient had a noncontributory deformity—hypospadias). Infection in 6 of the 7 patients without associated anomalies was presumably due to fecal contamination through the fistula, and, in 5 of these patients, no colonic washouts were given after the colostomy. The seventh patient had a urethral stricture following operation.

In recto-bulbar fistulae, although 8 patients possessed associated urinary tract anomalies, 7 did not develop infection because the anomalies were not a significant cause of urinary stasis (hypospadias, 5; a small nonobstructing urethral diverticulum, 1; reflux into a normal caliber ureter, 1). The one infected patient had bilateral reflux. The one infected patient without urinary tract abnormalities developed infection after an inadequate perineal exploration with recurrence of the urethral fistula.

The importance of upper urinary tract stasis in producing infection in its own right is further supported by the figures in Table 20 of rectal and anal deformities which do not communicate with the urinary tract. Only 12 of 138 patients developed infection; 10 of the 12

TABLE 20.—RELATION OF RECURRENT URINARY TRACT INFECTION TO ASSOCIATED URINARY TRACT ANOMALIES IN RECTAL DEFORMITIES WITH AND WITHOUT RECTO-URINARY FISTULAE

TYPES OF DEFORMITY	ASSOCIATED URINARY TRACT ANOMALY	URINARY TRACT INFECTION	NO URINARY TRACT INFECTION
A. Recto-urethral fistula—31	Associated anomaly— 15	14	1
	No associated anomaly— 16	7	9
B. Recto-bulbar fistula—10	Associated anomaly— 8	1	7
	No associated anomaly— 2	1	1
C. Deformities without urinary fistula—138	Associated anomaly— 26	10	16
	No associated anomaly—112	2	110

TABLE 21.—URINARY TRACT INFECTION RELATED TO PRESENCE OR ABSENCE OF URO-ANOMALY

	INFECTED	NOT INFECTED
Uro-anomaly	16	12
No Uro-anomaly	8	10
Total	24	22

were in children with associated anomalies, and all 10 patients had upper urinary tract disease (megaureters with or without reflux, duplex system, or hypoplasia.) Only 2 of 112 patients without associated urinary anomalies became infected, and one of these had stasis as a consequence of neurogenic bladder from sacral agenesis. The relationships are illustrated in Tables 21, 22 and 23.

(III) INFECTION AS A CONSEQUENCE OF NEUROGENIC BLADDER DISEASE.—Stasis due to neurogenic bladder is a potent source of urinary infection. Sacral agenesis and hemisacral deformities are common in rectal deformities and in at least 8 patients were responsible for the paralyzed bladder; 8 patients had a spinal myelomeningocele, the bladder being paralyzed in all. The urological features of these neurogenic states have been reviewed previously (Smith, 1959, 1965 and 1966). Both lesions result in a lower motor neurone type of paretic bladder, with a patulous bladder neck, but in some, especially sacral lesions, there may be outflow obstruction in the external sphincter zone due to spasticity in the urethral musculature. Both lesions are commonly associated with upper urinary anomalies, and persistent urethral obstruction and infection eventually cause serious parenchymal damage.

TABLE 22.—URINARY TRACT INFECTION, RELATED TO TYPE OF COMMUNICATING DEFORMITY AND PRESENCE OF URO-ANOMALY

TYPE	NO.	No. Infected	INFECTION Uro-anomaly	Types
Recto-vesical	5	1 (4 died perinatally)		
Recto-urethral	31	21	14	Reflux Megaureters Duplex Horseshoe Hypoplasia (1) Hypospadias
Recto-bulbar	10	2	1	Reflux
Total	46	24	15	

TABLE 23.—URINARY TRACT INFECTION IN NON-COMMUNICATING DEFORMITIES

	Infected		Not Infected
Uro-anomaly	10	Reflux Megaureters Duplex	16
No Uro-anomaly	2	(1 neurogenic bladder)	110
Totals	12		126

A neurogenic bladder may also result from operative damage to the bladder neck or to the pelvic parasympathetics during the performance of rectoplasty. In 4 patients referred to us after extensive perineal exploration elsewhere (for recto-urethral fistulae), the bladder neck or urethra was damaged; in 4 other patients, incontinence is attributable to too extensive dissection in the pelvis during abdominal mobilization. All these patients developed urinary infection at some stage. Spence (1954), Scott *et al.* (1960) and Partridge and Gough (1961), all report bladder neck obstruction from neurogenic injury.

(IV) INFECTION FROM OPERATIVE DAMAGE TO THE URETHRA.—A metal sound in the urethra is a vital precaution during dissection through the pelvis, especially if operating in the sacro-coccygeal ap-

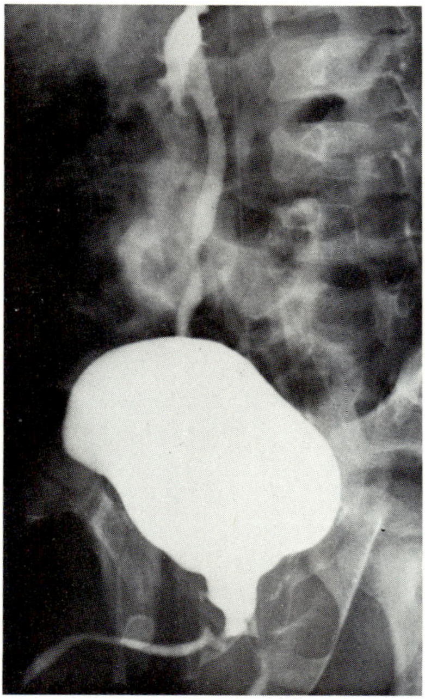

Fig. 138.—Patient with recto-urethral fistula. Patulous bladder neck and distorted posterior urethra, probably from injury at operation. Cystogram showing continuous leakage. Patient had urinary infection. Note also vesico-ureteral reflux into right normal caliber ureter. (Reproduced with permission from Smith, E. D.: J. Pediat. Surg. 3:337, 1968.)

proach. Without this safeguard in dividing the fistula, part of the urethra may be injured by "tenting" it out. A further safety precaution for the urethra is to open the terminal rectum near its extreme end, in order to find the fistula promptly by identification, and probing and circumcising from within, rather than to dissect blindly in the precincts of the urethra in search of the fistulous tract. Urethral stricture resulting from urethral damage may result in bladder stasis and infection (Fig. 138). This is referred to, also, by Wallace *et al.* (1948), Partridge and Gough (1961), Katzen (1962), Trusler and Wilkinson (1962), Santulli (1963) and Kiesewetter and Turner (5 patients in 1963).

Infection may follow if too much of the fistula is retained. The fistula may result in a urethral diverticulum, especially if a part of the rectum is attached, and a calculus may form in it; Partridge and Gough (1961) report a similar calculus and Kiesewetter and Turner (1963) reported two urethral diverticulae after sacro-coccygeal rectoplasty. The presence of calculi, acting as foreign bodies, contributes to urinary infection.

Consequences

(i) Pyelonephritis.—Persistent urinary infection ultimately produces irreversible changes in the renal parenchyma. This is all the more serious if renal reserve is already reduced by varying degrees of hypoplasia and dysplasia. Pyelonephritis may rarely result in hypertension.

(ii) Calculus Formation.—Stasis, infection and sedimentation of cellular debris may initiate calculus formation in the bladder or kidneys. Once calculi have formed, infection persists until the foreign body is removed. Calculi occurred in 2 patients in this series, as also in the series of Partridge and Gough (1961).

Calculi may also form in the colon distal to the colostomy, partly from infected urine and purulent debris entering through the urinary fistula and partly due to fecal or barium concretions. One patient with a recto-cloacal fistula developed a soft stone in the vagina.

(iii) Hyperchloremic Acidosis.—A metabolic acidosis may result from poorly functioning kidneys, further compromised by urinary infection. However, an additional cause of acidosis is the reflux of urine through the fistula into the distal limb of the colostomy. Chloride ions from the urine are reabsorbed through the bowel mucosa. This has occurred in one of our patients, and attention was first drawn to it by Poth (1956) and later by Kiesewetter *et al.* (1964) and Shepherd and Kiesewetter (1966), who reported 2 patients with this complication. Each of these 2 patients had a wide fistula (1.5 cm.), and each had urethral obstruction (by a flap valve). Tank and Watts (1968) also report 1 case. A severe degree of acidosis due to this cause would necessitate division of the fistula, with or without completion of the rectoplasty.

Prevention and Management

As pointed out above, a significant source of urinary infection is by contamination of the bladder or urethra by fecal organisms through the intact fistula. We do not advocate neonatal rectoplasty to meet this threat but rather make strenuous efforts to clear out meconium and feces from the distal limb of the colostomy. Experience has shown that *in the absence of an associated anomaly in the upper urinary tract thorough cleansing of the colon distal to the colostomy will prevent or clear urinary infection; however, the chances of preventing urinary infection are less in the presence of stasis caused by an associated urinary malformation, and, in these patients, the cause of stasis may need to be eradicated directly.*

In the total of 31 patients with recto-urethral fistula, 16 had no associated urinary anomalies; washouts were given to 9 of these 16 patients, and infection occurred in only 1 patient; no washouts were given to 7 patients, and 6 became infected. These figures point to the effectiveness of colonic toilet in preventing urinary infection when the upper urinary tract is normal.

On the other hand, of 15 patients with some associated urinary anomaly, all except one became infected, including patients who had satisfactory colonic toilets.

The low pressure established in the colon distal to the colostomy may be sufficient to prevent fecal contamination of the urinary tract, especially if the distal colon is thoroughly cleansed. For this reason, we believe that, in the first place, even with the knowledge that an associated urinary anomaly exists, the conservative plan of neonatal colostomy and postoperative colonic toilets should be advocated.

Regimen of Colonic Clearance.—The colonic washouts commence on the operating table after completion of the neonatal colostomy. Provided the general condition of the baby is good, this procedure may take 15–30 minutes of irrigation of the distal colon with syringe and saline through a soft rubber catheter. Much fecal matter is irrigated away, and what is left is well softened. On the subsequent postoperative days, saline washouts are continued for at least a week, or until the rectum is clear. A little water-soluble radiopaque medium is then run in to check whether any filling defects of meconium persist, and, if so, the washouts are continued (see Fig. 113).

It is important that the technique of colostomy prevent spill-over of feces from the proximal to the distal loops.

Onset of Urinary Infection.—Once infection supervenes, despite colonic clearance, again a conservative policy is initially adopted. The colon is again checked radiographically. In the presence of retained feces, the colonic washouts are recommenced, supplemented by the instillation of 0.2% neomycin solution; parenteral antibiotics and chemotherapy are commenced, and the bladder is given a series of washouts with the same strength neomycin solution. A thorough trial of chemotherapy is continued. In the total of 41 patients with recto-urethral and recto-bulbar fistulae, the proportion of infected to noninfected patients was 23:18, but after instituting the above routine, control of infection altered this proportion to 11:30, the failures occurring in those with severe upper urinary tract stasis. With the elimination of infection, the rectoplasty may be deferred to the elective time.

Persistence of Infection.—The management of persistent urinary infection, despite the above regimen, may then take various directions, depending upon the type and severity of the associated urinary problem.

(i) If there is no stasis and no malformation to account for infection (infection being proved by suprapubic needle aspiration of urine from the bladder), a further course of chemotherapy and bladder washouts is justified since the infection is not likely to be carried up the ureters to the kidneys when the uretero-vesical valves are intact. However, if the baby fails to thrive and the urine does not clear, the fistula could be disconnected, or the date for recto- or protoplasty advanced. Disconnection of the fistula alone may result in scarring, making a second exploration for the rectoplasty more difficult, and in general it would seem better to complete the rectoplasty in one stage. Much would depend upon the general condition of the baby and the age at which intervention was required. This decision has not had to be made yet by us, but, probably if the infant was over 6 months of age, we would endeavor to complete the rectoplasty in one stage.

(ii) If reflux and stasis are present but the ureters are of normal or near normal caliber (Fig. 138) and the baby is thriving, extra efforts with chemotherapy and bladder washouts for a limited period may succeed. However, if the baby is not thriving, the fistula should be disconnected forthwith (under 6 months of age) or the rectoplasty performed (over 6 months of age and normal weight for age). Division of the fistula, and antibiotics, have controlled infection in one 4-month-old infant in this series, despite the presence of ureteral reflux.

(iii) If the stasis is caused by reflux into megaureters (Fig. 139), then temporary ureterostomy may be the best method of improving the health of the baby. A unilateral megaureter with good or equivocal function may clear itself of infection once free drainage is

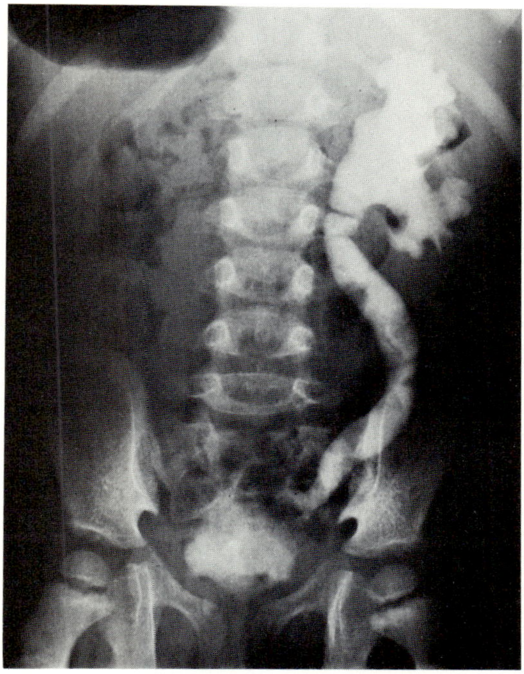

Fig. 139.—Patient with recto-urethral fistula. Left megaureter, vesico-ureteral reflux and hydronephrosis. Persistent infection required ureterostomy and eventual nephroureterectomy. (Reproduced with permission from Smith, E. D.: J. Pediat. Surg. 3:337, 1968.)

achieved by cutaneous ureterostomy. Ureteral collections and analysis of urine may subsequently establish the usefulness of this kidney, thus providing the evidence required either to counsel nephrectomy or reimplantation of the ureter after the rectal procedure has been completed (2 patients).

In bilateral gross megaureters with reflux (Fig. 140), it may be lifesaving to perform bilateral cutaneous ureterostomies. Following rectal operation at the elective age and assessment of renal function three procedures are advised: (1) the ureterostomies may be closed, and the patient perform multiple micturition; (2) an antireflux vesicoureteroplasty may be performed; or (3) reinsertion of one ureter, and nephrectomy for a poorly functioning opposite side (3 patients).

(iv) If stasis is associated with reflux and a derelict kidney with absent or negligible renal function, the kidney and ureter should be excised (6 patients).

When temporary diversion of urine is required, we prefer cutaneous ureterostomies rather than suprapubic cystostomy or pyelos-

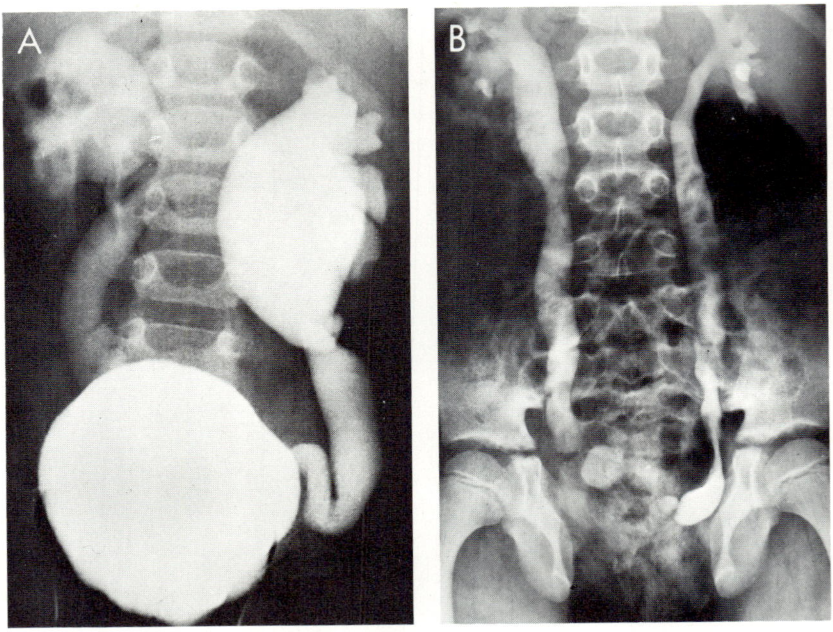

Fig. 140.—Stasis and infection in bilateral vesico-ureteral reflux. **A,** megaureters which required bilateral cutaneous ureterostomies to obtain control of infection prior to rectoplasty (recto-urethral fistula). **B,** infection controlled by parenteral antibiotics and neomycin bladder washouts (anterior perineal anus). (*A,* reproduced with permission from Smith, E. D.: J. Pediat. Surg. 3:337, 1968.)

tomy drainage. The former avoids drainage with an indwelling catheter, which only predisposes to further infection, and ureteral collections permit independent renal assessment, not possible with bladder drainage.

It is difficult to generalize, but, in the presence of a severe urinary anomaly such as given in the examples above, we believe it is preferable to achieve rapid control of infection by a primary nephrectomy or ureterostomy rather than to divide the rectal fistula or be precipitated into an early rectoplasty. With removal of the static field, colonic and bladder washouts may then achieve control of the lower urinary tract. Rectoplasty may then proceed at the optimal time in an unscarred field, followed later by corrective operation on the urinary tract.

When the type of urinary anomaly does not lend itself to corrective treatment and infection persists, the rectal fistula may need to be divided or an earlier rectoplasty performed.

When infection occurs uncomplicated by the presence of a recto-

or ano-urinary fistula, the cause of the infection is sought and treated by the appropriate urological principle in its own right, and no consideration need be given to interference with the optimal time for rectoplasty. Prolonged infection should be avoided to improve the health of the baby in preparation for the rectoplasty procedure.

Urinary Incontinence

Urinary incontinence in rectal and anal deformities may result from an associated anomaly, a neurogenic cause, or operative damage.

Causes and Treatment

(I) Associated Anomalies.—Most anomalies producing wetting (e.g., ectopia vesicae, epispadias, ectopic ureter, etc.) may be considered independently of decisions about the rectum, and their repair may follow the rectal operation.

A recto-cloacal malformation may produce incontinence because of the shortness of the urethra which issues into the cloacal canal or because of neural defects consequent on spinal cord and vertebral deficiencies, common in this group. Actually, our three surviving patients with recto-cloacal fistulae are all continent, but severe neurogenic incontinence would require permanent urinary diversion by ileo-cutaneous ureterostomy at a later date.

Finally, it should be remembered that wetting in childhood is most commonly not due to a structural "anomaly" but is of *functional origin* in a nervous, high-strung or sensitive child. In functional wetting, there are usually some periods of dryness, the bladder is not palpable and not expressible, and perineal sensation is normal (Smith, 1967). In the presence of sacral agenesis, it is particularly important not to proceed to urinary diversion on the assumption that this kind of wetting is due to a neurogenic bladder.

(II) Neurogenic Bladder.—The *causes* of neurogenic bladder have been discussed above (spinal myelomeningocele, sacral agenesis, operative damage to urethra and bladder neck and damage to pelvic parasympathetics during the rectoplasty operation).

Diagnosis of Neurogenic Bladder.—The diagnosis of a neurogenic bladder has a vital influence on the decisions regarding subsequent rectoplasty. *In the congenital spinal lesions, the integrity of the hidden levator ani, upon which continence depends, is indicated more by the behavior of the bladder than by any other factor.* The same sacral segments (2, 3 and 4) innervate levator ani, anal sphincters, bladder sympathetics and perineal dermatomes; an analysis of the latter functions provides information about the pelvic floor muscles. An overt spinal myelomeningocele or the radiographic appearance of a deformed sacrum may strongly suggest a neurogenic state, but the diagnosis finally rests on clinical grounds.

The chief features suggesting the neurogenic state relate to (1) the history of incontinence, (2) expressibility of the bladder and (3) lack of perineal sensation. These features, more fully discussed by one of us elsewhere (Smith, 1969, 1966 and 1967), are included here in summary form.

1. Clinical History of Incontinence.—The wetting from neurogenic defects of innervation is constant and permanent; a neurogenic basis cannot be entertained if there are definite periods of days or weeks when the child has normal control. Such intermittent wetting is usually functional in origin. Two clinical voiding patterns occur in the neurogenic-bladder patient:

(i) Almost continuous dribbling, every few minutes, in small volumes, aggravated by exertion; absence of sensation of fullness or of voiding and inability to stop the stream.

(ii) Overflow leakage; dribbling at less frequent intervals, but without sensation (except when the bladder is very full) and with inability to control the stream.

2. Bladder Expressibility.—The most constant and useful confirmatory sign of the paretic bladder is its expressibility by manual pressure. The bladder of a normal infant or child cannot be expressed. Two patterns of expressibility are observed:

(i) In the majority, the bladder is soft and not easily palpable, and urine can be expressed easily with manual pressure on the lower abdomen. The urethra has practically no resistance to flow.

(ii) In a minority, the bladder may be firm and readily palpable and strong pressure is required to expel urine; the discomfort engendered by the forceful pressure may cause the child to resist, thus initially suggesting that expression is not possible. However, some urine will be expelled, even if only during the transient relaxed period of inspiration.

3. Perineal Sensation.—The neurogenic bladder of myelomeningocele patients is almost always accompanied by perineal anesthesia of the saddle type. Of 130 surviving patients with myelomeningocele reviewed by one of us (Smith, 1960 and 1966), 126 have some disturbance to the bladder. In all but two of these patients with disturbed bladder, repeated examinations show anesthesia in the perineum.

Conversely, Smith has never observed a normal bladder in these patients in the presence of perineal anesthesia. An important clinical rule may, therefore, be formulated—if perineal anesthesia is present, bladder disability is to be expected. The elicitation of perineal sensation in infants and children is an important prognostic sign. On the other hand, as indicated by the two exceptions above, if perineal sensation is normal, this does not always indicate a normal bladder.

By contrast with the findings in myelomeningoceles, Williams and Nixon (1957) and one of us (Smith, 1959) have pointed out that in sacral agenesis there is not nearly so constant a relation between perineal anesthesia and bladder disability. In Smith's (1959) review of 26 patients with sacral anomalies (17 surviving), 4 patients who lacked urinary control were anesthetic in the perineum; 3 patients, also incontinent, had some perineal anesthesia but not exactly corresponding in extent to that expected from the sacral deficiency. These discrepancies are accounted for by the fact that occasionally some sacral peripheral roots may be present, even in the absence of corresponding vertebrae, e.g., the presence of perineal sensation in agenesis of 3d, 4th and 5th sacral segments, and the presence of foot muscle innervation and dermatome sensation of the 1st and 2d sacral divisions in patients exhibiting defective development of the first two segments of the sacrum.

Significance of Sacral Anomalies.—In the present series of 246 anal and rectal deformities, 51 patients had a sacral anomaly. Many of these were minor, but in 12 patients the extent of the sacral anomaly was sufficient to produce a neurogenic state. The anomalies are usually more significant if whole segments of sacrum are deficient (sacral agenesis), but even hemisacral defects may occasionally be responsible for defective innervation. By comparisons with dissections of the levator ani and analysis of the clinical effects, the following conclusions regarding these sacral defects were made:

(i) Deficiencies of the 4th and 5th sacral vertebrae usually allow normal innervation of the bladder and levator.

(ii) Deficiencies of the 3d, 4th and 5th sacral vertebrae are accompanied by variable innervation to bladder and levator, but most patients are incontinent.

(iii) Deficiencies involving the first or second segments have always been associated with incontinence in this series, and the levator ani was not only defective in its innervation but also poorly developed.

(iv) Innervation accompanying hemisacral defects is unpredictable: defects of more than the 4th and 5th sacral segments are associated with defects of innervation of bladder and levator ani.

It is emphasized, however, that these predictions must always be related to the clinical tests for neurogenic incontinence above. The diagnosis of a neurogenic state is strictly a clinical one, and the x-rays only put the surgeon on guard as to the possibility. This is because, in sacral agenesis, the sacral nerve roots may occasionally develop even in the absence of the bones (see Figs. 109 and 110).

The bladder dysfunction in sacral anomalies can be divided into two types:

(1) The paretic bladder with relaxed incontinent sphincters, expressible bladder and constant dribbling. All the sacral agenesis group and 1 patient with an hemisacral deformity exhibited this form of dysfunction. Manual expression was of little assistance in extending the periods of dryness.

(2) The paretic bladder accompanied by some degree of urethral sphincter spasm produces an unsatisfactory pseudocontinence. This occurred in 2 patients only, both with hemisacral deformities.

Significance of Spinal Myelomeningocele.—The second most common neurogenic disturbance in rectal anomalies is spinal myelomeningocele, and there were 8 affected infants in our series. All 8 patients were totally incontinent. The clinical patterns of wetting followed the classical patterns of neurogenic disturbance described above. There were no special features about these myelomeningocele lesions, which were identical with those of the 300 patients reviewed by one of us (Smith, 1965 and 1966) previously.

Management of Neurogenic Bladder.—In the management of neurogenic bladder lesions (sacral agenesis, spinal myelomeningocele), we have abandoned conservative training methods as being of no avail. Most patients have had surgical diversion of urine as being the only realistic method of management. The patients did not achieve useful periods of dryness, and the method was time consuming and demanding. The urine almost inevitably became infected eventually, jeopardizing the health of the upper urinary tract, especially in patients with neurogenic urethral obstruction. The child frequently remained in apparent good health in the presence of persistently infected urine, providing no clue to the progressive pyelonephritic damage proceeding inexorably in the kidneys. The risk of infection increased considerably during the second year of life.

The following scheme is suggested for the management of neurogenic bladder incontinence (Smith, 1966).

From birth to 2 years

(a) Investigations
  (i) Intravenous pyelography in the neonatal period and again in the second year
  (ii) Cystourethrography with I.V.P. in the first year
  (iii) Regular microscopy and culture of urine
(b) Protection of the perineal skin and reduction of residual urine by daily manual expression of the bladder

(c) Relief of neurogenic urethral obstruction by transurethral resection of longitudinal strips in the spastic zone or pudendal neurectomy
(d) Diversion by ileal conduit if deterioration occurs

At 2 years

(a) In boys, a penile urine-collecting apparatus may be fitted, unless voluntary voiding has been achieved; in girls, the urine should be operatively diverted from the bladder
(b) Boys with a penile bag should continue with expression of the bladder twice a day, and specimens of urine should be cultured frequently

Operative diversion of the urine is indicated for the following:

(a) All girls at 2 years of age, as the only realistic method of ensuring dryness.
(b) Smouldering or recurring urinary infection of more than 3 months duration, despite chemotherapy and regardless of clinical state or age or normal pyelographic appearances and especially if vesico-ureteral reflux is present.
(c) Increasing dilatation of the upper urinary tract.
(d) Progressive deterioration in renal function. This indication should seldom arise when infection of the urine has been detected early and the warning promptly heeded.

If the ureters are very large and tortuous, a double-nipple cutaneous ureterostomy can be fashioned to the right of the umbilicus (Smith, 1965), but with normal or only moderately dilated ureters an ileo-cutaneous ureterostomy at this site is the best method of urinary diversion. At present, one of us (Smith) has performed 145 ileal conduits, with one death; results have been satisfactory.

Influence of the Neurogenic State on Decisions Concerning Rectal Management.—When the neurogenic bladder is recognized in the neonatal period, its presence does not influence the initial decision to perform anoplasty for an anal deformity. Surgical correction of the anal canal is a relatively minor matter, and the fecal incontinence becomes a matter for later management. Most patients with myelomeningocele, with an incontinent anus, ultimately learn to keep themselves quite clean by daily evacuation, provided the feces are kept firm, and this is preferable to an abdominal colostomy.

Neurological defects associated with a rectal deformity, however, probably preclude complicated rectoplasty procedures. The colostomy performed in the neonatal period should therefore be a left iliac one, and fashioned to be permanent. If urinary diversion is subsequently required, the urinary stoma can be brought out to the right of the umbilicus. Two separated stomata are certainly difficult for the patient but are still preferable to twin stomata, or the "wet colostomy" of ureterosigmoidostomy and colostomy; the latter is subject to dangers of skin excoriation, ascending renal infection, hyperchloremic acidosis and difficulties of retaining the collecting appliance. The only alternative to two stomata is to carry out the rectoplasty later and establish what is virtually a perineal colostomy. In the case of myelomeningocele patients, this is not so unreasonable as may at first appear. Despite the patulous sphincters in this lesion, adequate cleanliness is maintained by most of these patients by the late years of childhood and thereafter. The stool is naturally a constipated one, and, by the judicious balance of diet and laxative and/or suppository or enema, abdominal muscle contraction can ensure complete evacuation. A compromise has to be found between feces sufficiently firm not to ooze out and so hard as to invite fecal impaction. Our experience with stool control in patients with sacral agenesis, however, is not nearly so encouraging. These patients much more frequently have soft and unformed stools, and soil repeatedly; in these patients an abdominal colostomy is preferable.

When the neurogenic bladder is recognized at a later period after the rectoplasty has been established, the management of the bladder is as above described, i.e., usually terminating in an ileal conduit. If the rectum is also incontinent from the same neurogenic cause, attempts to improve fecal control by the methods suggested should be tried over a number of years before resorting to a left iliac colostomy.

(iii) Operative Damage.—When the pelvic dissection has been too wide or extensive, the pelvic parasympathetics may become disrupted and result in neurogenic-bladder incontinence. Scott (1959) has shown that the pelvic plexus and nerves converge from posterolaterally towards the midline at the front of the fistula behind the bladder; the dissection must keep well posteriorly until the pelvic floor is reached, and only then come forward to penetrate the puborectalis anteriorly, keeping very close to the fistula.

Further, in perineal dissections the urethra, bladder neck or its sphincters have been injured directly, resulting in incontinence quite apart from injury to nerve supply.

Scott *et al.* (1960) reported wetting in 12 patients, 7 in high anomalies and 5 in low anomalies; sacral agenesis was responsible in 3, urethral stricture in one, and the remainder probably resulted from operative interference with nerve supply. Of 35 type 3 cases reported by Trusler and Wilkinson (1962), urinary control was impaired in 5 of 15 rectal anomalies (2 had sacral agenesis, and 2 had injury from multiple operations).

Unlike the neurogenic bladder lesions of sacral agenesis and myelomeningocele, that from operative nerve damage is not always permanent and may recover after a period of manual expression together with chemotherapy. Permanent neurogenic damage is difficult or impossible to correct. One boy who had had multiple procedures through the perineum for recurrent recto-urethral fistula eventually gained improved urinary control after plication of urethral musculature and levator ani behind the urethra in front of rectum. In another boy, forcible dilatation of a rectal stricture had disrupted the bladder neck completely, and bladder-neck plasty has restored improved, although not perfect, control.

Absent Bladder, Urethra and Genitalia

Absence of bladder and/or urethra may occur with or without renal agenesis. Three deaths occurred in our series with these associations. All three had high rectal imperforation without fistulae. One male infant lacked urethra only; in one female, the bladder and urethra were absent, but the kidneys were present; in one female, there was total absence of kidneys, ureters, bladder, urethra and external genitalia.

Genital Malformations

Some of the complex urethro-vaginal malformations associated with and without rectal abnormalities have been discussed by one of us (Stephens, 1966 and 1968). Reference should also be made to the description of the vagina and cloaca in the various rectal lesions (Chapt. 4).

Except in the presence of hydrometrocolpos, the vaginal malformations do not call for any urgent treatment and should be left until long after the rectal repair has been completed. To place these lesions in the perspective of development of the whole uro-genital sinus area, we include a description of several of them, some not found in association with anal abnormalities. In the female, the associated anal malformation is one in which the anal orifice is situated further forwards in the anterior perineal or vestibular situation.

Normal Development.—The müllerian ducts emerge on the wolffian ridges closely applied to the wolffian ducts which precede and guide their actively growing caudal ends to the uro-genital sinus. As far as the brim of the pelvis, the müllerian ducts lie lateral to the pilot ducts, but, in the pelvis, they turn medially, cross anteriorly to the wolffian ducts, meet and migrate side by side to the sinus. They penetrate the uro-genital sinus between the two openings of the wolffian ducts on the site of the müllerian tubercle at about the 35–37-mm. stage (Frazer, 1931). This eminence in the sinus is then excavated by small paired sino-vaginal protrusions which are separated from the müllerian canals by a thin septum, the hymen (Fig. 141).

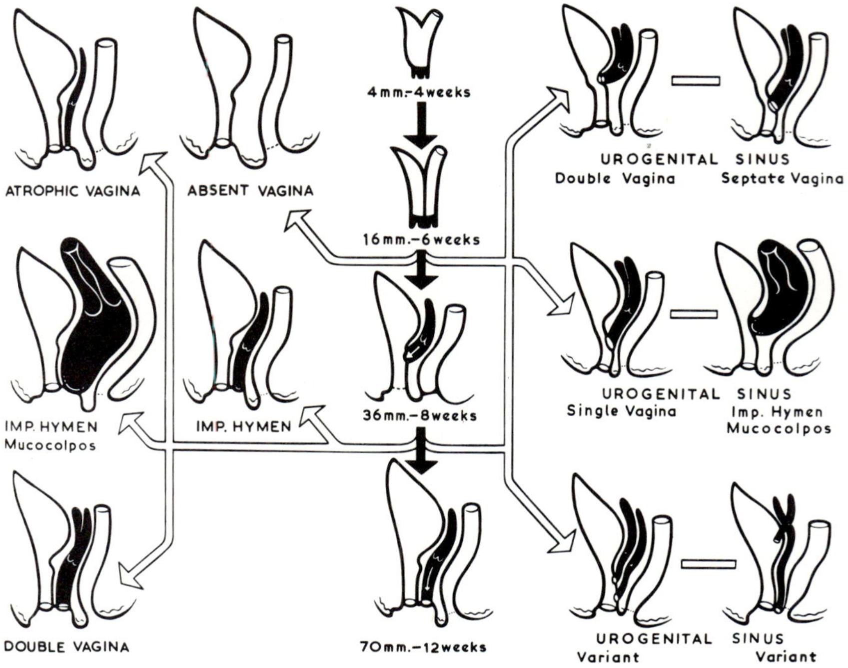

Fig. 141.—Utero-vaginal canal malformations. Anterior perineal or vulvar anus may occur in combination with any of the illustrated uro-genital defects. Schema shows the stages at which it is presumed that arrests of development occur. Black arrows indicated normal stages, and white arrows depict the corresponding defects. (Reproduced with permission from Australian & New Zealand J. Surg. 5:64, 1966.)

The uro-genital sinus is initially a tubal structure which explicates, becomes less deep and widens to form the vestibule as the embryo grows. The urethral and vaginal orifices descend caudally as a result of this change and issue externally. The hymen at first separates the epithelium of the sinus from that of the vagina, but eventually it disintegrates and the two structures become confluent. In the view of Koff (1933), sinus epithelium streams into and lines the vaginal wall in the distal two fifths of its extent, but other embryologists regard the hymen as the epithelial demarcation line. Our studies of deformities lead us to side with the latter view.

The wolffian ducts after piloting their müllerian sisters to their destination undergo atrophy in the female. Sometimes they persist temporarily or permanently in part or whole, as Gärtner's ducts, which are incorporated within the walls of the vagina. The orifices of persisting wolffian ducts, according to Frazer (1931), issue on to the outer aspect of the hymen.

INTRINSIC GENITAL DEFORMITIES.—Aberrations of fusion may lead to any degree of craniocaudal septal partition of the uretero-vaginal canal, varying from the most mild degree affecting the uterine lumen only—uterus subseptus unicollis, without any external evidence of the deformity in the uterus—to uterus didelphys with double vagina (Patten, 1947).

One or both müllerian ducts may fail to develop or, once started in their migration, may be arrested at any point on the course. Absence of both ducts occurred in 1 patient aged 4 years who lacked a vagina and whose solitary kidney was located in the pelvis.

The ducts which form the vagina may migrate in the normal manner but develop only as epithelial tubes, the walls of which may fuse but fail to maturate or grow to size. One stillborn baby exhibited this epithelial anlage of the vagina which was identified histologically from serially cut sections of the pelvic organs. No muscle was present in its walls which lay in a matrix of mesenchymal connecting tissue.

The hymen, a septum which should undergo atrophy, may remain imperforate. This may pass unrecognized until puberty when menstrual pains, absence of "period" blood flow and a mass caused by hematocolpos bring the child to the doctor for treatment. Occasionally, it may cause symptoms in the newborn infant. Then mucocolpos, a giant expansion of the vagina and uterus caused by excess mucus secreted by the cervical glands, compresses and partially obstructs by pressure the urethra and bowel and is readily detected by rectal and lower abdominal palpation.

Uro-Genital Deformities

The uro-genital sinus is similar in the male and female fetus at the 36-mm. stage, the urethra, the wolffian ducts and the müllerian ducts, all converging on the cranial aspect of the common outlet. Further development in the male is characterized by atrophy of the müllerian system, the wolffian ducts becoming the ejaculatory system, while the uro-genital sinus remains to become the posterior urethra. In the female, the müllerian ducts undergo rapid development, the wolffian ducts atrophy, the uro-genital sinus explicates, and the urethral orifice and the hymen, at first deeply situated, surface in the newly formed vestibule.

PERSISTENCE OF THE URO-GENITAL SINUS.—Arrest of the evolution from sinus to vestibule may occur at any stage. Five patients exhibiting such arrest have been observed and studied over periods ranging from 3 months to 13 years. All display major malformations representing arrests in the earlier stages, but several other trivial and insignificant departures from the normal, representing errors arising in the latest stage of development, have been noticed in other children (Fig. 142).

A variant on the sinus theme was seen in two stillborn infants, in each of whom the two vaginae were entirely separate. In the first, two separate vaginae were arranged in line down the back of the sinus; in the other, the müllerian ducts were widely separated: one of these stopped short of the bladder, and the other, being hypoplastic, was very fine and issued between the urethra and the sinus which lay adjacent to the vestibule.

SURGICAL SIGNIFICANCE OF URO-GENITAL SINUS MALFORMATIONS. — Urinary incontinence, double vaginae in tandem order, blind sacs, the small caliber of the sinus and urinary tract disorders were some of the serious problems which required further investigations.

(a) Incontinence. — Two children were continent and two incontinent, the former exhibited a longer length of urethra with a small sinus and in the latter these findings were reversed. The "long" urethra which in one girl measured only 1.5 cm. at the age of 14 years, apparently contained a sufficiently complete muscle wall to implement control of micturition. The short urethra associated with the long "sinus" was presumably insufficiently endowed with muscle because of its shortness and because of the fact that it was further hindered by the deficiency in its posterior wall caused by the wide aperture of a single vagina or double vaginae. No histological studies of the urethral musculature were undertaken. Operation was re-

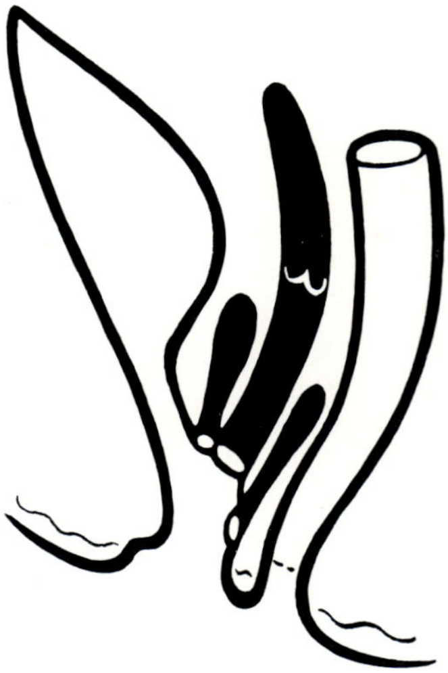

Fig. 142. — Anterior perineal anus associated with urogenital sinus deformity. The short urethra and vagina issue into the uro-genital sinus together with two additional blind sinuses. The anus lies close to the posterior wall of the vestibule.

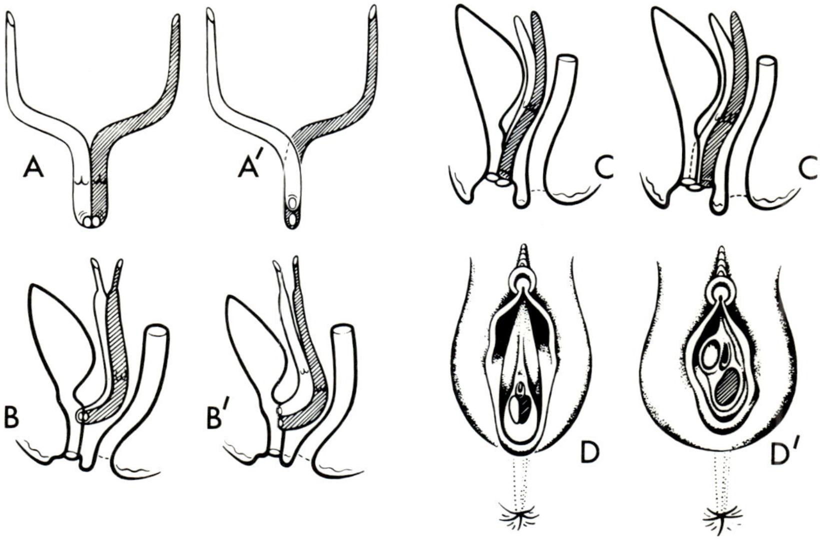

Fig. 143.—Tandem arrangement of double vaginae. Presumed explanation of fore-and-aft disposition of the lumens of double vaginae which are sometimes associated with recto-cloacal fistula and recto-vestibular fistula. **A–D,** usual disposition with side-by-side vaginae. **A′–D′,** abnormal craniocaudal arrangement of double vaginae in the uro-genital stage, and final fore-and-aft disposition in the vestibule.

quired, not for the sinus deformity per se but to counter incontinence by diversion of urine.

(b) Double Vagina.—Müllerian malformations are liable to occur. In 1 patient, two vaginae separated by a septum issued into the sinus, and, in another patient, it was presumed (because of absence of one kidney) that the single vagina originated from a single müllerian duct (Figs. 143, 144 and 145).

The septum of the double vaginae may need to be excised, but prior to adolescence it causes no inconvenience.

The tandem arrangement of the two components of the double vaginae is an interesting variant from the expected side-by-side disposition. Either the müllerian ducts on meeting in the coronal plane turn caudally but undergo a spiral turn towards the sagittal plane, or they meet tangentially, one lying anterior to the other. Once the müllerian ducts have spiraled, the two orifices, if they remain separated, will lie askew or tandem on the back wall of the uro-genital sinus. Should the sinus explicate in the normal fashion, it is likely that the urethral orifice will be slewed to one side, and the vaginal orifices to the other, as was seen in 1 patient who exhibited a uro-genito-rectal deformity (see Fig. 144).

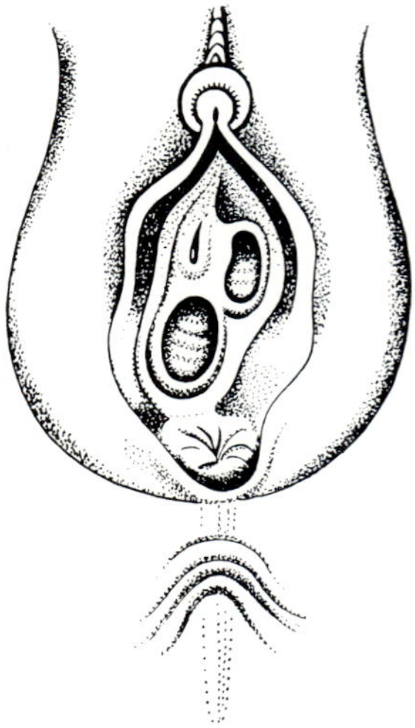

Fig. 144.—Vulvar anus showing associated double vaginae abnormality with fore-and-aft arrangement of the vaginae.

Vaginoplasty to widen the lumen of the external orifice or to excise a septum should be deferred till after puberty, when growth has ceased, and natural development and enlargement of the passage makes it unnecessary in many cases. Two postnatal processes may occur as shown by two of the patients described above. Firstly, the sinus may continue to explicate, bringing the urethra and vaginal orifices closer to the exterior. Secondly, the sinus may undergo considerable expansion at the time of puberty to resemble in caliber that

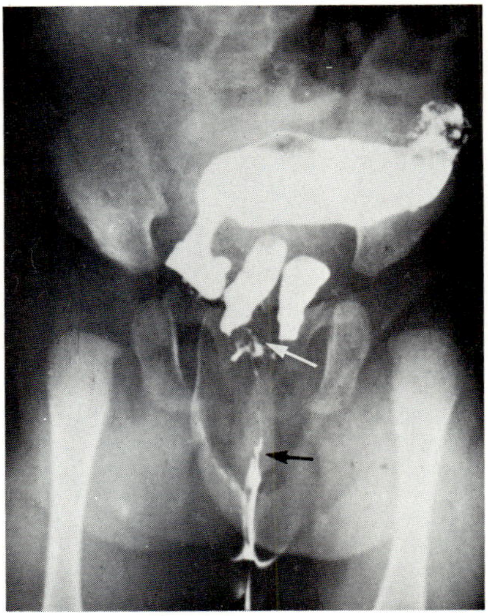

Fig. 145.—Recto-cloacal canal. Flushing fistulogram. Associated double vaginae—rectum issues into the cloacal canal between the two short vaginae (*white arrow*). External orifice of cloacal canal indicated by black arrow.

of a normal vagina. It seems from this evidence that treatment should be withheld until girl becomes woman.

Uro-Rectal-Genital Deformities

If the cloaca remains undivided, the rectum and urinary tract open to the exterior through a common outlet. The müllerian ducts superimpose themselves upon this cloaca, which then resembles the uro-genital sinus with a narrow rectal communication added to it. This uro-recto-genital deformity, termed recto-cloacal fistula, together with other recto-vaginal and recto-vestibular fistulae, has already been described in detail in Chapter 4.

Having now witnessed the progress and postnatal development of the congenital uro-genital sinus up to and beyond puberty in several children, it is our opinion that operation is not required to enlarge the lumen of the sinus and that, if continence of urine is satisfactory, no further reconstructive procedure is necessary. It seems, therefore, that if the rectum is detached from the recto-cloacal fistula and rerouted to the perineum in the fashion described to conserve the sphincteric control of the levatores ani muscles, the remaining uro-genital sinus may develop and enlarge in future years. One patient whose bowel was first treated by a defunctioning colostomy for a year has now had an appropriate reconstruction and has achieved a satisfactory measure of rectal continence. She is currently under observation at the age of 11 years. With operation, the visceral anatomy is made to match that of the congenital uro-genital sinus, and natural development should be observed until well after puberty, in the hope that the changes of adolescence are similarly favorable.

The rerouted rectum is unlikely to be quite as efficiently controlled as that of a child exhibiting a congenital uro-genital sinus, but if the pubo-visceral sling of the levator muscles is conserved, a high order of continence should be achieved (Stephens 1963 and 1965).

Hydrometrocolpos

Accumulation of mucus in the genital apparatus may occur behind an imperforate hymen, from vaginal atresia or from cervical obstruction. Cervical obstruction has been found particularly in cloacal malformations. Gough (1959) described cases of recto-cloacal fistulae with mucocolpos presenting as abdominal tumor. Moore and Lawrence (1952) had a patient with recto-vaginal fistula and hydrometrocolpos. Snyder (1966) described a hydrometrocolpos due to atresia of the midportion of the vagina, and Mahoney and Chamberlain (1940) had 1 patient with imperforate rectum and hydrometrocolpos due to a tranverse vaginal septum.

The abdominal tumor may be confusing in diagnosis. Even by those who normally advocate neonatal rectoplasty, hydrometrocolpos, because of its interference with the pelvic dissection, is taken as an indication to perform only colostomy. The diagnosis should become clear at laparotomy. The management of cases with vaginal atresia requires a vaginoplasty, but so few patients have survived that principles have not been established.

The uterine malformations require no treatment. The incidence of fertility and childbearing in patients with duplex müllerian systems associated with ano-rectal deformities is not known by the authors.

CHAPTER 13

Rare Complex Malformations

THE HINDGUT ANLAGE ultimately gives rise to the terminal ileum, cecum, colon and cloaca, the last becoming subdivided into rectum posteriorly and bladder and urethra anteriorly. Based upon the hypothesis of some early aberration of the primitive hindgut anlage, a number of very complex anomalies affecting all the hindgut derivatives, in varying degree, have been described. Two general groups of anomalies result. In one group, a split or twinning process of the anlage results in duplication of the terminal gut, with or without duplication of the genito-urinary structures; in a second group, an exstrophic process affects the anlage, resulting in ano-rectal agenesis associated with exstrophy of the ileo-cecal region and/or of the genito-urinary apparatus. Other structures are concurrently affected, either as part of the primary error or secondary to the hindgut malformations, so that anomalies of development are frequently seen in the müllerian, wolffian and genital fold structures—uterus and vagina, kidneys and ureters and external genitalia.

In the present context, we describe these anomalies, primarily in relation to the rectum and anus as (1) duplication of rectum and anus and (2) vesico-intestinal fissure, which is usually associated with ano-rectal agenesis.

Duplication of Rectum and Anus

We exclude from this discussion, duplication of the colon alone, of which there are many recorded cases; such "duplications" may be either spherical or tubular, affecting whole lengths of colon, but are more properly considered as "duplication cysts," "enterogenous cysts," etc. They are not associated with either anal or genito-urinary duplications. We have also seen three enterogenous cysts of the rectum (Smith, 1968), but these are similarly excluded from the discussion.

True duplication of the rectum and anus is a rare condition, and, including two previously unrecorded cases of our own, only 40 cases are recorded (Smith, 1969). The number of hindgut duplications of all kinds is slightly greater, but some series include cases with genito-urinary and genitalia duplication but with a single anus (e.g., in 9 of 37 cases reported by Beach *et al.*, 1961, and in 3 of those reported by Breen and Weinberg, 1965).

Of those with probable duplication of rectum and anus, we exclude from analysis the single case reports of the following papers for various reasons: Gleiss, 1904 (double anus and genitalia, but report unavailable), Gemmell and Patterson, 1913 (double recta and genitalia, but ani not recorded), Greig, 1934 (double colon but ani not recorded), Patterson and Maxwell, 1939 (double genitalia and urethra but ani not recorded), Kratzer *et al.*, 1951 (a complex parasitic twin), Judy, 1957 (a single anus, but two recta diverging 2 cm. from the anus; double colon, but single normal female genitalia), Christensen, 1959 (excision of a duplication cyst presenting in the perineum then revealed two ani; normal single female genitalia) and Abrami and Dennison 1961 (the paper presents an illustration of an infant with two ani in line in the natal cleft, but no details are recorded). Thirty-two cases remain for study (for references to 1968 see Tables 26, 27 and 28). The most extensive previous reviews are those of Ravitch (1953), notable for its detailed graphic illustrations of the 20 recorded cases to that time, and of Beach *et al.* (1961), with an extensive bibliography.

An analysis of these 32 cases indicates that there are three patterns of anatomical arrangement, each presenting a somewhat different therapeutic problem. (1) two separate perineal ani opening externally, (2) two ani, but one or both terminating in a fistula to the genito-urinary tract and (3) one external anus and one imperforate in the pelvis.

The sex and age of presentation are shown in Tables 24 and 25.

(I) DOUBLE PERINEAL ANI.—The detailed associations of 12 cases are shown in Table 26, including our own 2 cases. In all except 1 patient, the ani lay on either side of the midline, in line with their corresponding genitalia (Fig. 146). In 1 patient (Van Zwalenburg, 1952), the ani were only separated by a septum; in addition, although not included in Table 26 is the illustrated case of Abrami and Dennison, 1961, in which the ani are both in the midline, one behind the other. Our two cases are as follows:

TABLE 24.—SEX INCIDENCE OF DUPLICATED ANI

SEX	2 PERINEAL ANI	2 ANI WITH FISTULAE	2 ANI 1 IMPERFORATE	TOTAL
Male	2	2	6	10
Female	10	9	3	22
TOTAL	12	11	9	32

TABLE 25.—PERIOD OF LIFE OF PRESENTATION OF DUPLICATED ANI

PERIOD	2 PERINEAL ANI	2 ANI WITH FISTULAE	2 ANI (1 IMPERFORATE)	TOTAL
Newborn	7	6	2	15
Child	–	5	5	10
Adult	5	–	1	6
Not Recorded	–	–	1	1

(1) Baby P. (Figs. 63, B, 146 and 147) presented as a thriving infant with no other anomalies than genito-recto-urinary duplication. Below a midline soft-tissue mass is a widened pair of labia majora, within which are two normal looking complete vestibules, each consisting of clitoris, labia minora and urethral and vaginal orifices (Fig. 146). Urine issues from each urethra, and the infant is continent through both. In line with each vulval apparatus is a normal anal orifice, the two orifices being separated by approximately 1.5 cm. Each anal orifice issues feces, and each is continent. A series of radiographs with dye introduced into each anus, urethra and vagina (Fig. 147) show complete duplication of rectum and colon as far as the ascending colon where the colon is single, two separate bladders and urethrae, and two separate vaginae and cervices uteri. An intravenous pyelogram indicates a horeshoe kidney, with at least three separate pelvic systems. The infant is now 9 months old and thriving, and treatment is described below.

(2) Our second case became available for dissection of the sphincter anatomy which illuminated the bearing that this anatomy has on treatment. Baby K. (Fig. 148), fully reported by Beischer and Fortune (1968), was a stillborn female infant weighing 3,100 Gm. and was a double-headed fetus (dicephalic dipus dibrachius), with a single trunk formed by side-to-side union commencing at the necks. The heads were separate, the heart single, although abnormal, with two vertebral columns converging below to a single pelvis. The right diaphragm was deficient. The entire alimentary tract was duplicated, with close fusion of the two elements consisting of a common external muscle coat and fused inner coats. There were only two kidneys and ureters, and a single normal bladder and urethra. There was a single normal genital system (Fig. 148). Dissection of the pelvis by one of us (FDS) showed a rudimentary tail behind the vaginal orifice, containing a large nerve plexus which could be traced backwards to the termination of the spine, passing between the two separated anal canals. Two recta were apposed to one another, with a continuous longitudinal muscle coat surrounding both recta, but the circular coat was fused along the adjoining walls down to the perineal body. The anal canals were quite separate below the perineal body, diverging towards

TABLE 26.—Reported Colon Duplications with Two Separate Perineal Ani

Author	Sex	Age of Presentation	Colon	External Genitalia	Internal Genitalia	Bladders	Urethrae	Kidneys and Ureters	Associated Anomalies	Treatment and Results
Piccoli (1892)	F	Newborn	Double 2 caeca 2 appendices	1 vulva 1 clitoris 2 vaginae	2 uteri (unicornuate) 1 tube and ovary each side	Exstrophy of single bladder	Single exstrophy	N/R	Omphalocele	Died 24 hours after repair of omphalocele
Smith and Boulgakov (1926)	M	Stillborn	Double alimentary canal (septum)	1 penis 1 scrotum	–	1 divided by septum	2 becoming one	2 kidneys 2 ureters	Double-headed monster double spine	Stillborn
Bruni (1927)	M	35	N/R but "forked rectum"	2 penes 2 scrota	–	2	2	N/R	–	Died of extraneous causes
Lesbre (1927)	F	Adult	Double from terminal ileum 2 caeca 2 appendices	2 vulvae 2 vaginae	2 uteri 1 tube and ovary each side	2	2	N/R	Double spine from L2	No treatment, alive
Hinckle (1928)	F	62	Double 2 caeca 2 appendices	2 vulvae (1 pair of labia majora, 2 clitorides) 2 vaginae	2 uteri 1 tube and ovary each side	2	2	N/R	N/R	No treatment, alive, normal urination, defecation and menses through each of double orifices
Van Zwalenburg (1952)	F	52	Double from terminal ileum 2 caeca 2 appendices	1 vulva 2 clitorides septate vaginae	1 uterus	2	2	N/R	Meckel's diverticulum polyp in colon	Anal septum divided, alive (polyp removed)
Bornstein (1957)	F	Newborn	Double	1 vulva 1 clitoris 1 vagina	N/R	2	2	N/R	Spina bifida and myelomeningocele	

Beach *et al.* (1961)	F	Newborn	Double from terminal ileum 2 caeca 2 appendices	2 vulvae (1 pair of labia majora) 2 clitorides 2 vaginae	2 uteri 1 tube and ovary each side	2	2 (1 normal 1 opens to right vagina)	2 kidneys 2 ureters	Spina bifida and myelomeningocele, talipes, peritoneal septum	Myelomeningocele excised. R. colon divided inferiorly (leaving a stump to vagina) and anastomosed to L. colon. Alive, feces through L. anus–some urinary incontinence
Breen and Weinberg (1965)	F	20	Double from caecum	2 vulvae 2 clitorides 2 vaginae	Uterus didelphys	2	2	2 kidneys 2 ureters	–	No treatment, alive, simultaneous normal urination, defecation and menses through each of double orifices. Coitus in R. vagina, 3 infants born per vaginum
Beischer and Fortune (1968)	F	Stillborn	Double alimentary canal	1 vulva 1 clitorides 1 vagina	1 uterus 2 tubes and ovaries	1	1	2 kidneys 2 ureters	Double-headed monster, double spine single pelvis	Stillborn
Smith (1968) Present report	F	Newborn	Double from caecum	2 vulvae 2 clitorides 2 vaginae	2 uteri	2	2	Horseshoe 3 ureters	–	Alive, normal continence with simultaneous voiding and defecation through each of double orifices. Alive, aged 9 months
Rowe *et al* (1968)	F	Newborn	Double from rectum	2 vulvae 2 clitorides 2 vaginae	2 uteri 1 tube and ovary each side	2	2 (1 urethra ran an ectopic course)	2 kidneys 2 ureters	Hemivertebrae 4 lower limbs omphalocele	Repair of omphalocele. Colon resection and ileo-colostomy. Colostomy. Excision of 2 lower limbs

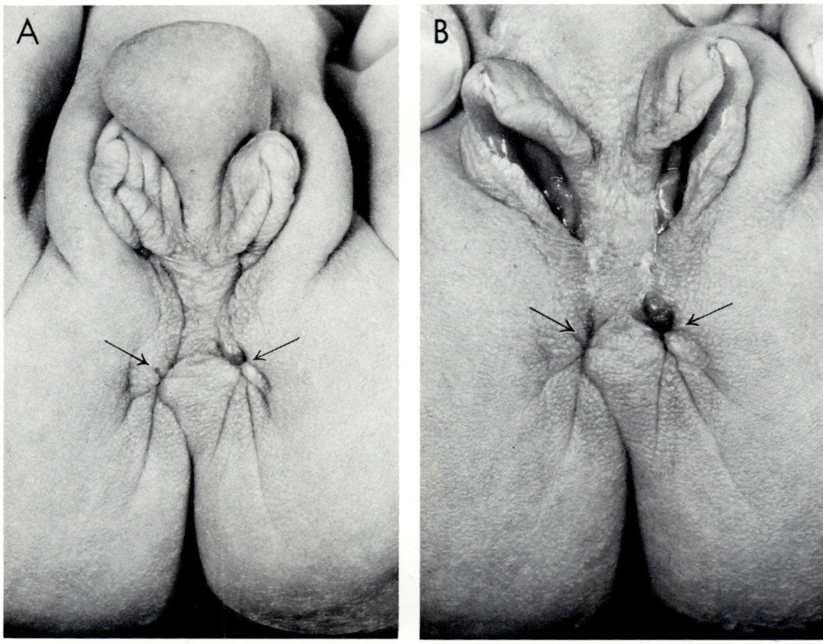

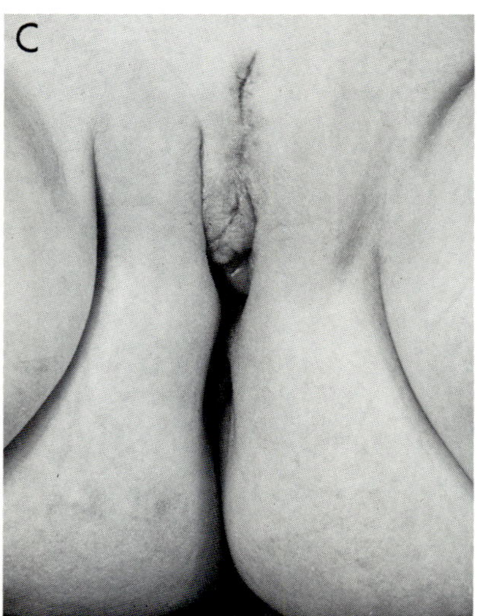

Fig. 146.—Double anus and duplication of vulva. **A** and **B,** the ani are side by side (*arrows*), and both function normally and simultaneously; baby now aged 9 months. Within each vulva is a normal urethra and vagina. Micturition occurs simultaneously through urethrae. The central mound between the paired vulvae proved to be fat only. **C,** appearance 3 weeks after operation. The central mound of fat has been excised, together with the medial two labia minora, and partial clitorectomies. The lateral minora have been sutured in the midline. The two urethrae and two vaginae remain in the now single vestibule, the external appearances beginning to simulate those of a normal vulva.

the skin where the orifices lay 1.5 cm. apart. Each was lined by normal anal canal epithelium. Each anal canal had its own complete internal sphincter and longitudinal muscle. The external sphincters were arranged so that the main mass of voluntary muscle passed around both of the anal canals, joining in front, but no voluntary muscle passed between the two anal canals. The pubo-rectalis and levator ani muscle were single and passed around both anal canals.

Only two of the 12 recorded cases are males. These patients present only because of their abnormal external appearance and are symptom-free, apart from associated disease. Of the 4 deaths, two were stillborn, 1 died aged 24 hours, after repair of omphalocele (Piccoli, 1892), and 1 died at age 35 years of extraneous causes (Bruni, 1927). The remainder survived with anal and urinary continence (Table 26). All patients had a double colon, including duplication of the terminal ileum in 5, although the details of the colon are not clear in Bruni's case (1927). One male patient had two penes and scrota (Bruni, 1927).

The external genitalia in the female patients varied, but in the majority the structures were duplicated – complete double vulvae, clitorides and vaginae in 4, double vulvae or clitorides and vaginae, but within a single pair of labia majora in 3, a single vulva with double vaginae in 1 and single vulva, clitoris and vagina in 2 patients.

In the urinary tract, there was an exstrophied single bladder and urethra in 1, a single normal bladder and urethra in 1, but the remaining 10 patients had double bladders and urethrae. The state of the upper urinary tract is not recorded in 6, our patient has a horseshoe kidney with three pelves and ureters, and the remaining 5 patients each have two normal kidneys and ureters.

Associated anomalies occurred frequently, being present in 8 of 11 recorded findings. Two stillborns were double-headed monsters with double spines, one other patient had a double spine, caudal to the 2d lumbar vertebra; in 2, there was a spina bifida with myelomeningocele, 1 patient had an omphalocele, and 1 patient had omphalocele and four lower extremities (Rowe *et al.*, 1968).

Management. – Excluding the 4 patients who died of extraneous causes, and 1 in whom the outcome is not recorded, the remaining 7 patients are alive and well. In Van Zwalenburg's patient (1952), a 52-year-old female, an anal septum was divided, but no treatment was necessary for the ani in the remainder, defecation being controlled and simultaneous through both ani. The case reported by Beach *et al.* (1961) was complicated by the presence of a myelomeningocele and by the unexplained later development of a fistula from the right rectum to the right vagina, so that some neurogenic incontinence might be expected. In this patient, the right colon was di-

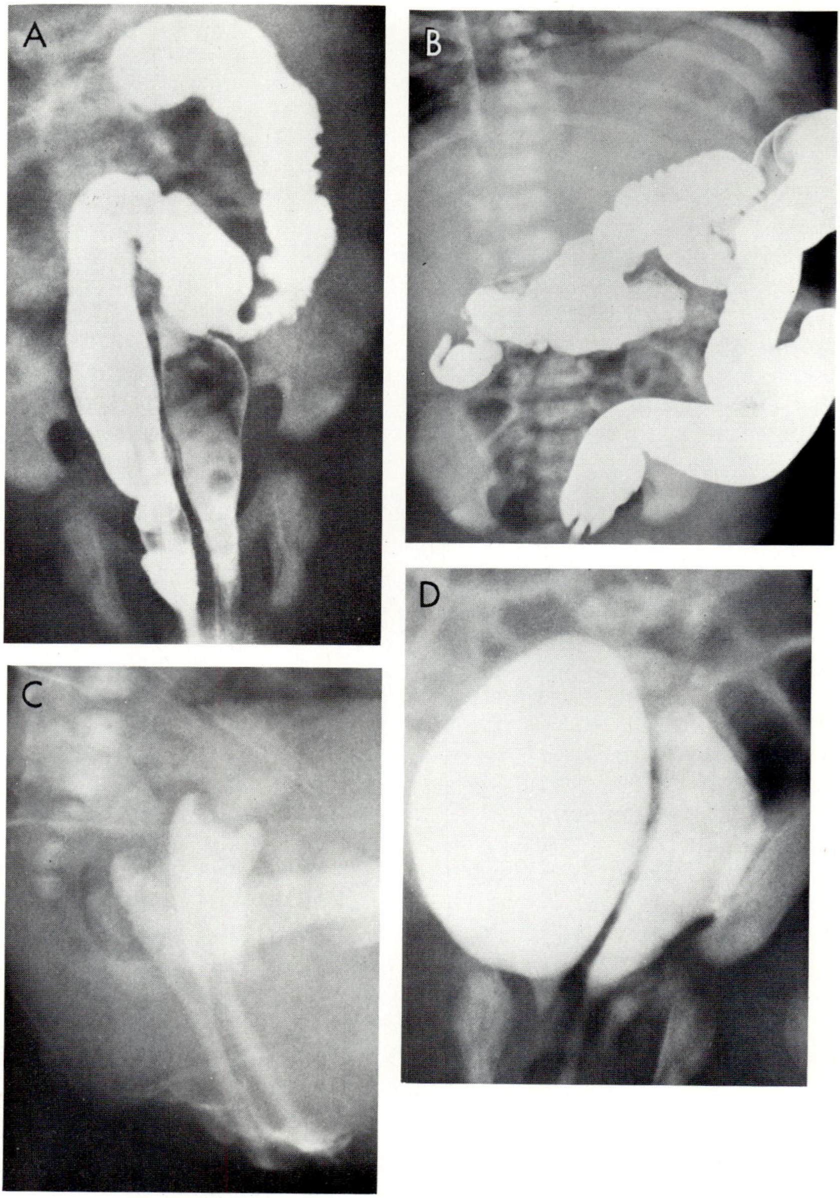

Fig. 147.—Duplication of anus, rectum, colon, and genito-urinary tract. **A,** right rectum and colon filled; left rectum partially filled with contrast medium. **B,** left rectum and colon filled and separate as far as the ascending colon. At this point, the medium demonstrates the junction of the two colons, the right colon just

vided inferiorly and anastomosed to the left colon (leaving a rectal stump draining into the right vagina).

All the recorded patients appear to urinate simultaneously and with control through their double urethrae (apart from neurogenic paralysis from spina bifida in the case of Beach *et al.* 1961). In the 4 adult females, simultaneous menses occurred through each vagina. Parturition is recorded in only 1 patient (Breen and Weinberg, 1965) and this was normal, following coitus through the right vagina. Only in 1 patient (our own Baby P.) has any local operative treatment to the genitalia been attempted.

Provided there is no neurogenic element, as from spina bifida, it appears that continence and normal function can be expected through both the ani and urethrae. This finding, taken in conjunction with the fact that both recta appear to lie within the same single pubo-rectalis muscle sling, and within a single external sphincter (dissection of Baby K.), suggests that it may be best to accept the two ani permanently. Normal continence might be jeopardized by attempting to excise one rectum from the other. As the levator and sphincter muscles are mesodermal structures and not related to hindgut development, it is reasonable to assume that they will al-

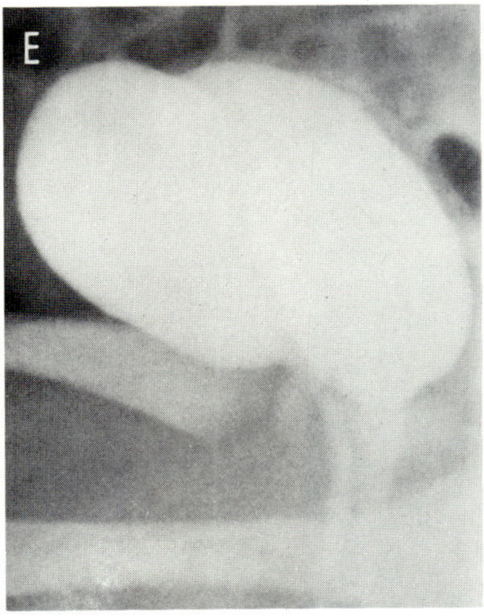

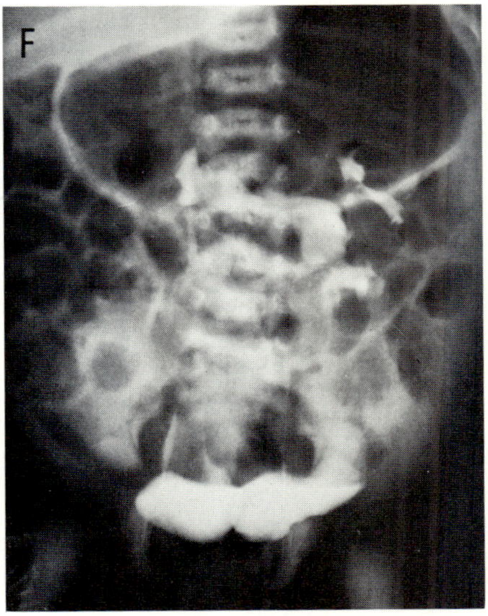

beginning to fill from the left. Note the single caecum and appendix. **C**, double vaginae, each with filling defect produced by the cervix. **D** and **E**, micturition cystourethrogram (catheter to each urethra) demonstrates two separate bladders and urethrae and normal bladder necks. **F**, intravenous pyelogram showing at least three renal pelvicalyceal systems (possibly horseshoe kidney). Two ureters visible also both bladders. Note normal spine.

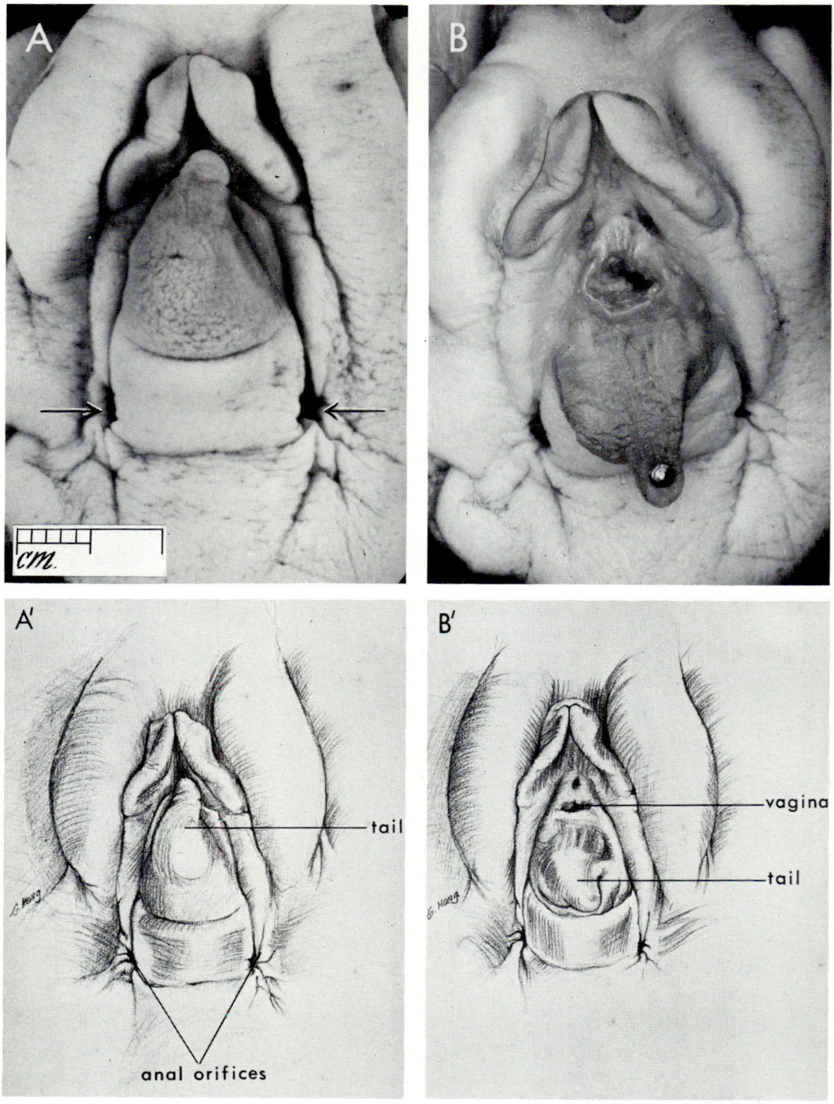

Fig. 148.—Duplication of anus with single vulva. **A, A′** and **B, B′** stillborn infant perineum. Double ani side by side in line with labia minora. Single urethra and vagina. Vagina partially hidden by a rudimentary tail containing a nerve plexus. (See text for internal anatomy.) (After Beischer, N. A., and Fortune, D. W.: Obst. & Gynec. 32:158, 1968.)

ways be single, except if the spine and sacrum be duplicated. Should some obstructive complication occur in the double colon, one could be excised, but its lower rectal stump should be left in situ through the sphincters. Alternatively, it might be conceivable to evaginate the mucosa of the rectal stump to achieve its nonfunction, by a technique similar to that described by Babcock (1947), Ravitch (1948), Bacon (1949), Romualdi (1960 and 1961) and Soave (1964).

Should intervention be necessary, Beach *et al.* (1961) have shown that in double colons associated with duplication of genitalia, the two colons are usually not fused and have separate blood supply, so that resection of one colon from the other should be possible. In the recorded cases, including our own Baby P., both colons appear to function normally, and there seems no compelling reason to wish to intervene electively, provided the double ani do not appear to be a social embarrassment to the patient in later life.

For the same reason, there seems to be no special case to remove or close over one urethra in the female, unless the siting of one of them interferes with vulval reconstruction. The simultaneous continent urinary streams should prove no great disadvantage, especially if they can be masked by reconstructing a single vulva.

Duplication of the vagina has been shown to be no disadvantage to menses, coitus or parturition, unless there is stenosis.

The principal problem would appear to be the cosmetic one of duplicated penile and vulval anatomy. No patient in these series (prior to our Baby P.) has had any reconstruction operation, the adult patients apparently accepting their disability. However, in Baby P., the labia have been reconstructed by excising the central fatty mound and the two medial labia minora, joining the two lateral labia minora centrally. This provides an external appearance of a single vulva, within which the two urethrae and two vaginae open unimpeded (see Fig. 146, *C*).

(II) Double Ani Terminating as Fistulae.—In 11 patients (Table 27), either one or both of the ani terminate as a fistulous communication into either the genital or urinary tract. All the colons were duplicated caudal to the ascending colon, and, in five, the duplication commenced in the terminal ileum; 1 patient had an additional duplication cyst in one colon. In 6 patients, 1 rectum opened to a normal anus in the perineum, the second rectum terminating in the vestibule (3), the vagina (2) and the male urethra (1). In the remaining 5 patients, both ani terminated ectopically into vestibule, vagina, cloaca, bladder or urethra (Table 27). Although many of these patients also possessed abnormal genitalia, the majority presented clinically because of a complication to the bowel, quite unlike those above with two separate perineal ani. All patients in this group consequently presented in early infancy or childhood, none reaching adult life

TABLE 27.—Reported Colon Duplications with Fistulae

Author	Sex	Age of Presentation	Colon	Ani	External Genitalia	Internal Genitalia	Bladders	Urethrae	Kidneys and Ureters	Associated Anomalies	Treatment and Results
Suppiger (1876)	F	Newborn	Double from caecum	1 recto-vaginal 1 recto-vestibular	2 vulvae 2 clitorides 2 vaginae	2 unicorn-uate uteri 1 tube and ovary each side	2	2	2 kidneys 2 ureters	Double spine from L3	Died from intes-tinal obstruct-ion at age 1¾ yr. No treatment
Grohé (1900)	F	10	Double 2 caeca 2 append-ices	1 normal 1 recto-vestibular	1 vulva 1 clitoris septate vagina	N/R	1	N/R	N/R	N/R	Excision of septum between recta; division of vaginal septum. Alive
Volpe (1903)	M	29 days	Double from caecum	1 recto-urethral 1 recto-vesical	2 penes	–	2	2	Horseshoe with 1 ureter to left bladder	N/R	Died of intes-tinal obstruct-ion. No treatment
Aitken (1912)	F	Newborn	Double from terminal ileum 2 caeca 2 append-ices	1 normal 1 recto-vestibular	1 vulva	1 unicorn-uate uterus	N/R	N/R	N/R	Omphalocele	Died at aged 24 hours. No treatment
Ballance (1930)	F	10	Double from ascend. colon	2 recto-vaginal (into one vagina)	1 vulva 1 vagina	1 uterus 1 tube and ovary each side	1	1	N/R	–	Several attempts to repair recto-vaginal fistulae excision of double colon. Alive
Ombredanne (1936)	F	2	Double from terminal ileum	1 normal 1 vestibular anus	2 vulvae 2 clitorides 2 vaginae	Uterus didelphys	N/R	1 urethra on right 1 blind urethra left	N/R	N/R	Died at aged 10 weeks. No treatment

Brunschwig *et al.* (1948)	F	7	Double from terminal ileum	1 normal 1 recto-vaginal	1 vulva	1 uterus 1 tube and ovary each side	N/R	N/R	N/R	–	Two colons anastomosed; colon to recto-vaginal fistula divided, leaving a mucous sac to the vagina. Alive
Aitken (1950)	F	Newborn	Double from terminal ileum	2 recto-vestibular	2 vulvae bifid clitoris 2 vaginae	1 bicornuate uterus	N/R	1 at root of bifid clitoris	N/R	Omphalocele	Omphalocele repaired only. Alive
Van Velzer *et al.* (1956)	F	11	Double from caecum	1 normal 1 recto-vaginal	1 vulva	1 uterus 1 tube and ovary each side	1	1	1 right kidney absent left kidney	–	Fistula closed, colons anastomosed. Alive
Mysorekar *et al.* (1967)	F	Newborn	Double from terminal ileum 2 caeca 2 appendices (Right colon also had duplication above the cloaca)	1 recto-cloacal 1 recto-vestibular	2 vulvae laterally (a) Right: 1 labium majorus 1 clitoris 1 cloacal opening (b) Left: 1 labium minorus 1 clitoris 1 urogenital opening	2 unicornuate uteri, each with single tube and ovary	2	1 to right cloaca 1 to left vagina	1 right duplex with bifid ureters 1 single left kidney	2 hemi-livers, double spine from L1, Absent sacrum anterior myelomeningocele	Died at aged 1 month. No treatment
Cohen (1968)	M	Newborn	Double from hepatic flexure	1 normal 1 recto-urethral	Bifid penis bifid scrotum	–	2	2	2 kidneys 2 ureters	–	Operated on but no details. Alive

without operation. All 5 patients not treated died of intestinal obstruction.

The genitalia were more variable in type than in the previous group, duplicated systems being not quite so common. Although both the males had duplication of the penes, only 4 of the 9 females had duplication of the external genitalia, one had a single vulva with a septate vagina, the remaining 4 patients possessing a single normal vulva and vagina. The most complex arrangement was the patient of Mysorekar *et al.*, 1967 (Table 27).

Information about the urinary tract is not well documented, with no records available in 4 patients. In 4, the bladder was duplicated and single in 3. With the duplicated bladders, the urethrae were also double to the perineum, but, in Mysorekar's patient, one urethra opened to a cloaca, the other to a common uro-genital canal. In an additional patient (Ombredanne, 1936) in whom the state of the bladder is not recorded, one urethra was blind. In 5 patients in whom the upper urinary tract is documented, there were two normal kidneys in each of 2 patients, but abnormalities in the other 3 patients (horseshoe with one ureter, 1; absence of one kidney, 1; and renal duplex on one side with bifid ureters, 1).

Associated anomalies were present in 4 of the 8 cases in which this feature was recorded (omphalocele, 2; double spine, 2). In Mysorekar's patient with duplicated spine caudal to the 1st lumbar vertebra, there was also an anterior myelomenigocele and bifurcated liver.

Management.—The only patients who survived in this group of ani with fistulae were those 6 patients operated upon. In the presence of one normal anus, the successful operation was the anastomosis of the two colons together to permit defecation through this anus, the other fistulous anus being divided (3 patients). In 1 other patient with one normal anus (Cohen, 1968), the details of operation are not provided. Two other operative survivals are those of Ballance (1930), who excised both colons following unsuccessful attempts to close both recto-vaginal fistulae, and of Aitken (1950), who repaired an associated omphalocele but in which the recto-vestibular fistulae persist without obstruction.

Unlike the previous group of patients with two separate perineal ani, this group with fistulae obstruction to one or both colons forced operative intervention; operation was successful in all to whom it was offered, even in Grohé's patient in 1900.

No operation has been performed in any patient for the genito-urinary malformations, but the comments made above in group (I) probably apply to the present group also.

(III) DOUBLE ANI, ONE IMPERFORATE.—In 5 of 9 patients (Table 28), there was one normal anus, and the second rectum was imperforate in the pelvis. In 1 patient, both the recta were imperforate (Bar and De Kervilly, 1909); in 2 patients, the colon was terminally triplicate, so that there were three recta to be disposed. In Gray's patient (1940), the middle colon opened to the perineum, the lateral colon was imperforate and the medial colon opened into the middle rectum. In Leon-Diaz's patient (1951) two colons ended blindly, and one terminated in the bladder. The colons in all the remaining patients were double (Table 28). As in the previous group, these patients presented mainly because of obstruction in one colon in infancy. However, one female did not present until the age of 27 years, when she developed acute appendicitis in one of the appendices.

Unlike the previous groups, duplication of the genitalia was the exception, only one female having double vulvae and vaginae, and only one male having a bifid glans penis. One patient had no external genitalia.

However, in all recorded cases, either the bladder or urethra or both were double. Three bladders were septate, and one was exstrophied. Table 28 indicates some of the complex arrangements of the urethrae. In the upper urinary tract of 5 recorded cases, one kidney was absent or atrophic in two cases.

Management.—These patients did more poorly than either of the two previous groups. Of the 10 patients whose course is recorded, 2 died in infancy without treatment, and 6 had operations, of whom 3 died—1 after colostomy, 1 after transrectal incision of colonic septum and 1 after total colectomy and ileo-anal anastomosis. Three patients survived total colectomy. The operative experience supports the contention of Beach *et al.* (1961), that when the external genitalia are single the double colons tend to be intimately fused, so that colonic resection of both colons together is necessary.

The bladder septum has been excised in 2 patients, but the remaining patients died without treatment of their urinary abnormalities. No record is available of the management of the patient with double vulvae. As Table 28 indicates, this group did not present a cosmetic problem because the external genitalia were almost all normal.

Reference to Tables 26, 27 and 28 shows that, although there are exceptions, the derivatives of the müllerian and wolffian systems are generally not duplicated. In all cases, there is only one tube and ovary on each side, and although some uteri are double or bicornuate this probably only represents nonfusion or partial fusion of the müllerian ducts which are normally paired structures. In most patients, similarly, there is a single kidney on each side. These systems are not part of the hindgut-cloacal anlage and are thus not affected by the malformation.

TABLE 28.—Reported Colon Duplications with One or Both Ani Imperforate

Author	Sex	Age of Presentation	Colon	Ani	External Genitalia	Internal Genitalia	Bladders	Urethrae	Kidneys and Ureters	Associated Anomalies	Treatment and Results
Chiarleoni (1894)	F	?	Double	1 vestibular anus 1 imperforate	2 vulvae 2 vaginae	N/R	1	2	N/R	N/R	N/R
Bar and DeKervilly (1909)	M	14 days	Double from caecum	1 imperforate at sigmoid 1 imperforate on bladder wall	1 penis bifid scrotum	–	2	2 1 at glans 1 on ventral surface of penis	2 kidneys 2 ureters	Spina bifida and myelomeningocele	Died at 14 days after colostomy
Asai (1933)	M	1	Double from terminal ileum 2 caeca 2 appendices	1 normal 1 imperforate at sigmoid	1 penis 1 scrotum	–	N/R	2 on penis but one blind	N/R	–	Died aged 1 year after trans-rectal incision of colonic septum
Gray (1940)	F	9 months	Triple from caecum	1 anterior anus (from middle colon) 1 colo-rectal fistula (medial colon to middle rectum) 1 imperforate rectum (from lateral colon)	No genitalia	1 uterus (rudimentary) 1 tube and ovary each side	1 exstrophy	1 exstrophy	N/R	–	Died at aged 9 months with constipation. No treatment
Menten and Denny (1945)	M	4 months	Double from caecum	1 normal 1 imperforate rectum	1 penis	–	2 septate	N/R	2 kidneys 2 ureters	–	Died at aged 4 months with fecal impaction.

			2 caeca 2 appendices								No treatment
Weber and Dixon (1946)	F	27	Double from terminal ileum 2 caeca 2 appendices	1 normal 1 imperforate rectum	1 vulva	2 uteri 1 tube and ovary each side	N/R	N/R	1 left kidney, absent right	–	Acute appendicitis in one appendix, excision of colons and anastomosis after excision of spur. Alive
Allard *et al.* (1949)	M	$4^1/_2$	Double from terminal ileum 2 caeca 2 appendices	1 normal 1 imperforate rectum	1 penis 1 scrotum	–	N/R	1	N/R	–	Excision of colons, septum crushed, ileo-sigmoidostomy. Alive
Leon-Diaz (1951)	M	Newborn	Double from caecum 2 caeca 1 appendix (one colon double again at termination)	1 recto-vesical 2 ended blindly	1 penis 1 scrotum	–	2 septate	1 left (right bladder – no urethra)	2 kidneys 2 ureters	Omphalocele	Died at 7 weeks after colostomy, repair of omphalocele and excision of bladder septum (stage 1); and (stage 2) total colectomy and ileo-anal anastomosis
Ravitch and Scott (1953)	M	$4^1/_2$	Double from terminal ileum 1 appendix	1 normal 1 imperforate rectum	1 penis, with bifid glans 1 scrotum	–	2 septate	2	2 kidneys (but left atrophic)	–	Excision of colon and anastomosis, bladder septum excised and left bladder neck closed; left nephrectomy. Alive 3 years later

Vesico-Intestinal Fissure

This complicated anomaly has been variously called "vesico-intestinal fissure" (Schwalbe, 1909), "ectopia cloacae" (Williams, 1958) and "exstrophy of the cloaca" (Johnston and Penn, 1966). It was first described by Meckel (1812), and Keith (1908) collected 14 cases. Some of the common features are described by Johnston and Penn (1966) as follows*:

An exstrophic hemibladder with a ureteric orifice lies on each side of the midline and between them is a zone of intestinal mucosa with an upper and a lower orifice, the former discharging intestinal contents. Dissection reveals that the exstrophic bowel is the ileocaecal region, the upper opening being the terminal ileum, which commonly prolapses, whilst the lower leads to a 2 to 3 inch length of large intestine which ends blindly in front of the sacrum. A third orifice, that of the vermiform appendix, may be visible on the exposed mucosal surface and occasionally there are paired appendices (Russell, 1939). A broad exomphalos containing small intestine and often a portion of the liver is usually present immediately above the exstrophy. The anus is imperforate but a surface dimple may be present [Fig. 149].

Abnormalities of the upper urinary tract and the internal and external genitalia are very common. Soper and Kilger (1964) reviewed fifty-seven recorded cases, twenty-nine male, twenty-four female and four in which the sex was either not determined or unspecified. Of thirty children in whom the urinary tract was described, fifteen showed gross unilateral or bilateral anomalies such as renal aplasia or hypoplasia, multicystic disease, hydronephrosis, hydro-ureter, ureteral stenosis, ureteral atresia and anomalous ureteral termination. Union between the ureter and the vas deferens occurred in one of our three cases of classical cloacal exstrophy and a similar persistence of the original mesonephric duct was recorded by Bryce (1895), Emrys-Roberts and Paterson (1906), and Wood-Jones (1912).

In the male the phalli are usually duplex, one on each side, but the occurrence of a single midline penis was described by Bartels (1868), Steinbuchel (1900) and Spencer and Geer (1967). The phalli have been epispadiac in all recorded cases except that of Hall *et al.* (1953), in which each of the two phalli contained a small central urethra. Bilateral cryptorchidism has been present in all cases with the exception of two of Bartels' (1868) in which the testes were normally descended.

In twenty-two of the twenty-four female cases recorded (Soper and Kilger, 1964) the uterus was bicornuate, and in fourteen the vagina was duplex; absence of the vagina occurred in six cases.

In one of our patients, of undetermined sex, there was no external genitalia; a similar state of affairs has occurred both in the female (Dietrich, 1904), and in the male (Russell, 1939). The most common of the many coexistent but unrelated abnormalities is spina bifida which has been present in thirty-two of the fifty-seven cases recorded by Soper and Kilger (1964).

---

*Reprinted with permission from Johnston, J. H., and Penn, I. A.: Brit. J. Urol. 38:302, 1966.

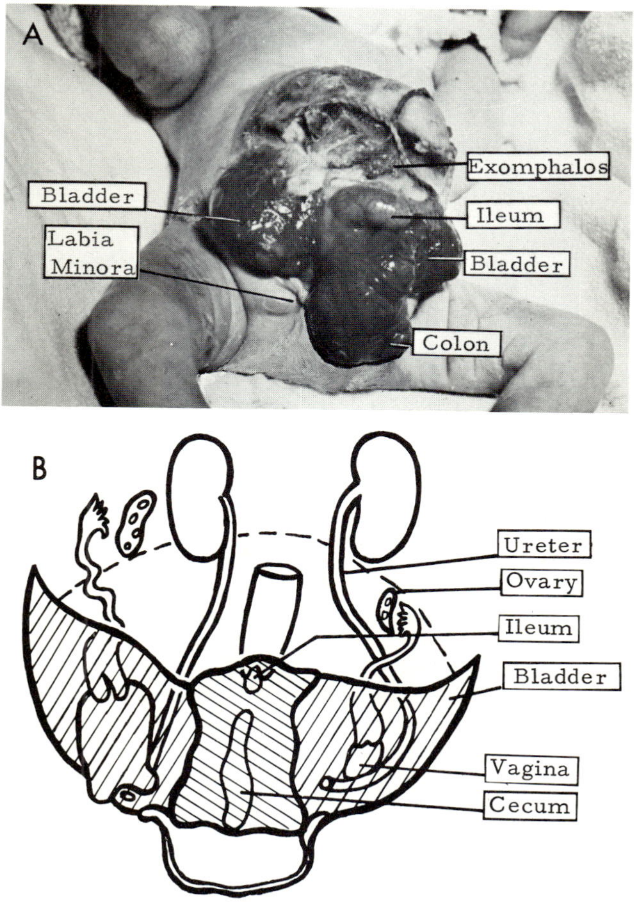

Fig. 149.—Vesico-intestinal fissure (female). **A** and **B,** exomphalos, bladder exstrophic and divided, the two lateral halves separated by intestinal epithelium. Absence of hindgut and anus.

We have encountered 11 patients in the Melbourne series with spina bifida, 7 males and 4 females.

In our Melbourne experience, all the female specimens showed defects of müllerian development, absence, deficiencies of distal segments of the ducts, imperforate terminations, mucocolpos or free passage through the vesical wall, but all showed complete separation of right and left systems. The vaginal part of the müllerian duct was always shorter than normal.

These patients all possessed the common features described above. As in the majority of recorded cases, the rectum ended blindly in 9 of our patients. However, in 1 patient, there was a recto-cloacal fistula and in 1 other patient a covered anus with a "bucket-handle" raphe in the perineum. The cystogram appearances of this patient are shown in Figure 150, *A*. These patients with terminal fistulae represent intermediate types of the anomaly. Magnus (1969) describes the nine imperforate specimens in detail (Fig. 150, *B*).

Management.—We have operated upon 3 patients, with one survival. The survivor is a boy whose rectal problem was minimal (a

Fig. 150.—**A,** partial vesico-intestinal fissure (male.) Double bladder, left vesico-ureteral reflux and left hypoplastic kidney shown by cystography. This baby also exhibited double penis, widely separated pubes, hypoplasia of the muscles of the abdominal wall and exomphalos. **B,** dissection of the bowel component of nine specimens of vesico-intestinal fissure; *a* represents the anatomy as it should occur, in the commonly accepted theory of Johnston (1913) of formation of ectopia cloacae; and *b–j* represent the bowel anatomy in the nine specimens. (See text.) (Reproduced with permission from Dr. R. Magnus: J. Pediat. Surg. 4:511, 1969.)

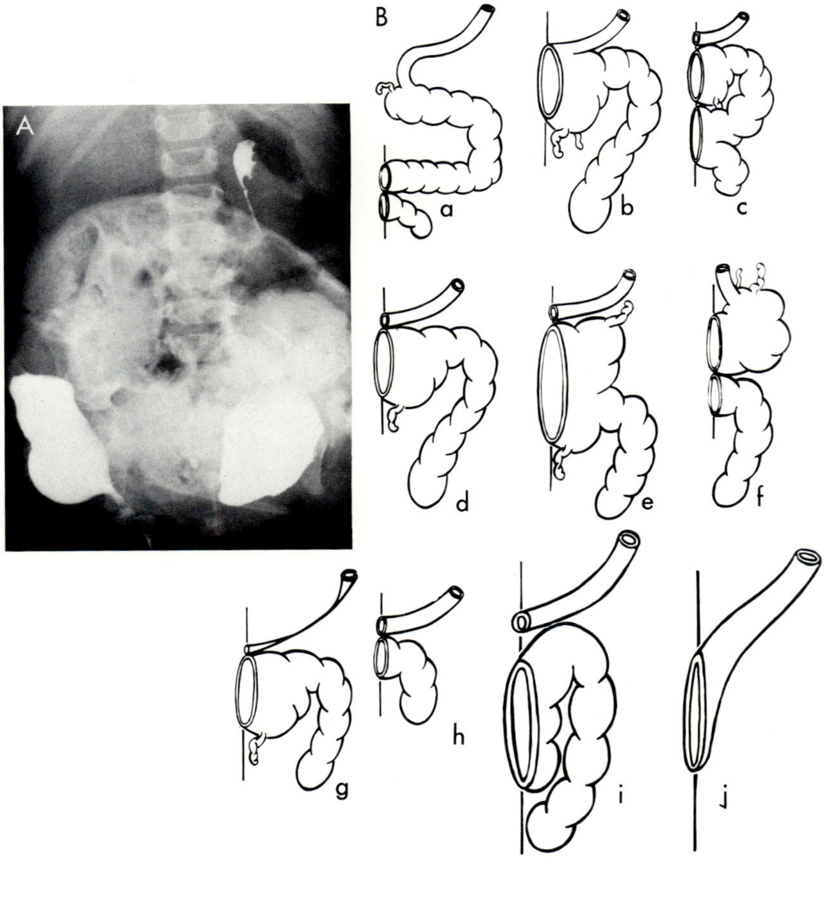

"bucket-handle" covered anus) and whose malformation does not represent the full picture. He is still living after (1) anoplasty, (2) laparotomy and closure of exomphalos and (3) excision of one half bladder and establishment of a single urethra to the remaining half. The child exhibits rectal and urinary incontinence. In 1 patient, in 1962, the exomphalos was repaired, a rectoplasty performed and an ileostomy established, but the infant died 2 weeks later from broncho-pneumonia; in 1 patient, in 1954, an ileostomy was performed, with repair of the exomphalos, but the infant died 1 week later.

In the remaining 8 patients no treatment was attempted.

The first successful surgical result was achieved by Rickham (1960), who described 4 patients, 3 of whom were operated upon, with one survival. This last patient survived after (1) closure of the everted caecum and colon (2) coloplasty to the perineum and (3) repair of exomphalos; later the bladder was excised, the two penes were joined and an ileal conduit urinary diversion was performed. At the time of the report (child aged 22 months), there was no fecal continence.

Zwiren and Patterson (1965) described another patient who was operated upon and survived; they reviewed the embryology. There are further reports of the anomaly by Veal and McFetridge (1934), Swan and Christensen (1953) and Van Geldern (1960). Louw (1965) has encountered 15 cases, but details are not provided in his report. Chisholm (1966) has operated upon 5 of 7 patients, with two deaths. The 3 survivors have varying lengths of colon present, and all 4 deceased patients had no colon.

Embryology of Vesico-Intestinal Fissure

The embryology of the developmental aberration is discussed by Rickham (1960), Zwiren and Patterson (1965), Johnston and Penn (1966) and Magnus (1969). The usual theory advanced to explain the abnormality is that by Johnston, in 1913, explained by Johnston and Penn as follows:

> It represents the same basic anomaly as vesical exstrophy but the dehiscence of the cloacal membrane and its infra-umbilical extension occurs earlier, before the formation of the urorectal septum, at the 5 mm. stage (Johnston, 1913). Exstrophy occurring at this phase causes the formation of a central bowel field between two bladder fields. An objection to this hypothesis is that exstrophic bowel does not involve the termination of the gut, but the ileocaecal region, an area which does not normally enter into the formation of the cloaca. Johnston (1913), however, pointed out that the hindgut, which he believed to begin at the usual site of a Meckel's diverticulum, would be greatly restricted in growth by its involvement in an exstrophy. He suggested that

the exposed bowel represents an extremely short hindgut and that the distal blind length of intestine is the persistent postanal or tail gut.

Magnus (1969), however, presents convincing evidence by a study of nine dissected specimens that only one specimen is adequately explained by Johnston's theory (Specimen *a* in Fig. 150, *B*), in which the large bowel opened by the cranial orifice and the caudal opening could be presumed to be persistent tailgut. In the other eight specimens it was the terminal ileum, not large bowel, which formed the cranial opening, and the only large bowel present opened at the caudal opening; further, in 5 specimens, the caecum (which develops from midgut, not tailgut) opened at the caudal orifice.

Magnus proposes that the midgut loop of terminal ileum and caecum, supplied by a common artery on a single mesentery (present in all specimens) prolapses through the deficient abdominal wall and then becomes strangulated by the closing abdominal wall. This would explain the number of orifices seen (depending upon the number of loops strangulated); the position of the caecum being either cranial or distal (depending upon the part of gut strangulated); and the length of bowel present (depending upon the length of bowel strangulated). Magnus does not offer an explanation for the double bladder fields or the imperforate rectum, but the evidence that the bowel malformation is an acquired catastrophe to the blood supply is convincing. We adhere to her suggestion of the name "vesico-intestinal fissure" as a purely descriptive term rather than "ectopia cloacae," which infers an embryological basis which may be fallacious.

Johnston and Penn (1966) point out that vesico-intestinal fissure is the grossest expression in a spectrum of exstrophic lesions; the most minor degrees are epispadias and superior vesical fissure; next in severity is vesical exstrophy. Intermediate types occur between vesical exstrophy and cloacal exstrophy (3 patients of Johnston and Penn) in which the exstrophic bowel lies caudal to a single bladder field; in these 3 intermediate cases, only 1 patient exhibited a rectal atresia.

A further intermediate type was described by Spencer and Geer (1967), in which, in addition to the classical features of the bowel and exomphalos, there was no bladder exstrophy. Rather there were two closed intra-abdominal bladders, one of which opened to a wide perineal orifice, the other bladder possessing a single penis (with hypospadias).

CHAPTER 14

Results and Complications and Assessment of Continence

THE PRINCIPAL DIFFICULTY in comparing the results of treatment between different series is the lack of agreement on classification and terminology. It is not always clear for which comparable anomaly a particular treatment is advocated. This is especially so in those series using the original Ladd and Gross classification of type 3 cases – a group consisting of both simple anal anomalies and difficult rectal deformities – in which a statement of "results in type 3" can have no significance. Similar confusion arises in comparing results of treatment of "recto-vaginal fistulae," for such a term frequently fails to distinguish between orifices into vagina, vestibule or posterior vulva, each of which carries a different prognosis.

Further, a combined case series from a number of surgeons within a particular hospital includes varying techniques and alternative operative choices, even where there is agreement on the type of anomaly. If an ill-advised perineal approach has been performed for a high rectal anomaly, with consequent sphincter damage, this unfairly depresses the over-all results of high rectal anomalies.

Finally, results must bear relation to the presence of associated anomalies and the complications of treatment. Apart from those anomalies which threaten life or complicate treatment (such as urinary stasis), the preoperative assessment of the sacral nerve outflow to the sphincters is fundamental. Rectoplasty performed on a child who lacks appropriate sacral innervation through sacral agenesis and is thus certain to be incontinent is an unfair disadvantage to the operation of rectoplasty. Some investigators using undamaged autopsy specimens of the pelvis may include these subjects in the over-all mortality series, which should be separate from the operative mortality.

For these reasons, in discussing the operative mortality, complications and functional results in this chapter, we do so primarily on those patients treated personally (167 patients), with briefer comment on the remaining patients in the series attending this center (94 patients) and on those reported in the literature.

Mortality

Fifty-seven of our 167 patients are dead (34.1%). This figure comprises both fatalities caused by accompanying serious deformities and operative complications.

Relation of Mortality to Type of Deformity and to Sex

The mortality statistics in relation to the type of rectal or anal deformity in our cases are shown in Table 29. These include deaths resulting from associated kidney defects or accompanying cardiac, tracheoesophageal fistula or other lesions; in some of these cases, the patients were operated upon for the rectal deformities or the accompanying deformities or both.

Type of Deformity.—The seriousness of risk in rectal deformities is apparent in Table 29—45.5% of the patients are dead (31 of 68 patients), whereas only 28.7% with anal deformities are dead (20 of 70 patients). As will be seen, the high mortality in rectal cases is due to the frequency of serious associated anomalies, these being less frequent in the anal cases.

Sex.—The high mortality risk is more marked in the males with rectal deformities (50.9% or 27 of 53 patients are dead) and less so in females with rectal deformities (26.7% or 4 of 15). In anal deformities, males also appear to be at a disadvantage (26.2% or 16 of 61 are dead) compared with females (13.8% or 4 of 25).

The over-all mortality for all levels of deformity in males is 38.7% (46 of 119) and in females 22.9% (11 of 48).

The figures relating to individual lesions are probably too small for analysis, although it is significant that a high proportion of rectovesical fistulae were necessarily fatal because of associated anomalies, and the risk is very high in ano-rectal agenesis without fistula. On the other hand, the anal stenosis group carries a particularly good prognosis but, surprisingly, somewhat less so in the covered anus groups.

Relation of Mortality to Treatment

Many of the patients who died possessed such severe associated or other accompanying visceral malformations that treatment was not indicated for the rectal or anal deformity; most of these patients died within a few hours of birth. Sixteen patients died following some

TABLE 29.—MORTALITY IN RELATION TO TYPE OF RECTAL OR ANAL DEFORMITY

MALE Deformity	Alive	Dead	FEMALE Deformity	Alive	Dead
Recto-urethral fistula	22	15	Recto-cloacal fistula	4	1
Recto-vesical fistula	–	4	Recto-vesical fistula	–	1
Ano-rectal agenesis	4	7	Recto-vaginal fistula	2	–
Rectal atresia	–	1	Recto-vestibular fistula	5	1
			Ano-rectal agenesis	–	1
			Rectal atresia	–	–
Rectal cases	26	27	*Rectal cases*	*11*	*4*
Anterior anus	–	–	Anterior anus		
Covered anus			(a) Perineal	2	–
(a) Ano-cutaneous fistula	18	8	(b) Vulvar	2	–
(b) Recto-bulbar fistula	8	5	Ano-vestibular fistula	11	3
			Perineal groove	1	–
Anal agenesis	5	–	Perineal canal	1	–
Imperforate anal membrane	–	1			
			Covered anus		
			(a) Ano-cutaneous fistula	2	1
			(b) Ano-vulvar fistula	4	–
Anal stenosis					
(a) Covered anus type	11	1	Anal agenesis	–	–
(b) Anal membrane stenosis	3	–	Imperforate anal membrane	–	–
(c) Ano-rectal stenosis	–	1	Anal stenosis		
			(a) Covered anus type	1	–
			(b) Anal membrane stenosis	1	–
			(c) Ano-rectal stenosis	–	–
Anal cases	*45*	*16*	*Anal cases*	25	*4*
Rare anomalies			Rare anomalies		
Vesico-intestinal fissure	1	3	Vesico-intestinal fissure	–	3
Urethro-anal fistula	1	–	Duplication of anus	1	–
TOTAL	73	46	TOTAL	37	11

	Alive	Dead
Total rectal cases	37	31
Total anal cases	70	20
Rare anomalies	3	6
TOTAL	110	57
	167	

form of operative treatment, but in only 2 patients was death related in any way to treatment. In 1 male with recto-urethral fistula, a colostomy was performed at birth, and death occurred at 10 months of age from meningitis and hydrocephalus; 1 female patient with a long recto-vestibular fistula died 7 days after rectoplasty (at 15 months of age) from necrosis and secondary hemorrhage of the terminal rectum. In our series of 167 patients, this was the only death directly due to an operative complication. The other 14 deaths following treatment were all due to unrelated severe associated anomalies or concurrent illness (Table 30).

CAUSES OF DEATH.—Analysis of the autopsy material clearly indicates that death is almost entirely due to the presence of severe associated anomalies of heart, brain or kidneys. As discussed above and shown in Table 30, only 2 patients died as the direct result of an operative complication, and only one of these was due to a technical error. Apart from the 16 deaths included in Table 30 (causes of death listed), all 41 deaths in patients for whom surgical treatment was not offered occurred in the first 2 weeks of life from severe associated anomalies, unrelated to the type of rectal or anal deformity. Many of these patients lived only a few hours.

The anomalies present were usually multiple and included congenital heart lesions of various types, renal agenesis, hypoplasia or dysplasia, renal vein thrombosis, myelomeningocele, esophageal and alimentary atresia, biliary atresia, pulmonary atelectasis, exomphalos, Down's syndrome, and severe prematurity.

COMPARISON WITH OTHER AUTHORS.—Up to the period ending in 1949, the operative mortality rate (i.e., death from any cause in the immediate postoperative period) varied between 19.0–46.0% (with one notable exception, that of Berman, 1938, 6.6%), but it is not always clear to what extent associated anomalies contributed to these early deaths.

Comparable figures since 1950 of both over-all mortality and operative mortality rates are shown in Table 31, together with the incidence of associated anomalies and the percentage of deaths due to associated anomalies.

It appears that over-all mortality has altered little in the last 20 years, the constant factor being the presence of associated anomalies beyond our therapeutic capacity. Operative mortality is probably also unchanged over this period, at present varying from 1 to 3%, but the information in some of the earlier series is not always clear as to whether "operative mortality" includes patients dying from associated anomalies in the immediate postoperative phase. For example, the figure of 6.8% in the London Hospital for Sick Children series (Partridge and Gough, 1961) includes death from any cause "at operation or before discharge from hospital"; conversely, where the deaths due to associated anomalies are specifically excluded from the operative mortality, the figure is low (e.g., Bradham, 1958, 2.3%), comparable with more recent series. In our own series, the figure of 1.2% operative mortality specifically refers to death due to a complication of treatment exclusive of that produced in the immediate postoperative phase by an associated anomaly. In fact, if the latter deaths were included in our operative mortality, the figure would be

TABLE 30.—MORTALITY IN RELATION TO TREATMENT—ANALYSIS OF 16 PATIENTS WHO DIED*
(Authors' 167 Cases)

DEFORMITY	PATIENTS	TREATMENT	CAUSE OF DEATH	AGE AT DEATH
Recto-urethral fistula	1†	Colostomy	Meningitis and hydrocephalus	10/12
Recto-vesical fistula	1	Colostomy	Hypoplastic kidneys and pyelonephritis	2 yrs 10/12
Ano-rectal agenesis	1	Colostomy	Vent. septal defect	16/12
Recto-vestibular fistula	1†	Colostomy and rectoplasty	Necrosis and hemorrhage of terminal rectum	10/12
Ano-cutaneous fistula	5	Cutback	Congenital heart disease and renal anomalies	5 days
		Cutback	Congenital heart disease, bronchopneumonia	5 days
		Cutback	Multiple anomalies	1 day
		Cutback	Exomphalos and multiple anomalies	2 days
		Dilatation	Megaureters, renal dysplasia, bronchopneumonia	20/12
Recto-bulbar fistula	1	Colostomy	Myelomeningocele and Congenital heart disease	1 day
Ano-vestibular fistula	2	Cutback	Congenital heart disease	5 yrs
		Colostomy	Congenital heart disease Down's syndrome	3/12
Anal stenosis (covered)	1	Cutback	Congenital heart disease Down's syndrome	6/12
Ano-rectal stenosis	1	Cutback	Viral pneumonia	10/12
Vesico-intestinal fissure	2	Ileostomy and rectoplasty	Multiple anomalies	2 days
		Ileostomy and repair of exomphalos	Multiple anomalies	7 days

*No treatment was offered in 41 patients. All died from associated anomalies. Treatment was given to 126 (alive 110; dead 16).
†Death related to treatment.

TABLE 31.—COMPARATIVE TABLE OF MORTALITY

AUTHORS	NUMBER OF CASES	OVER-ALL MORTALITY (%)	OPERATIVE MORTALITY (%)*	ASSOCIATED ANOMALIES (% OF CASES)	DEATHS DUE TO ASSOCIATED ANOMALIES (%)
Mayo and Rice (1950)	165	9.1	6.7	44.0	26.7
Bacon and Sherman (1952)	111	–	6.4	29.0	–
Moore and Lawrence (1952)	120	42.0	8.4	–	–
Brayton and Norris (1955)	93	25.8	9.7	53.7	64.0
Potts *et al.* (1954)	51	17.6	4.0	–	77.8
Palmer (1956)	100	45.1	25.7	37.0	43.2
Bradham (1958)	130	32.6	2.3	48.0	92.8
Scott *et al.* (1960)	63	12.7	4.8	55.0	62.5
Partridge and Gough (1961)	323	17.9	6.8	40.8	–
Forshall (1962)	83	30.0	–	37.7	–
Katzen (1962)	41	31.7	14.6	46.3	54.0
Lynn and Arcari (1962)	58	29.3	5.2	30.0	70.6
Swenson and Grana (1962)	112	14.2	5.4	38.6	62.5
Trusler and Wilkinson (1962)	147	27.0	12.2	38.0	–
Santulli (1963)	220	11.8	–	31.8	–
Kiesewetter *et al.* (1964)	146	19.1	6.2	47.9	68.0
Somerschild *et al.* (1964)	35	14.0	–	–	–
Louw (1965)	110	16.4	2.7	52.2	–
Rehbein (1967)	70	11.4	–	–	–
Swenson and Donnellan (1967)	54	11.1	3.7	40.7	–
Cozzi and Wilkinson (1968)	133	20.0	2.7	55.6	89.0
Present Authors (1968)	167	34.1	1.2	60.6	94.8

*Exclusive of the effects of associated anomalies but see text for qualifications.

6.2%. It is clear that the overriding determinant of death is the association of other severe visceral malformations; in their absence, the risk of death is negligible, even following major rectoplasty for rectal deformities, and should not exceed 1%.

A point of considerable controversy has been the relative mortality risks of neonatal rectoplasty versus a staged program of neonatal colostomy and later rectoplasty. Prior to the paper by Rhoads *et al.*, in 1948, the mortality from multiple procedures for high rectal anomalies varied from 50 to 100%. These deaths were due to septic complications of colostomy and to sepsis following the frequent complications of perineal explorations. The initial survival of Rhoads' two infants following neonatal abdomino-perineal rectoplasty excited interest because it avoided secondary procedures. Similarly Norris *et al.* (1949) pointed to the 18–25% mortality from colostomy and other complications of secondary procedures and successfully performed abdomino-perineal rectoplasty on 4 neonates, although 2 subsequently died from associated defects. In 1953, Butcher reported six newborn rectoplasties, without mortality, and Brayton and Norris (1958) had three deaths of 22 neonatal abdomino-perineal operations compared with three deaths of 11 patients who had colostomy only.

Superior as was the Rhoads' neonatal operation to the disastrous results of perineal surgery for high rectal anomalies, in more recent years several surgeons report a decreased mortality by a staged program. Trusler and Wilkinson (1962), in 42 type 3 cases (Ladd and Gross classification) reported 4 deaths of 13 primary abdomino-perineal rectoplasties, as compared with 3 deaths of 25 staged operations. Louw (1965) had 2 deaths in 6 neonatal reconstructions, but no deaths in 27 staged operations. Cozzi and Wilkinson (1968) had only 1 death after 48 staged rectoplasties (and that from an associated anomaly), and in our own series there has been 1 death in 47 major reconstructions by a staged program.

The mortality risk of colostomy is difficult to assess because in many series the basis of selection for colostomy is not defined, e.g., in Partridge and Gough's series (1961) 20 of 36 patients (55%) died following colostomy as neonates, but this figure almost certainly includes patients with severe associated anomalies. In our own series of 49 colostomies, only 5 patients died during the period of their colostomy (1 from meningitis, and 4 from associated anomalies), but an additional 41 died without treatment, in some of whom other surgeons might have elected to perform colostomy. In Cozzi and Wilkinson's series (1968) 12 of 44 patients (27%) died following neonatal colostomy, and 8 of 9 patients died in Louw's series (1965) from ano-rectal agenesis when treated by colostomy only (4 from associated anomalies and 4 admitted *in extremis*). On the other hand, Louw had no mortality after colostomy in 30 patients who underwent rectoplasty months later. The mortality risk of colostomy, exclusive of associated anomalies, is thus probably very small (1–2%), although not negligible, as all surgeons report deaths from time to time from colostomy complications (peritonitis either before or after closure, septicemia, meningitis and bowel obstruction).

Prematurity rates high in all series as a major determinant of death. Forshall (1960) in reporting results in 53 rectal lesions found that in 29 patients without a severe associated anomaly there were 6 premature babies, of whom 4 died, and in 24 patients with an associated anomaly there were 14 premature babies, all of whom died.

Cozzi and Wilkinson (1968) similarly found a high mortality in premature infants with birth weight below 1.8 kilograms. They suggest a useful classification of mortality risk based upon birth weight and associated mild or severe anomaly, irrespective of the type of ano-rectal malformation. For example, group A (weight greater than 2.5 kg., with no other anomaly), mortality was 3.8% in 26 patients. Group B (weight 1.8–2.5 kg., with no anomaly, or greater than 2.5 kg., with mild anomaly), mortality was 3.7% in 27 patients. Group C (weight less than 1.8 kg., with no anomaly, or 1.8–2.5 kg., with mild anomaly, or greater than 2.5 kg., with severe anomaly), mortality was 55% in 38 patients.

In Trusler and Wilkinson's series (1962), 9 of 39 deaths were due to prematurity alone.

Complications of Treatment

Complications of treatment (exclusive of urinary complications—see Chapter 12) contribute a significant morbidity in all series. Complications involving the bowel itself frequently necessitate multiple operations (e.g., secondary anoplasties for stricture or redundant anal mucosa, etc.), each carrying further risks of sepsis, anesthesia, etc.

Reference to the extensive literature of operations enables a compilation of almost every complication encountered in surgery. These are listed in Table 32, together with those of our own series of 126 operations (exclusive of those complications due to associated congenital anomalies of other organs).

Complications of Colostomy.—In our series of 49 colostomies, complications occurred in 17 patients as listed in Table 32. Although 5 of these patients died, death was not directly due to the colostomy (except possibly in one who died of meningitis—the remaining 4 patients died of associated anomalies). However, in 13 patients, the complication necessitated additional operation upon the colostomy. Comment has been made in Chapter 9 on the relevance of this colostomy morbidity to the operative decisions for the rectal anomaly. Apart from technical considerations in the construction of the colostomy, adequate postoperative colostomy washouts are essential to remove fecal matter from the distal limb and to prevent urinary infection in the presence of a recto-urinary fistula (see Chapter 12).

Anal and Rectal Stricture.—Stricture is prone to occur following any operative procedure involving an ano-cutaneous suture line. After simple cutback such stricture as occurs is short, at the anal verge, but following rectoplasty the stricture may be longer. Factors in stricture formation are inadequate postoperative supervision of dilatation, peri-anal sepsis and scarring, multiple perineal operations and ischemia of terminal rectum from inadequate mobilization and tension. Stricture has often necessitated secondary anoplasty (16 patients).

Prolapse of Rectal Mucosa.—Prolapse of excess rectal mucosa has been common after rectoplasty, having occurred on 15 occasions (Fig. 151). In a further 3 patients, the anal mucosa was excessive after a simple anal repair. In an effort to avoid tension and sloughing of the rectum, we have tended to mobilize the rectum well down, but frequently after 2–3 weeks this results in some descent of excess

TABLE 32.—COMPLICATIONS OF TREATMENT

COMPLICATIONS	INCIDENCE IN AUTHORS' CASES	
General complications		
Fluid and electrolyte disturbance, "shock"	1	
Pulmonary sepsis, atelectasis	–	
Distant sepsis—septicemia	–	
meningitis	1	
osteomyelitis	1	
Postoperative intestinal obstruction	4	
Sclerema neonatorum	–	
Anemia	–	
Complications of colostomy		
Severe excoriation	7	in 49 colostomies
Hemorrhage	–	
Prolapse	6	
Retraction	–	
Stenosis	3	
Sloughing	1	
Evisceration or herniation	1	
Colo-colic fistula	2	
Dysfunction	–	
Fecal or barium impaction	–	
Hyperchloremic acidosis	2	
Following closure—stricture	–	
small bowel obstruction	1	
peritonitis	–	
fecal fistula	–	
incisional hernia	–	
Direct ano-rectal complications		
Dehiscence of recto-cutaneous junction	–	
Necrosis of rectum	1	
Ano-rectal stricture	16	
Prolapse of rectal mucosa	18	
Recurrent fistula	8	
Sepsis—peritonitis, pelvic abscess	–	
peri-anal abscess	1	
Mucous discharge from rectal pouch in vagina or cloaca	2	
Rectal inertia and secondary megacolon necessitating rectosigmoidectomy	2	

mucosa. Even though secondary anoplasty is required and skin flaps are laid up into the anal canal at this procedure, we believe this is preferable to the more serious effects of stricture from incomplete mobilization of the rectum. Secondary mobilization of extra rectal length results in further scarring and places the pubo-rectalis sling at great risk.

RECURRENT FISTULA.—This complication now rarely occurs since the abandonment of the perineal approach to rectal lesions. Prior to

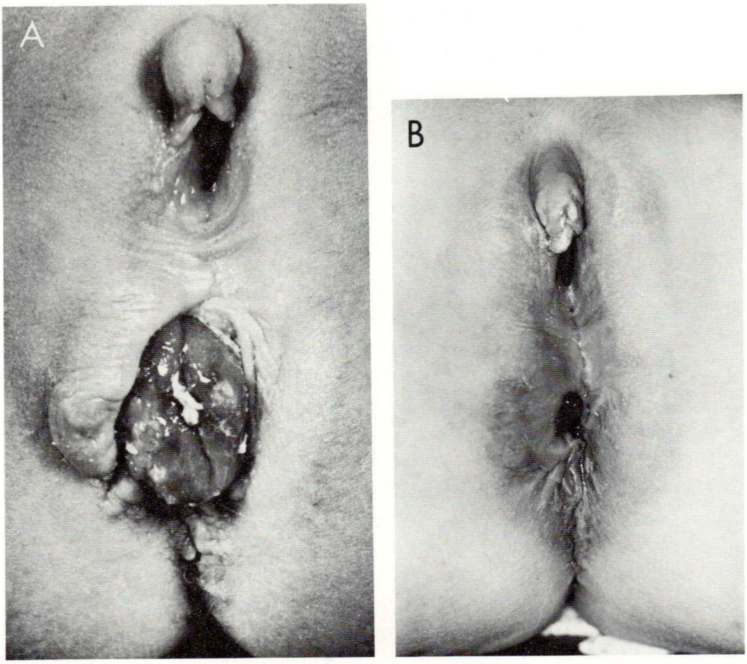

Fig. 151.—Rectal prolapse after rectoplasty—recto-cloacal fistula. **A,** prolapse of rectal wall after rectoplasty. **B,** after trimming of rectal prolapse.

abdomino-perineal rectoplasty, or its variants, recurrent fistulae were common, leading to many secondary perineal explorations and their attendant morbidity of scarring and sphincter damage to both anal canal and urinary tract. All eight recurrent fistulae in our series resulted from such perineal explorations prior to referral to us (for anal agenesis (1), recto-urethral fistula (2), recto-bulbar fistula (4) and recto-cloacal fistula (1)).

Mucous Discharge from Vagina or Cloaca.—On two occasions following rectoplasty for recto-cloacal fistula, patients have presented with a mucous discharge due to a retained terminal stump of rectal mucosa opening into vagina or cloaca. These stumps have required sleeve resection as a relatively minor procedure, beginning with circumcision of the orifice, circummural dissection and enucleation.

Rectal Inertia and Secondary Megacolon.—Proper management of the bowel after anal or rectal surgery is vital to ensure maximal continence. Constipation may be due to obstruction from stricture, to dietary and training mismanagement, to operative interference with nerve supply, to neurogenic states (e.g., sacral agenesis) or, rarely, to Hirschsprung's disease. Established constipation seriously interferes with continence and results in fecal overflow. This troublesome leakage causes much diagnostic confusion with incontinence from suspected sphincter damage.

Acute constipation may be entirely relieved by bowel softeners taken orally or introduced per rectum and by adjustment of diet.

The chronic state of secondary megacolon needs more radical measures. The evacuation of fecal accumulation should be instituted. This requires daily soap and water enemas, followed, after evacuation, with saline bowel irrigation washouts to remove the residue from the rectum and sigmoid colon. On rare occasions, these hard masses may need manual removal under an anaesthetic. Because the overdistended rectum and colon do not evacuate completely by natural efforts, further washouts are necessary until rectal tone returns; three times a week for 3 weeks, twice a week for 2 weeks, and once a week for several weeks. This should be done, even though normal stools are passed in the intervals.

Softening of bowel content by aperients should also be carried out to prevent the reformation of hard stools and to stimulate the overdistended bowel to contract. Appropriate laxatives in adequate dosage should be given daily during the course of washouts and continued for several months; parents usually become adept in assessing the timing and dosage. Purgatives that failed prior to the evacuation of the fecal accumulation will usually act effectively in smaller dosage, once the overloading is relieved.

A system of bowel training should be practiced. Regular daily "potting" is necessary after the first few bowel washouts.

Prevention of Relapses.—It has been noted that even though normal bowel habits may return quickly after this treatment the overdistention and enlargement of the rectum and colon takes many months or years to revert to normal dimensions. For this reason, relapses may occur, especially during periods of mild or severe intercurrent illnesses. Prevention of such relapses can be ensured by temporary increase in aperients or by instituting bowel washouts during and after the illness.

On two occasions, the extent of rectal dilatation has been such that, after many months of strenuous medical treatment and failure, rectosigmoidectomy has been performed, leaving a generous anal segment for anastomosis to the colon. Both children were boys who presented some months after infancy with long-standing untreated anal stenosis, and both required a prolonged regimen of aperients and enemas before the habit and efficiency of defecation were established.

Functional Results

Reference has already been made to the difficulty in comparing functional results in different series because of the lack of agreement on classification. We, therefore, detail only the results of treatment of our own cases, so that one important variable has been eliminated, namely, multiplicity of control. Further, the follow-up has been performed by the same team, thus ensuring continuity in evaluation over many years.

An initial problem is to select adequate criteria on which to judge results. Most series define results as "good," "fair" or "poor," but frequently such terms incorporate multiple parameters which lead to difficulties in interpretation. For example, in Partridge and Gough's paper (1961), in low anomalies, "good" refers to "when bowel control is normal without the use of regular laxatives," "fair" is "when continual supervision is needed to avoid recurrent constipation or anal stenosis" and "poor" is "when a state of severe colonic inertia or incontinence exists." This does not distinguish between the factors contributing "control" by the sphincters and factors responsible for the type of stool. Although the child is frequently incontinent from colonic inertia with overflow, it must be remembered that incontinence has other more serious causes. A child with good sphincters may be converted from a fair to a good result by treatment of colonic inertia, but if the sphincters are impaired by operative damage or nerve lesions, no amount of bowel correction will make the child continent. It is therefore necessary to analyze each variable of the total result separately. The parameters we have assessed in our follow-up are as follow:

(i) Continence of the fecal stream
(ii) Staining or smearing of the anus
(iii) Rectal sensation
(iv) Stool consistency
(v) Appearance of the anus
(vi) Sphincter contraction on digital examination
(vii) Miscellaneous factors, such as age, mentality and social and parental adequacy

(i) Continence.—The term was reserved for the sphincteric control of the fecal stream through the anus in the prevention of accidents, and the ability to postpone evacuation and then initiate it at the appropriate time and place. Separate inquiry was made for control of solid feces, liquid feces, and flatus, as more critical control is required for the last two evacuates. A patient may be "good" under normal conditions, but "poor" if the stools are loose, as after emotional upsets or dietary indiscretion.

Continence is a function of the sphincters themselves—their development or operative integrity, their innervation and the effects of later stresses upon them, such as the overfull rectum or diarrhea.

In assessing continence, we recorded a point score devised by Kelly (1968) as follows:

Score 2—Normal control under all circumstances, with no accidents.
Score 1—Occasional escape of feces or flatus, with occasional major accidents.
Score 0—No control, or frequent accidents (more than 50% of the time).

Scharli and Kiesewetter (1969) recently provided an important paper on the manometric assessment of continence.

(ii) Staining and Smearing of the Anus.—A distinction needs to be made between "incontinence" on the one hand and "smearing" or "staining" on the other. A patient may be fully continent, in that the sphincters may provide control of the main fecal stream, so that complete evacuation can be achieved on demand or the fecal stream restrained till an appropriate time, yet such a patient may have a small mucous stain on the underclothes because of the exposed anal mucosa below the levator ani (in the absence of internal and external sphincter components). Further, the stain may be fecal as well if the sphincteric occlusion of the canal is incomplete or if the patient has not learned various "toilet tricks," e.g., not cutting off the stool in midstream, which causes arrest and subsequent seepage of fecal fragments from the canal distal to the sphincter. Meticulous cleaning inside the anus after defecation is important to avoid staining. "Continence" refers to confident and effectual voluntary and involuntary control of the fecal flow by the sphincters, and "staining" is reserved for the minor degrees of soiling resulting from incompletely occlusive sphincters or from postsphincteric seepage; staining is related either to leakage or seepage.

Patients scored points as follows:

Score 2—Always clean
Score 1—Occasional stain
Score 0—Always stained

(iii) Rectal Sensation.—The term refers to awareness of oncoming stool or flatus and to the strength and adequacy of warning. It is closely related to continence. We have also frequently recorded physical sensation in the skin-lined anal canal and the immediately adjoining margin of rectal mucosa to pinprick, but in the context of clinical follow-up the term "rectal sensation" is here referred to as the subjective feeling of the patient for oncoming stool and flatus.

(iv) Stool Consistency.—Stools may be hard, soft or liquid. The bowel habit may be regular and normal, with stool consistency alternating from hard to soft, accompanied by a corresponding tendency to constipation and diarrhea. The obstinate constipation of rectal inertia may necessitate bowel washout or enema management.

Stool behavior is related to parasympathetic nerve supply, to obstruction by stricture, to the effectiveness of bowel supervision in stenotic cases before treatment and for several years after anal and rectal surgery, and perhaps to abnormal gut above the atresic segment.

(v) Appearance of Anus.—The anus may be closed or open and patulous with exposure of varying amounts of mucosa. Mucosal exposure induces staining and is mainly dependent on external sphincter anatomy and partly on surgical technique.

(vi) Sphincteric Contraction on Digital Examination.—Careful rectal examination with the finger, and the patient cooperating by "squeezing" on the finger, provides information about the various sphincter components. Particular attention is paid to the following:

(a) The effectiveness of the "sling action" of the pubo-rectalis, detected by its posterior to anterior pull
(b) The side-to-side action of the remaining portion of the levator diaphragm
(c) Any circumferential squeeze below the levator ani and between it and the anal verge

Squeeze assessment is not always easy to interpret because the child may not cooperate or may be too young to understand. However, even in the crying child, contraction can often be assessed.

The examination is of considerable prognostic significance and has been found reliable, e.g., in distinguishing between simple overflow from constipation and soiling from damaged sphincters.

Score 2—Effective strong squeeze of pubo-rectalis
Score 1—Weak or partial squeeze of pubo-rectalis
Score 0—No contraction detectable

(vii) Miscellaneous Factors.—Although not subject to measurement, comments on continence must always be qualified by reference to the age of the patient, length of follow-up, adequacy of parental discipline, encouragement and training, social opportunity or neglect and the child's own mental, intellectual and emotional development. Given adequate surgery, improvement is usually noticeable within a few weeks but the factors enumerated may delay the final outcome for months or years.

The Clinical "Score"

Kelly (1968) developed the notion of a clinical "score" in the recording of functional results, thus enabling a partial quantitative assessment. He found that the major assessment could be made on the basis of three parameters—continence, staining and sphincter squeeze—defined with the scores described above. Stool consistency, sensation, anal appearance and miscellaneous factors, all contribute, but for simplicity are added as qualifications to the score. Thus, the maximal score attainable by a child with normal continence, no staining, and strong sphincter squeeze is 6 points, the minimal score by a totally incontinent child, 0 points, with variable figures in between. This method of assessment has permitted some quantitative comparison of the results of surgical procedures in various ano-rectal lesions.

Detailed Analysis of Functional Results

In the results which follow, we use the clinical score of 6, with a separate comment on 25 patients analyzed by Kelly with both clinical and radiographic analyses.

As an approximate comparison with other authors, clinical scores of 5–6 are "good," 3–4 are "fair," and 0–2 are "poor" results. The numerical system of points permits more realistic interpretation, because often a patient can fluctuate between the levels determined by stressful circumstances, e.g., constipation, dietary imbalance, social pressures, etc. We have tended to allocate scores for "average" circumstances for the patient, although a number of patients can do better than their scores indicate when under more concentrated supervision or as they themselves learn to understand their problem with advancing age. These qualifying circumstances may make a difference of up to 3 points on the clinical score, but we have deliberately recorded them conservatively so as not to inflate the general impression. Some will eventually do better than indicated.

The analysis of results is complex because in some patients now under our care the initial, often definitive, procedure was performed "elsewhere." Some patients are lost to follow-up and some are within 18 months of their definitive procedure and thus too recent to assess; the clinical scores of those followed-up represent results of all children more than 18 months after their definitive operation.

Analysis by Type of Deformity

The over-all results are indicated in Table 33, which includes all patients treated *ab initio* by ourselves, or in whom we have carried

TABLE 33.—OVER-ALL SURVEY, ACCORDING TO TYPE OF DEFORMITY (167 PATIENTS)

Type of Deformity	Number of Patients	Deaths: No Treatment Offered	Deaths: Treated Patients	No Follow-up or Too Recent	Followed up	Clinical Score: 0	1	2	3	4	5	6	Permanent Colostomy	Colostomy Awaiting Rectoplasty	No Treatment Yet
Supralevator (rectal)															
Recto-urethral fistula	37	14	1	2	20	2	1	2	5	2	2	3	3		
Recto-vesical fistula	5	4	1												
Recto-cloacal fistula	5	1			4			1	1	1	1				
Recto-vaginal fistula (high and low)	2			1	1						1				
Recto-vestibular fistula	6		1*	1	4					1	1	1		1	
Rectal atresia	1	1													
Ano-rectal agenesis (no fistula)	12	7	1	1	3				1	1	1				
Anal agenesis (no fistula)	5				5		1			1	2	1			
Recto-bulbar fistula	13	4	1	3	5			1	1	1	1	1			
TOTAL	86	31	5	8	42	2	2	4	8	7	9	6	3	1	
						"Poor"			"Fair"		"Good"				
Translevator (anal)															
Anterior anus	4				4		1				1	2			

Covered anus – ano-cutaneous fistula	29	4	5	3	17		1	2	6	8	
Covered anus – ano-vulvar fistula	4			1	3			1		2	
Ano-vestibular fistula	14	1	2	3	8				3	5	
Perineal groove	1				1					1	
Perineal canal	1				1					1	
Imperforate anal membrane	1	1									
Anal stenosis – covered anus	13		1	3	9			1	1	7	
Anal stenosis – anal membrane stenosis	4				4			2		2	
Anal stenosis – ano-rectal stenosis	1		1								
TOTAL	72	6	9	10	47	1	1	6	11	28	
						"Poor"	"Fair"		"Good"		
Rare complex anomalies											
Vesico-intestinal fissure	7	4	2		1		1				
Urethro-anal fistula	1				1						1
Duplication of ani	1				1					1	
TOTAL	9	4	2		3		1			1	1

*The only death directly related to operation; the remaining deaths in this column were in patients with colostomies but dying from other anomalies.

out a secondary procedure after initial operation elsewhere. These "elsewhere" procedures were frequently damaging ones (Table 34), so that the over-all results in Table 33 tend to be somewhat depressed. Although anal agenesis (no fistula) and recto-bulbar fistulae have been classified embryologically in our text as predominantly "anal" lesions, in respect of treatment their intermediate relation to the pubo-visceral sling requires a supralevator approach, and hence are listed only in that group in Table 33.

In the 42 supralevator lesions followed-up and treated by a variety of techniques, good results (scores of 5–6) and fair results (scores of 3–4) occurred with equal frequency, and a smaller number had poor results (scores 0–2), the numbers of patients being 15:15:8, respectively. Three patients have permanent colostomies, two following multiple perineal procedures elsewhere for recto-urethral fistula resulting in levator or neural injury, and one following abdomino-perineal rectoplasty performed elsewhere, with similar injury.

The proportion of good results was far higher in translevator anal lesions (39) compared with fair results (7) and poor results (1).

Recto-Urethral Fistula (Excluding Recto-Bulbar Types).—There were 37 patients seen. Fourteen died of severe associated malformations without treatment, and 1 died of heart disease after colostomy only. Two patients are too recent to review following sacro-perineal rectoplasty.

The results of the remaining 20 patients are "good" 5, "fair" 7, "poor" 5, and 3 permanent colostomies. However, these patients must be analyzed separately for those treated primarily by ourselves, and for those in whom the initial definitive operation was performed elsewhere.

In 11 patients, the primary rectoplasty has been performed by ourselves *ab initio*, all at 12–16 months of age and following newborn colostomy. Sacro-perineal or sacro-abdomino-perineal operations were performed on 10 patients, 3 of whom scored 6 points, 2 scoring 5, 1 scoring 4, 3 scoring 3 and 1 scoring 0 points, i.e., 5 "good," 4 "fair" and 1 "poor" results. One other patient scored 0 after a straight abdomino-perineal pull-through operation. The factor causing lack of points from a full score of 6 was most commonly a degree of staining of mucus or feces from the exposed sleeve of unprotected mucosa below the level of the pubo-visceral sling in a degree greater than in anal anomalies. This can be reduced by teaching "toilet tricks" as described above or perhaps by more effective skin lining the anal canal. The next factor was the tendency to constipation, present intermittently in 5 of these 10 sacral repairs, and at times the "fair" scores rise to "good" when the stools are kept at normal consistency. All but 3 of these 10 patients scored the full 2 points for continence and control; 1 patient scored 0 points because of almost certain muscle or neural damage, for there was no sphincter squeeze in this patient; 2 other patients scored 1 point because of occasional accidents, especially with loose stools or flatus, although their sphincter squeeze was strong. Most patients may drop a point with episodes of liquid stools, and only 3 patients can be said to be totally continent all the time for solid, flatus and liquid.

In 9 patients the initial definitive operation was performed elsewhere; of these 9 patients, 3 had extensive perineal dissection during the neonatal period; secondary sacro-perineal repair was performed in 1 patient who now scores 3 points, and 2 others have permanent colostomies; in 6 patients, abdomino-perineal rectoplasty had been performed. Of these 6 patients, the rectoplasty had been performed in the neonatal period in 2, and both had low scores of 0 and 2, respectively; in 4 others, the rectoplasty had been performed later in infancy, but because of fecal incontinence, these 4 patients were referred to us for secondary repair of the levator ani muscle. On re-exploration by the sacro-abdomino-perineal route, all 4 patients had either partial rupture of the pubo-visceral sling or eccentric routing of the rectum off the midline of the sling. As a result of our secondary repair, the clinical scores improved to 2, 3 (2 patients) and 4, respectively. In none of these 9 "elsewhere" patients was a "good" result (score of 5 or 6) obtained.

Seven of the 20 patients required secondary anoplasty, 4 for excessive prolapse of anal mucosa, and 3 for anal stricture. Qualifying factors of stool consistency, diet, mental, emotional and social status may improve or depress the clinical score up to 3 points.

Ano-Rectal Agenesis (No Fistula).—The incidence of severe associated anomalies accompanying ano-rectal agenesis appeared to be excessively high, no less than 8 of the 12 patients dying, 7 without treatment and 1 after colostomy. The remaining 4 patients gave clinical scores similar to recto-urethral fistula (3–5 points); 1 of these who had had an abdomino-perineal rectoplasty elsewhere, with resulting complete incontinence, was elevated to 4 points after secondary sacro-perineal repair.

Other Rectal Deformities.—The results in 9 additional patients followed-up (recto-cloacal fistula, 4; recto-vaginal fistula, 1; and recto-vestibular fistula, 4) showed similar clinical scores to recto-urethral fistula, being in the range of 3–6 points. One additional patient awaits rectoplasty, and our one fatality resulting from technical error in 126 treated patients occurred in this group (necrosis of terminal rectum).

Anal Agenesis (No Fistula) and Recto-Bulbar Fistula.—The results in 10 patients with these two similar lesions showed a wide scatter over the whole range of clinical score, but with 5 patients scoring 5–6 points. Poor results were recorded in 1 patient with anal

TABLE 34.—TREATMENT SURVEY OF SUPRALEVATOR DEFORMITIES (55 PATIENTS)

TYPE OF PROCEDURE		NUMBER OF PATIENTS	DEATHS	NO FOLLOW-UP OR TOO RECENT	FOLLOWED-UP	CLINICAL SCORE 0	1	2	3	4	5	6	Permanent Colostomy	Colostomy, Awaiting Rectoplasty
Treatment by FDS Unit Throughout†*														
Perineal rectoplasty		2			2				1			1		
Abdomino-perineal rectoplasty		2			2		1	1						
Sacro-perineal rectoplasty		17		6	11	1				3	5	2		
Sacro-abdomino-perineal rectoplasty		12	1‡	1	10				3	1	4	2		
Colostomy only		5	4		1									1
TOTAL		38	5	7	26	1	1	1	4	4	9	5		1
						"Poor"			"Fair"		"Good"			
*Definitive Procedure Elsewhere, Secondary Procedure by FDS Unit**														
"Elsewhere" Initial Procedure	FDS Unit* Procedure													
Perineal recto-plasty	nil	1			1		1							
Perineal recto-plasty	Sacro-perineal rectoplasty	3			3				1			1	1	

Perineal recto-plasty (some multiple)	Sacro-abdomino-perineal rectoplasty	2		2			1	1			
Perineal recto-plasty (multiple)	Abdomino-perineal rectoplasty	1		1							1
Perineal recto-plasty	Closure of fistula	1		1					1		
Abdomino-perineal rectoplasty (neonatal)	nil	2		2	1		1				
Abdomino-perineal rectoplasty (infant)	Closure of fistula	1		1							1
Abdomino-perineal rectoplasty (infant)	Sacro-abdomino-perineal rectoplasty	5		5			1	2	2		
No treatment	No treatment	1	1								
TOTAL		17	1	16	1	1	3	4	3	1	3
					"Poor"			"Fair"		"Good"	

*FDS Unit - The Chief Surgeons in the Unit are F. D. Stephens, Robert Fowler and E. Durham Smith.
†In 4 patients the initial colostomy was performed prior to transfer to us, but no definitive rectal repair.
‡The only death directly related to operation; the remaining colostomy deaths in this column were from associated disease.

agenesis following a perineal dissection elsewhere, and in 2 patients with recto-bulbar fistula, both after extensive perineal dissection, including multiple attempts to close a fistula. Sacro-perineal proctoplasty gave the best results in these lesions. The remarks concerning other qualifying factors (constipation, diet, mental status, etc.) resemble those relating to recto-urethral fistula.

Translevator Deformities.—The results in this wide group of anal lesions are considered together as there are insignificant differences in results between individual types. The one poor result, in anterior anus, occurred in a child with neurogenic incontinence from associated spinal myelomeningocele. The seven fair results (scores of 3–4) were as follows: in 4 covered anus type of patients, the loss of points was associated with some overflow and staining with constipation, and all 4 can score 5 or 6 in periods of normal stool behavior; 2 patients persisted with established secondary megacolon (1 following delayed treatment of anal membrane stenosis) and eventually required rectosigmoidectomy for this, but both now still stain and have occasional accidents with overflow despite a fully developed sphincter squeeze; 1 patient, with ano-cutaneous fistula, scored only 3 points because of staining and occasional accidents from irregular stool behavior, and this patient attends a psychiatrist for a very disturbed emotional state.

Thirty-nine patients scored 5 or 6, indicating the excellent control established in the majority of translevator lesions for both solid and liquid stools, and flatus. Some mucous staining occurs in the 5-point scores, but this is less of a problem than in the supralevator lesions. All patients have a strongly contracting and low-placed levator ani, but most show no ringlike contraction of any muscle below the levator ani. In 8 patients, however, the anus lies closed, and in these there appear to be some longitudinally running muscle fibers which pucker the peri-anal area on one or both sides. Although some deep external sphincter muscle is apparently present and is sufficient to partially close the canal, it does not close the anal orifice, it is not in the form of a complete ring superficially and does not always prevent mucus or fecal staining. Mucous staining is minimal in degree and is often no more than a slight stain once or twice a month. The length of exposed mucosa responsible for this staining is very short, varying from only 1 or 2 mm. to 1 cm. in length; this is attributed to the fact that the deep part of the external sphincter may be preserved in anal anomalies, and also because the levator ani has a lower insertion than its main pubo-rectalis fibers by reason of longitudinally running penetrating fibers to the anal wall.

In 3 children with ano-cutaneous fistulae, the definitive anus has remained slightly anterior to the normal site, and these 3 patients all possessed long fistulae either to the midscrotum (in 2) or to the penile shaft (in 1). This follows the general rule that the more forward the fistula, the less well developed is the perineum and therefore the more ectopically placed will be the final location of the anus after the fistula is laid open.

Following treatment of ano-vestibular fistula by cutback, the anal orifice remains in the fourchette or at the posterior rim of the vulva, and a collar of mucosa is constantly exposed, no sphincter being palpable below the levator ani. Despite this, only 3 children of a total of 11 have any staining – 2 have a minute amount of mucous discharge from the mucosa and 1 a tiny amount of fecal and mucous staining. These children naturally keep themselves clean, although some require the normal careful attention to the area after defecation. The ectopic site of the orifice rarely provides any difficulties in normal perineal hygiene as the fecal stream is not directed into the vulva or vagina. Anal transplantation has been considered necessary only on one occasion to date.

Constipation, excess mucosa and anal stricture remain the greatest threats to a full score in the anal group of deformities. Despite early and adequate treatment in the majority of patients 12 of them were cutback incompletely, necessitating dilatation of the temporary stricture of the anus. Ten responded to repeated dilatation, but 2 patients required secondary anoplasty for stricture. Two additional patients needed a similar operation for redundant mucosa.

Analysis According to Type of Treatment

Supralevator Deformities. – Table 34 summarizes the statistical information of 54 patients who received treatment.

In 38 of these patients treatment has been supervised by ourselves throughout, apart from 4 infants who had their initial colostomy performed before transfer to us. All the major definitive repairs have been performed in our own unit, so that some idea of the efficacy of the sacro-perineal and sacro-abdomino-perineal approach can be studied. Of the 5 deaths in the series, 4 died of associated anomalies after colostomy, and our only operative fatality was from hemorrhage following necrosis of the terminal rectum after repair of a long recto-vestibular fistula. Seven patients are not included in the follow-up as their procedure has been performed too recently; 1 patient awaits rectoplasty. In the remaining 25 patients the proportion of good:fair:poor results is 14:8:3.

In 2 patients with recto-bulbar fistula, the rectum was mobilized by the perineum directly; both these patients had a relatively thin perineum, and reasonable access was obtained with identification of the fistula, bulb and pubo-rectalis sling. One of these patients is now fully continent (score 6), but a recurrence of a fine recto-bulbar fistula required closure at 11 years of age; the other patient was involved in a car accident and is hemiplegic, hydrocephalic (V–A shunt), and mentally retarded (score 3). However, we believe that when the perineum is of normal thickness better access is obtained in recto-bulbar fistula and anal agenesis by the sacro-perineal route; in five such operations, the scores were 6 points (1 patient), 5 points (3 patients) and 4 points (1 patient).

Our experience with abdomino-perineal rectoplasty has been negligible, and the poor results recorded in both patients operated upon is not a fair comment on the technique. One of these patients has some neurogenic disturbance from sacral agenesis, and one has an obscure recto-cloacal fistula with partial features of vesico-intestinal fissure.

Thirty patients have had sacro-perineal or sacro-abdomino-perineal rectoplasty, as described by Stephens (29 in Table 34 and 1 in Table 35). The results in 22 patients followed-up are 6 points (5 patients), 5 points (9 patients), 4 points (4 patients), 3 points (3 patients) and 0 points (1 patient), i.e., a proportion of good:fair:poor of 14:7:1. We believe that these figures compare more than favorably with those recorded in a series of patients operated upon for abdomino-perineal rectoplasty, and we attribute this to the better identification and preservation of the pubo-rectalis sling. The very poor result of 0 points in 1 patient who had a sacro-perineal rectoplasty for recto-urethral fistula was almost certainly due to too extensive an exploration, because there is now both a neurogenic bladder and absence of sphincter squeeze. Comments concerning the loss of points from a full score in the remaining 29 patients are identical with those described above for our 10 patients with recto-urethral fistulae operated upon by the sacral route. With improvement in some of the qualifying factors (constipation, "toilet tricks," training, age maturation and social and parental influences), the clinical scores will eventually be better than described and at periods approach them even now, of the order 18:3:1 for good:fair:poor, with at least half the good results having a score of 6 points. It is also significant that in the 30 sacral route operations, apart from secondary anoplasty for redundant prolapsed mucosa or anal stricture, no child has required a secondary intra-abdominal procedure, nor has a fistula recurred.

Analysis of those 16 patients of Table 34 in whom we have performed a secondary operation after definitive repair elsewhere is described below under secondary rectoplasty and repair of levator ani.

TRANSLEVATOR DEFORMITIES.—Table 35 indicates the methods of treatment adopted in 66 patients, and 63 of these were performed by ourselves *ab initio*, and 46 patients are currently available for follow-up. The results are good:fair:poor in the ratio 38:7:1, with 28 of these patients having scores of 6 points, indicating perfect control under all circumstances.

TABLE 35. – TREATMENT SURVEY OF TRANSLEVATOR DEFORMITIES (66 PATIENTS)

TYPE OF PROCEDURE		NUMBER OF PATIENTS	DEATHS	NO FOLLOW-UP OR TOO RECENT	FOLLOWED-UP	CLINICAL SCORE 0	1	2	3	4	5	6
Treatment by FDS Unit Throughout*												
Dilatation only		8	1		7		1					6
Anoplasty		49	7	9	33					5	8	20
Initial anoplasty, with later sacro-perineal transplantation		1			1						1	
Initial anoplasty, with later perineal transplantation		1			1						1	
Anoplasty, with later rectosigmoid-ectomy for secondary megacolon		2			2				1	1		
Colostomy, later sacro-perineal rectoplasty		1			1							1
No treatment required		1			1							1
TOTAL		63	8†	9	46		1		1	6	10	28
						"Poor"			"Fair"		"Good"	
*Definitive Procedure Elsewhere, Secondary Procedure by FDS Unit**												
"Elsewhere" Initial Procedure	FDS Unit* Procedure											
Colostomy	Anoplasty	1	1									
Anoplasty	Anoplasty	1			1						1	
Perineal transplant	Anoplasty	1		1								
TOTAL		3	1†	1	1						1	

*FDS Unit – The Chief Surgeons in the Unit are F. D. Stephens, Robert Fowler and E. Durham Smith.
†All from associated anomalies unrelated to treatment of the anus.

Seven patients were dilated only (anal stenosis, anterior anus); all except 1 scored 6 points. The one poor result was in a patient with myelomeningocele.

Thirty-three patients had anoplasties, most often a simple cutback of a fistula, and occasionally a minor incision of membrane or covering or slight mobilization of the terminal anal canal. Twenty patients scored 6 points. The loss of points from 6 in the remaining 13 patients was due to constipation and staining in 12, which reduced the "control" and "staining" scores by 1 or 2 points; 1 patient scored only 4 points because of occasional accidents and staining, but she is a disturbed girl in a broken home. All 33 patients scored the full 2 points for sphincter squeeze and have a normal sense of rectal awareness.

Only 2 patients have required secondary transplantation of the anus backwards. In 1 patient (ano-vestibular fistula), an initial cutback resulted in some vulval dirtiness, and the anus was transplanted directly via a perineal exposure; she now has a little mucus staining, thus reducing her otherwise normal state to a score of 5 points. A second patient had a large competent vulvar anus requiring no initial treatment. However, at 7 years of age, vulvar soiling necessitated transplantation. A perineal approach was first used, but a fistula developed between the new anal canal and the vestibular site due to insufficient mobilization of terminal bowel through the inadequate exposure afforded by this operative route. Re-exploration by the sacro-perineal method was then successful, and she also now scores 5 points, one point being deducted because of some mucus staining. Her pre- and postoperative appearances are shown in Figures 59, *E*, and 128.

Comparative Results with Other Authors

It is almost impossible to provide comparative statistics of results because of the confusion in terminology, the complexity of treatment regimens and the varying criteria defined as "good," "fair" or "poor." Many series classified under the Ladd and Gross classification do not indicate whether the lesions discussed in type 3 are supralevator or translevator, so that results have little meaning. For example, Mayo and Rice (1950) in 95 type 3 cases show 47% good result, 21% poor result; Brayton and Norris (1958) in 37 such cases show 62% good, 32% poor; Santulli *et al.* (1965) 54% good and 26% poor. But the texts of these papers refer to "recto-perineal fistulae," "fourchette fistulae," etc., indicating the inclusion of anal (translevator) types, in which good results can be almost guaranteed in the analysis.

Some reports, however, do make the distinction between a high and low level and provide the basis for Table 36.

TABLE 36.—COMPARATIVE TABLE OF FUNCTIONAL RESULTS IN REPORTS WHERE "HIGH" OR "LOW" IS INDICATED

AUTHOR	NUMBER OF CASES*	"GOOD"	"FAIR"	"POOR"
Supralevator Deformities				
Gross (1959)†	?	– (60%)	– (20%)	– (20%)
Scott *et al.* (1960)	19	4 (21%)	2 (11%)	13 (68%)
Partridge and Gough (1961)	63	21 (33%)	27 (43%)	15 (24%)
Swenson and Grana (1962)	21	5 (24%)	4 (19%)	12 (57%)
Swain and Tucker (1962)	13	4 (31%)	6 (46%)	3 (23%)
Trusler and Wilkinson (1962)	15	4 (27%)	3 (20%)	8 (53%)
Kiesewetter and Turner (1963)	39	– (38%)	– (15%)	– (45%)
Louw (1965)	22	7 (32%)	9 (40%)	6 (28%)
Swenson and Donnellan (1967)	22	14 (64%)	5 (23%)	3 (13%)
Present Authors (1968)				
Total cases	42	15 (36%)	15 (36%)	8 (28%)
Own cases only	26	14 (54%)	8 (31%)	3 (15%)
Sacral route only	22	14 (64%)	7 (32%)	1 (4%)
Translevator Deformities				
Scott *et al.* (1960)	19	17 (90%)	1 (5%)	1 (5%)
Partridge and Gough (1961)	150	130 (87%)	17 (11%)	3 (2%)
Swenson and Grana (1962)	23	14 (61%)	2 (9%)	7 (31%)
Swain and Tucker (1962)	18	12 (67%)	6 (33%)	–
Trusler and Wilkinson (1962)	20	16 (80%)	4 (20%)	–
Kiesewetter and Turner (1963)	43	– (72%)	– (11%)	– (17%)
Louw (1965)	31	25 (81%)	4 (13%)	2 (6%)
Swenson and Donnellan (1967)	21	20 (95%)	1 (5%)	–
Present Authors (1968)	46	38 (83%)	7 (15%)	1 (2%)

*Followed-up cases only.
†Quoted in Scott and Swenson (1959) "for babies who have a high rectum."

In Table 36, we have included only those children who have been followed-up and have excluded patients who died of other causes.

Except for those of our own and of Swenson and Donnellan (1967), it is seen that in supralevator deformities the "good" results in most series are approximately 33%, with "poor" results ranging from 23–68%. However, it should be pointed out that all series include patients operated on "elsewhere," with sometimes damaging procedures, so that the results are not necessarily those of the authors themselves. In our own total series, when we include patients only secondarily operated on by us, the results are comparable with the above figures. The superior results of our sacro-perineal operations (64% good results and only 4% poor results) and those of the careful sphincter-preserving technique of Swenson and Donnellan (64% good results and 13% poor results) are apparent in Table 36.

A further breakdown of these figures provides an assessment of the relative merits of the various types of rectoplasty. As regards neonatal abdomino-perineal rectoplasty, the best results are those of Swenson and Donnellan (1967), which are their 22 cases listed in Table 36, although it is not quite clear from the paper whether all these were actually performed in the neonatal period; and of Kiesewetter and Turner (1963), who show a good:fair:poor ratio of 8:1:2 on 11 patients. In 19 such operations reported by Partridge and Gough (1961) the good:fair:poor ratio was 7:9:3; in 7 cases of Moore and Lawrence (1952), 0:4:1 (with 2 deaths); in 3 cases of Louw (1965), 1:0:2. Many other authors have utilized this technique, but, as their figures are based upon the Ladd and Gross classification, "type 3," it is not always clear whether the cases include some translevator lesions as well. Louw (1965) has abandoned the neonatal operation "due to difficulties in defining the puborectalis in the newborn, and overstretching of the puborectalis at the time of surgery and during subsequent dilatations."

Delayed abdomino-perineal rectoplasty after colostomy in the newborn period provides results indicated by most of the figures in Table 36. Of 29 such operations reported by Partridge and Gough (1961) the good:fair:poor ratio was 7:14:8; of 6 cases of Louw (1965), 1:3:2; of 15 cases of Trusler and Wilkinson (1962), 4:3:8; and of 16 cases of Kiesewetter and Turner (1963), 7:2:7.

Neither the results in neonatal nor delayed abdomino-perineal rectoplasty, however, approximate those of the sacro-perineal operations in our series. Louw (1965) who previously used an abdomino-perineal approach comments that with this "the overall results have been poor . . . partly due to inadequate visualization of the puborectalis sling with consequent incorrect tunnelling through the levator behind the sling." He now prefers the sacral approach. In 18 sacral operations, he had only 1 poor result, and this child had sacral agenesis with deficiency of musculature. Kiesewetter and Turner (1963) and Kiesewetter (1966) also reported their experience with the Stephens technique in a follow-up of 22 patients. In 13 patients where the definitive operation was sacro-perineal or sacro-abdomino-perineal good or fair results were obtained in 7, with 6 poor results (4 had major lumbo-sacral anomalies); in 8 secondary such operations, the results were good or fair, 4, with 4 poor results (1 mentally retarded, 1 emotionally disturbed).

The results of the Rehbein procedure or the combination of the sacro-perineal approach with Rehbein procedure are too early to assess. Rehbein's (1967) own series of 42 cases showed a good:fair:poor ratio of 18:13:11, but there is no breakdown provided in the report to indicate which of these patients had supralevator or translevator lesions.

Discussion is not required in the translevator deformities. All authors agree on good results of 70–95% and a small sprinkling of poor results, generally because of some associated anomaly (Table 36).

TABLE 37.—CINEDEFECOGRAPHY PROCEDURE

NAME NUMBER DATE

In attendance -
Names of Doctors - - - - - - -
Nurses - - - - - - -
Technicians - - - - - -

Equipment—Six-inch image intensifier; spot films (2 only); Cine—less than 10 frames per second; defecography chair; rectal catheters 14 and 26 French gauges; long metal catheter holding tongs; liquid barium in graduated transparent flask, 600 cc. and connecting tubing and flow stopper.

Procedure—Position of child: lateral sitting on special chair.
Insert into rectum via 14 Fr. catheter, several milliliters of barium suspension.
Remove catheter, wait a minute and take - - - - - - - - Spot film.
Reinsert 14 Fr. catheter; fill to 400 milliliters or till sensation of fullness.
Volume - - - - - - - - milliliters.
If child is able to hold barium back then go on to Part 1 but if leakage to Part 2.

Part 1	*Part 2*
Read the following instructions and explain general procedure to patient.	
	If leakage occurs after removal of 14 Fr. catheter, insert 26 Fr. catheter and refill. If no leakage, proceed; if free leakage turn to Part 3.
(*a*) Instruct child to hold back barium. Record sensation of fullness yes/no and volume - - - - - - ml.	(*a*) See (*a*) Part 1 yes/no Volume - - - - ml.
If no sensation of fullness insert more until full - - - - - - ml.	See (*a*) Part 1 - - - - ml.
(*b*) Remove catheter and start ciné	(*b*) See (*b*) Part 1
(*c*) After few seconds, instructions given to defecate, then to stop yes/no	(*c*) See (*c*) Part 1 yes/no
(*d*) Instruct to restart almost immediately yes/no	(*d*) See (*d*) Part 1 yes/no
(*e*) Turn off ciné several seconds after (*d*) and take spot film during defecation -Spot film	(*e*) See (*e*) Part 1 - Spot film

Part 3
Leakage during filling with 26 Fr. catheter in anus; state whether procedure abandoned, yes/no.
Radiologist to compute functional and radiological assessment: The Kelly Code of Continence, Table 38.

Radiographic Analysis

In a separate study, Kelly (1969) has performed ciné "defecograms" in a wide variety of rectal conditions, including 25 patients

TABLE 38.—KELLY CODE OF CONTINENCE

Clinical Assessment

SCORE	ACCIDENTS	STAINING	SPHINCTER SQUEEZE
Normal 2 points each	Never	Never	Strong
Intermediate 1 point each	Occasional	Occasional	Weak
Inadequate 0 points each	Daily	Daily	Absent

Functional and Radiological Assessment

SCORE	OBSERVED FUNCTIONAL CAPABILITY		RADIOGRAPHIC APPEARANCE
	Catheter Size	Performance	
Normal 2 points each	No leakage around 14 French catheter	Sensation of fullness, retention and evacuation of normal volumes	Normal levator indentation and levator lift
Intermediate 1 point each	No leakage around 26 French catheter	Abnormal sensation, evacuation or volume	Defects in any of above
Inadequate 0 points each	Leakage around 26 French catheter	Retention not achieved	Absent levator indentation and lift

with ano-rectal deformities treated by ourselves and others in the Royal Children's Hospital, Melbourne. This radiographic assessment has provided a valuable objective adjunct to clinical assessment of both sphincter activity and rectal sensation. Details of the technique are provided in his paper and involved the cinefluoroscopic recording of the rectum and anal canal viewed from the lateral aspect, after filling with liquid barium through a catheter. In this view in the relaxed state, a normal continent child shows the ano-rectal angulation to lie opposite the level of the lowest limit of the obturator foramen; during defecation, the ano-rectal junction descends and the angle diminishes (see Fig. 9). The procedure is summarized in Table 37 and Figure 152, *A*.

Three parameters of measurement provide a radiographic score, similar to the clinical score already described and in Table 38. These are as follow:

1. The ability to prevent defecation or leakage around the catheter:
   Score 2—No leakage around 13/14-French-gauge rectal catheter and after removal of catheter

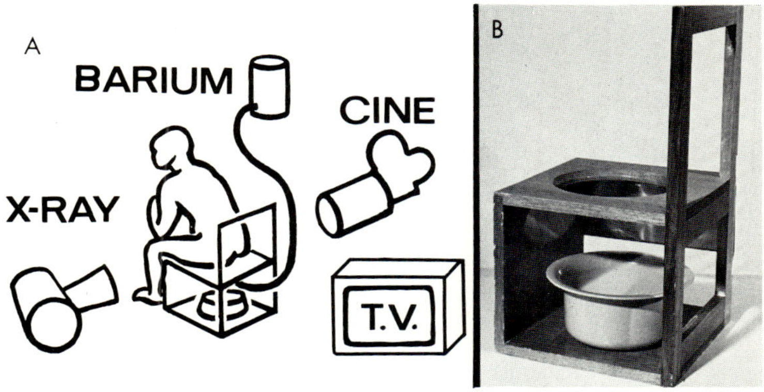

Fig. 152.—Cinedefecography procedure. **A,** posture and topography of equipment. **B,** radiolucent (wooden) chair with space provided between patient, seat and pot for maneuvering the catheter into the anus and for viewing the flow of barium.

Score 1—Leakage around 13/14-gauge, but not around 26-gauge catheter

Score 0—Leakage around 26-gauge catheter

2. Rectal sensation and detrusor function:
   - Score 2—Ability to appreciate filling after 100–400 ml. of barium, and to defecate on command
   - Score 1—Greater than 400 ml. to register filling and delay in defecating
   - Score 0—No sensation registered, and filling impossible because of leakage
3. Radiographic appearance:
   - Score 2—Maintenance of ano-rectal angulation during filling, diminution on defecation, and rapid restoration of the angle on command to stop
   - Score 1—Diminished angulation and movement
   - Score 0—No angulation or movement

Thus, a maximal defecogram score is 6, a minimal is 0, and, when added to the clinical score, a considerable degree of prognostic information is assembled. The demonstration of leakage around catheters of standard size indicates degrees of malocclusion of the lumen, and a normally contracting pubo-rectalis sling on the defecogram study may give encouragement that an apparently incontinent child may improve after more time and training, or after the elimination of some factor such as colonic inertia, stricture or redundant mucosa. Figures 153–157 show examples of various defecogram appearances after operation.

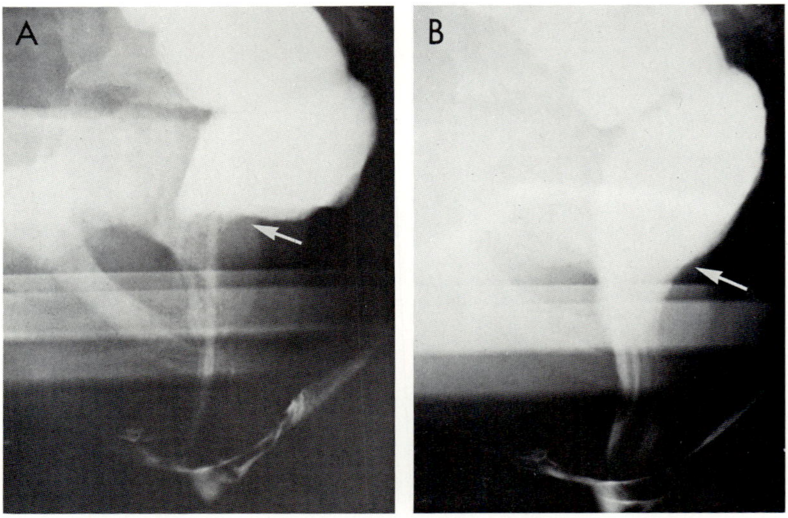

Fig. 153.—Post-rectoplasty defecogram. Repair of recto-urethral fistula—good functional result. **A,** high pubo-rectalis sling (*arrow*) holding back the barium with small caliber catheter in rectum (14F. gauge). **B,** defecating, showing relaxation of pubo-rectalis sling. The arrow indicates the lowered position of the sling in relaxation.

Fig. 154.—Post-rectoplasty defecogram. Repair of recto-urethral fistula—bad functional result. **A,** ineffectual and damaged pubo-rectalis muscle (*arrow*), with free leakage past large diameter catheter (26 F. gauge). Inadequate closure and angulation of the rectum. **B,** defecation, with relaxation of damaged sling (*arrow*).

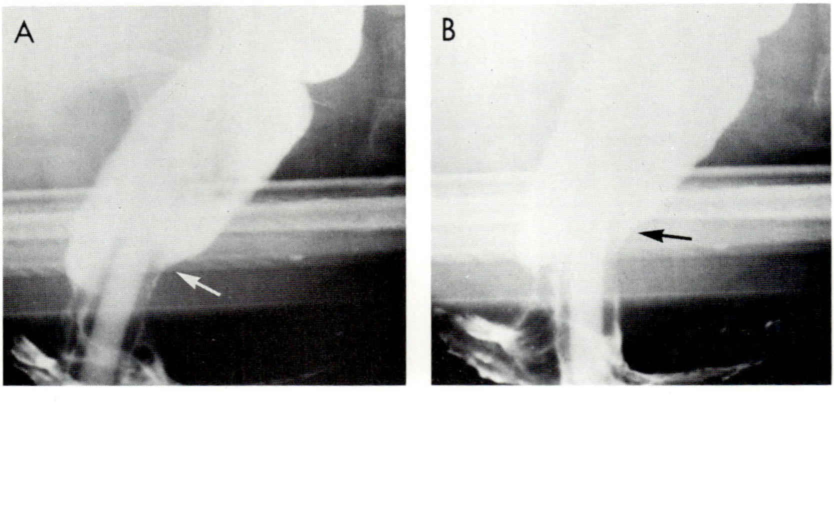

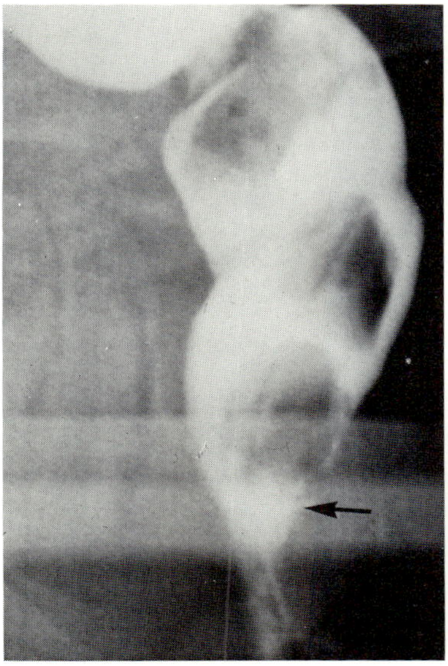

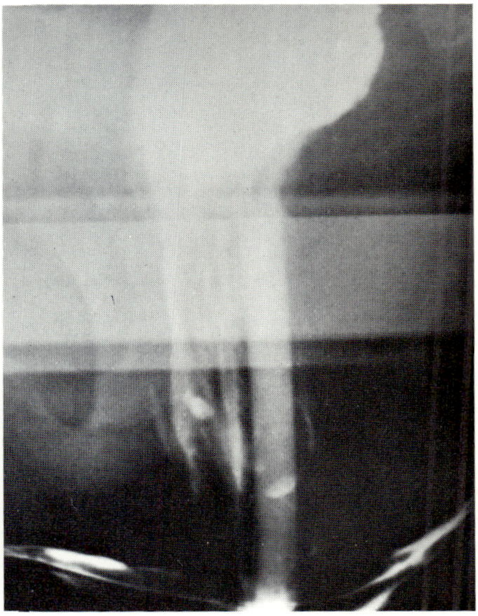

Fig. 155 (left). – Post-rectoplasty defecogram. Repair of recto-urethral fistula – impaired pubo-rectalis function, and fair result. Note shelving angulation (*arrow*); slight leakage of barium occurred around small sized catheter (14 F. gauge) when rectum full.

Fig. 156 (right). – Post-rectoplasty defecogram. Sacral agenesis and neurogenic rectal incontinence (deficiency of S3, 4 and 5). Rectum fills and empties without power to hold back, even with large diameter catheter (26 F. gauge) in anal canal. Radiograph shows a wide open anal canal.

Radiographic Results After Sacro-Perineal or Sacro-Abdomino-Perineal Operations. – The relation between clinical score and radiographic assessment is shown in Table 39.

TABLE 39. – Sacro-Perineal Technique with Radiographic Score in 12 Patients (Supralevator Lesions)

Cases	Clinical Score	Radiographic Score						
		0	1	2	3	4	5	6
8	5-6					1	2	5
2	3-4				1	1		
2	0-2	2						

The radiographic score paralleled the clinical score, the poorer results being associated with leakage past the catheter, diminished sensation and loss of ano-rectal angulation. The loss of radiographic points in the "good" clinical cases was due to constipation which abolished the ability to detect rectal fullness, but the ano-rectal angulation and levator movement were normal.

RADIOGRAPHIC RESULTS AFTER ABDOMINO-PERINEAL OPERATIONS. – The 5 patients who were operated upon were referred to us because of incontinence. In the radiographic assessment, all 5 children leaked with even the largest catheter, and none had sensation. Ano-rectal angulation was minimal or absent. All 5 scored 0 points.

RADIOGRAPHIC RESULTS AFTER MINOR ANOPLASTY OPERATIONS IN TRANSLEVATOR DEFORMITIES. – The 8 children with these deformities were fully continent, but 5 had some degree of anal staining (from constipation with overflow leakage). Two of the latter group, while constipated, lost radiographic points on sensation and initiation of defecation, but all 8 patients had normal ano-rectal angulation and movement (see Fig. 157).

As described by Kelly, dynamic radiography has several potential clinical applications. It may be used to (1) accurately assess the various factors in bowel control in patients with soiling problems, (2) predict the likely outcome after ano-rectal operations when the clinical state is obscured, as by a proximal defunctioning colostomy, (3) indicate the state of levator function when incontinence follows rectoplasty, particularly if secondary levator repair is contemplated and (4) make an objective comparison between the results of different types of operation for anal and rectal conditions.

Fig. 157. – Covered anus – ano-cutaneous fistula. Defecogram after cutback procedure. The anal canal is tightly closed around the 14 F. catheter, holding back the barium load in rectum without leakage.

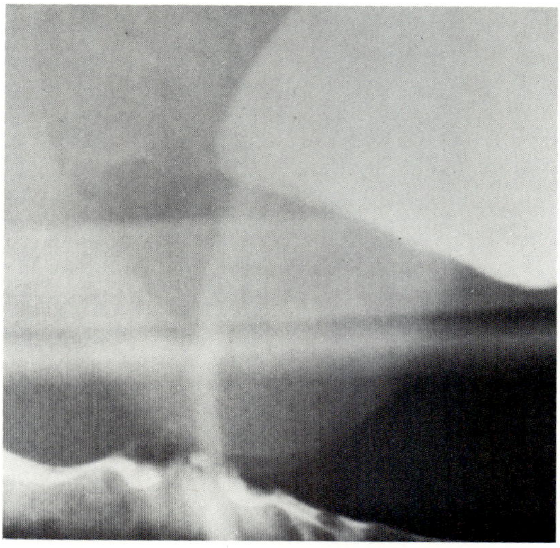

Secondary Rectoplasty and Repair of Levator Ani

Every surgeon who writes on ano-rectal malformations is at pains to point out that his over-all results tend to be depressed by the inclusion of cases operated on "elsewhere"! We are no exception to this and have listed our encounter with these cases separately in Tables 34 and 35. The results are poor, partly on the basis of selection, because this has been the reason for referral, partly because an ill-advised extensive perineal procedure has initially been performed.

Perineal rectoplasty for supralevator deformities has generally been disastrous, resulting in poor sphincter control, in all 8 such patients in our experience. Attempts to restore continence in these patients have proved to be the most difficult of all procedures, but the sacral exposure of the rectum and muscle has gained some success. Two case histories illustrate the problem:

In B. D. (aged 12 years, with recto-urethral fistula), a perineal approach was made in search of the rectum at 4 days of age in a country area. Following stricture of the new anal opening, sounds were passed which apparently went through the fistula into the bladder and ruptured the bladder neck. The child presented to hospital with urinary incontinence, anal stenosis and persistent recto-urethral fistula. Four attempts have been made to plicate the bladder neck, with only partial success, and, after defunctioning colostomy, a sacro-abdomino-perineal rectoplasty was performed at age 4½ years. Two subsequent attempts at levator ani repair have been performed. The new anus is a satisfactory one, with no stricture, and the child can remain almost clean on a routine of daily enemas. He is frankly incontinent for liquid stool and flatus but has just sufficient control of solid stools to make his present arrangements more acceptable than an abdominal colostomy. His levator ani contracts only weakly, a consequence of almost certain damage in the original perineal approach.

B. C. (aged 19 years) was born with recto-bulbar fistula and had a deep perineal exploration at birth. His fistula recurred, urinary infection supervened and defunctioning colostomy was required. One attempt at closure of fistula failed, and rectoplasty was reperformed at 10 years of age. Subsequently, two attempts at levator ani repair have achieved an acceptable degree of control, although he requires a daily enema to achieve this.

In 5 patients, abdomino-perineal rectoplasty had been performed in the neonatal period; all were incontinent with clinical scores of 0–1. In each, we have attempted restorative sacro-abdomino-perineal rectoplasty with repair of the levator muscle. Although the results are early and not fully acceptable, the clinical scores have been improved to 2 (1 patient), 3 (2 patients) and 4 (2 patients).

In all, sacro-perineal or sacro-abdomino-perineal re-exploration and levator repair have been carried out in 10 patients, the resulting clinical scores being improved from incontinence (0–1) to 2 (2 patients), 3 (4 patients), 4 (2 patients) and 6 (1 patient). In 1 patient, Kelly has had an opportunity to perform cinedefecography before and after the secondary repair. A preoperative radiographic score of 2 points has been improved to 5 points after repair, by the ability to hold back the barium column, and restoration of the ano-rectal angle and lift action of levator muscle.

Prior to intended repair, defecography in 5 patients has been of value in indicating, by complete or partial loss of ano-rectal angulation and movement, that the incontinence is indeed due to muscle inaction rather than some simply correctable factor such as constipation.

Fig. 158.—Secondary repair of levator ani muscle following inadequate rectoplasty. Rerouting the rectum from lateral tunnel in diaphragmatic to sphincteric parts of levator ani. **A,** perineal incision in natal cleft and around anus. **B,** rectum located in lateral tunnel in the levator diaphragm. **C,** levator incised in the line of the raphe. **D,** rectum then dissected from its tunnel through the levator muscle. **E,** rectum drawn up through the lateral tunnel. **F,** rectum rerouted through puborectalis tunnel; levator ani sutured in midline, lateral rent closed and anus resutured.

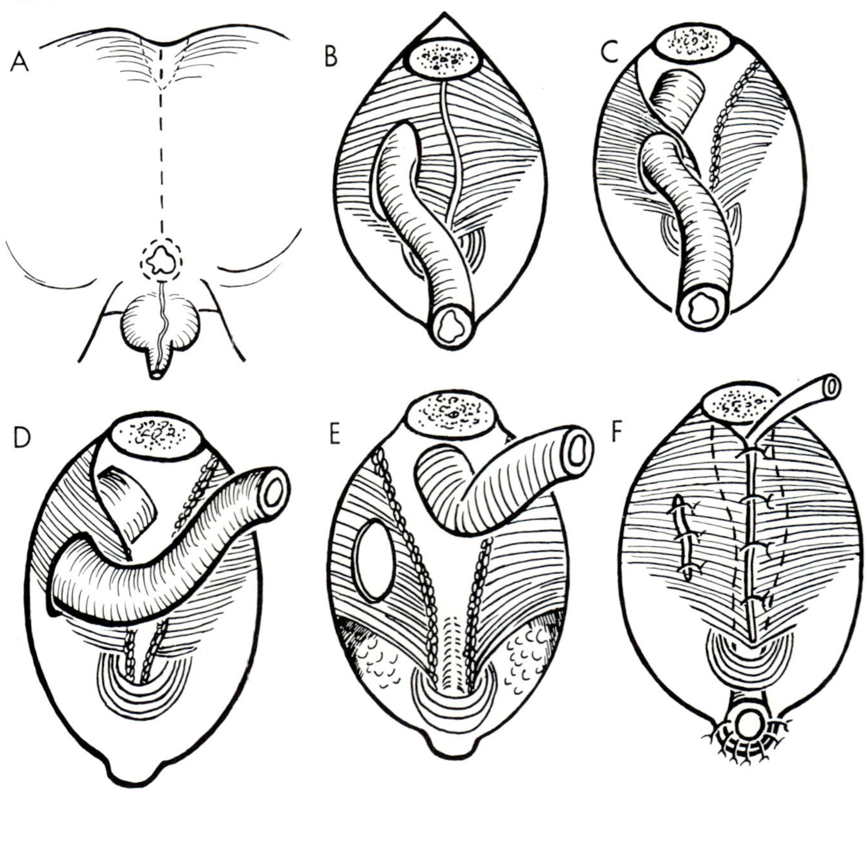

In these re-explorations, the common factors found have been wrong routing of the rectum through the levator or actual damage to the levator. Sometimes the rectum lies frankly behind the pubo-rectalis sling, either because of wrong placement or from rupture of the sling or else the rectum has been tunneled eccentrically through a lateral window in the diaphragmatic part of the levator. We believe that these risks are constantly present in the inadequate exposure of the pubo-rectalis sling from the abdominal route. The technique of repair is illustrated in Figures 158 and 159. Apart from the rerouting of the rectum well forward against the urethra or vagina, it is essential to repair the levator diaphragm and its sling in the midline.

Kiesewetter (1966) has also described the advantages of the sacral route in revision repairs. Four of his 8 secondary rectoplasties by this route have given good or fair results.

Kottmeier (1966) and Kottmeier and Dziadiw (1967) describe an operation to gain increased effectiveness of levator ani in secondary repair. Although the pubo-rectalis sling is relatively mobile, the pubo-

Fig. 159. – Secondary repair of levator ani muscle following inadequate rectoplasty. Rerouting the rectum from a posterior position in the sagittally divided levator ani muscle. **A,** rectum emerging from the split diaphragmatic part of the levator ani. **B,** liberation of rectum from the adherent levator muscles. **C,** levator ani incised in midline behind and around the rectum. **D,** rectum tucked closely against the urethra and the levator ani muscle, including the remains of the pubo-rectalis, approximated caudal to it. End of rectum resutured to the skin of the perineum.

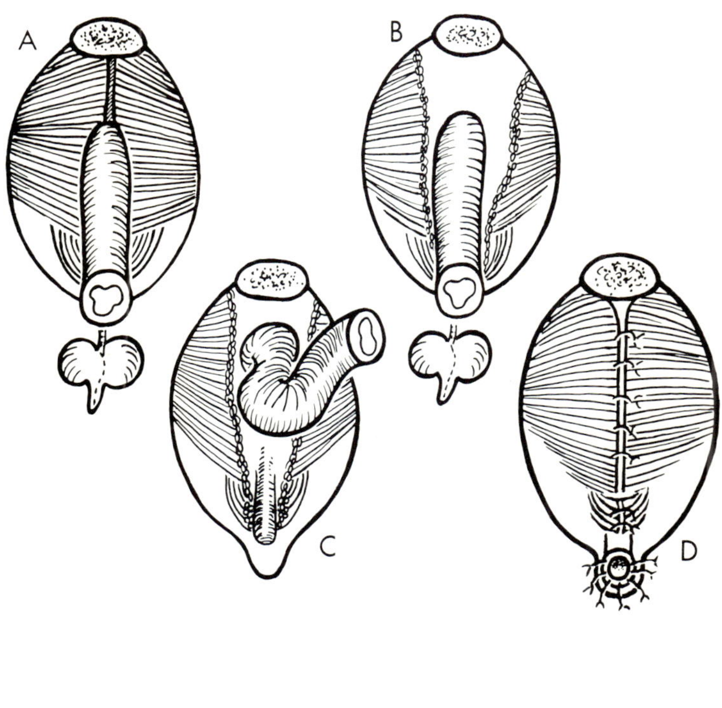

coccygeus and ileo-coccygeus components of the levator ani are fixed posteriorly and laterally by their attachments to the sacrum, coccyx and obturator line. By the division of these posterior and lateral attachments, the levator may move forwards and upwards to gain a slinglike sphincter action. Evidence is given of convincing clinical improvement, supported by cinefluoroscopic studies of increased ano-rectal angulation in 3 children after such levator release. They have recently extended the application of this procedure to the primary abdomino-perineal repair of high rectal cases, but the follow-up is not yet reported. It is remarkable that the nerve supply to the levator is not divided in this procedure; nevertheless, the accompanying radiographs show forward and backward movement of the muscle, with a considerable shutter effect on the rectal lumen.

Technique of Secondary Repair of Levator Musculature.—The purpose of the operation is to so place the "rectum" that it lies adjacent to the urethra or vagina, with the levator muscles drawn together behind it. The most anterior muscle bundles are approximated in the midline as far anteriorly as possible, preferably indenting the rectum to the point of occlusion.

The age of these patients is usually 3 years or older, and for this reason it is deemed unnecessary to perform a preliminary colostomy. Here the pelvis and the levator muscles are larger than in the newborn and are larger compared with the size of the collapsed rectum which is tucked up anteriorly against the urethra or vagina. Needless to say the bowel should be empty and pretreated with neomycin. The patient is anesthetized, a metal sound is tied into the urethra or a Hegar sound in the vagina, and the patient turned into the jackknife position. The anus is temporarily occluded with a circumanal stitch inserted in the mucosal layer.

The natal cleft incision is made from sacrum to anus, which is encircled by a circumferential racket extension. The incision is deepened in the midline through the fat, using a muscle stimulator to identify muscle as it comes into view. It is possible to detect activity and direction of muscle pull and so incise the pelvic diaphragm as close to the raphe as possible. The coccyx should be split or excised and the supralevator space dissected up under the tip of the sacrum. It is then possible to separate the tissues from the rectum from above down, within and without the supralevator space. In this way, the pelvic diaphragm is laid open, the rectum isolated from the levator muscles, and the route that the rectum has taken can be identified (Figs. 158 and 159).

The nerves to the levator muscles pass from the lateral pelvis wall towards the midline on or in the substance of the levator muscle. Midline operation with expansion of the window so created should not impair these nerves.

It may be necessary to incise the occluding stitch of the anus at this juncture in order to insert a metal obturator or gloved finger in the rectum to facilitate the isolation of the wall from the surrounding very adherent fibrous and muscular tissues.

The "rectum" and "anus" are cleared and thoroughly mobilized from the pelvis and perineum and replaced in a collapsed and empty state against the urethra or vagina, and the levator muscle, ragged and barely recognizable, partly obscured by fat and fascia, is sutured with silk in the midline as far anteriorly as possible to indent or if possible temporarily occlude the rectal lumen and so heal in this position.

The remainder of the diaphragm and the fat of the perineum are approximated and the anus, divested of any cutaneous cuff still adhering to the wall of the rectum, is resutured in its original site.

A drain tube is brought out of the incision in the vicinity of the coccyx.

A rectal tube is then passed into the rectum through the indented zone and is left in place for several days. Six hourly saline irrigations of the rectum are recommended to deflate the lumen and wash away feces as it accumulates. The tube may be removed on the fourth day and reintroduced three times a day for irrigations and deflations. In order to reduce residue, the patient should be given fluids by intravenous route and water only by mouth for at least 3 to 4 days and longer if tolerated after operation, and a low-residue diet is continued for at least 2 weeks postoperatively.

At 14 days, gentle dilatation of the indented zone of the rectum is then performed daily with the finger of surgeon or parent until the sling is softened and agile. This may take several weeks.

References

Abrami, G., and Dennison, W. M.: Duplication of the stomach, Surgery 49:794, 1961.

Aitken, A. B.: Case of doubling of the great intestine, Glasgow M. J. 78:431, 1912.

Aitken, J.: A case of colon and ileum duplex, Brit. J. Surg. 37:349, 1950.

Aldridge, R. T., and Campbell, P. E.: Ganglion cell distribution in the normal rectum and anal canal. A basis for the diagnosis of Hirschsprung's disease by anorectal biopsy, J. Pediat. Surg. 4:475, 1968.

Allard, C. A.; Ross, D. E., and Hopkirk, J. F.: Complete duplication of large bowel treated by subtotal colectomy, Ann. Surg. 130:249, 1949.

Allen, V. K.: Malformations of anus and rectum, Tr. Am. Proctol. Soc. 33:148, 1932.

Amussat, J. J.: Observation sur une opération d'anus artificial pratiquee avec succès par un nouveau procédé, Gaz. med. (Paris), 1835.

Anders, E.: Über das operative Verfahren bei congenitaler analer und rectaler Atresia, Arch. klin. chir. XIV:489 and 571, 1892.

Anderson, R. C., and Reed, S. C.: The likelihood of recurrence of congenital malformations, Journal-Lancet 74:175, 1954.

Arnheim, E. E.: Congenital malformations of the rectum and anus, Am. J. Surg. 81:538, 1951.

Asai, T.: Duplication totale du gros intestin, Arch. jap. chir. 10:592, 1933.

Ashley, J. D., Jr.: Congenital atresia of oesophagus with tracheo-esophageal fistula, Radiology 36:621, 1941.

Babcock, W. W.: Radical single stage extirpation for cancer of the large bowel, with retained functional anus, Surg., Gynec. & Obst. 85:1, 1947.

Bacon, H. E.: *Anus, Rectum and Sigmoid Colon: Diagnosis and Treatment* (Philadelphia: J. B. Lippincott Company, 1938), Chapter 3.

Bacon, H. E.: Cancer of the rectum, Surgery 26:584, 1949.

Bacon, H. E., and Sherman, L. F.: Surgical management of congenital malformations of the anus and rectum: Report of 111 cases, A.M.A. Arch. Surg. 64:331, 1952.

Ball, C.: *The Rectum and Anus. Their Diseases and Treatment* (London: Cassell & Co., Ltd., 1887).

Ballance, H.: Double colon, Proc. Roy. Soc. Med. 23:1570, 1930.

Bar, P., and De Kervilly, M.: Gros intestin duplex chez un enfant nouveau-né, Obstetrique 2:81, 1909.

Barnard, C. N.: Duplication of alimentary tract: Report of case of double uterus, vagina, large bowel and anus, Minnesota M. J. 40:257, 1957.

Barney, J. D.: The urological complications of imperforate anus, Tr. Am. A. Genito-Urin. Surgeons 21:393, 1928.

Bartels, M.: Über die Bauchblasengenitalspalte; ein bestimmte Grad der sogenannten inversion der Harnblase, Arch. Anat. Physiol., 1868, p. 165.

Beach, P. D.; Brascho, D. J.; Hein, W. R.; Nichol, W. W., and Geppert, L. J.: Duplication of the primitive hindgut of the human being, Surgery 49:779, 1961.

Beischer, N. A., and Fortune, D. W.: Double monsters, Obst. & Gynec. 32:158, 1968.

Bell, B.: Cited by Mastin in Surg., Gynec. & Obst. 7:316, 1908, from Bodenhammer (1860), q.v.

Berdon, W. E.; Hochberg, B.; Baker, D. H.; Grossman, H., and Santulli, T. V.: The association of lumbo-sacral spine and genito-urinary anomalies with imperforate anus, Am. J. Roentgenol. 98:181, 1966.

Berdon, W. E., and Baker, D. H.: The inherent errors in measurements of inverted films in patients with imperforate anus, Ann. radiol. 10:235, 1967.

Berdon, W. E.; Baker, D. H.; Santulli, T. V., and Amoury, R.: The radiologic evaluation of imperforate anus, Radiology 90:466, 1968.

Berman, J. K.: Congenital anomalies of rectum and anus, Surg., Gynec. & Obst. 66:11, 1938.

Bevan, A. D.: Imperforate anus, Surg. Clin. 4:21, 1920.

Bielowicz, A.: Review of congenital malformations of the anus and rectum, Polish Surg. Rev. 37:525, 1965.

Bill, A. H., Jr.: Pathology and surgical treatment of imperforate anus, J.A.M.A. 166:1429, 1958.

Bill, A. H., Jr.: Common denominators in rectal anomalies on both sides of the Atlantic, Arch. Dis. Childhood 39:149, 1964.

Bill, A. H., Jr., and Johnson, R. J.: Congenital median band of the anus: Report of 6 cases with results of surgical events leading to abnormality, Surg., Gynec. & Obst. 97:307, 1953.

Bill, A. H., Jr., and Johnson, R. J.: Failure of migration of the rectal opening as the cause for most cases of imperforate anus, Surg., Gynec. & Obst. 106:643, 1958.

Bill, A. H., Jr., Johnson, R. J., and Foster, R. A.: Anteriorly placed rectal opening in the perineum "ectopic anus": A report of 30 cases, Ann. Surg. 147:173, 1958.

Bodenhammer, W.: *A Practical Treatise on the Etiology, Pathology and Treatment of Congenital Malformations of the Anus and Rectum* (New York: Samuel S. and William Wood, 1860).

Bornstein, F. P.: Duplication of large intestine associated with multiple malformations, Arch. Path. 63:376, 1957.

Bourne, C. W.: Urethra-rectal fistula: Unusual case in 25 year old man, J. Urol. 96:65, 1966.

Bradham, R. R.: Imperforate anus: Report of 130 cases, Surgery 44:578, 1958.

Bradham, R. R.: Delayed correction of type III imperforate anus in the male child, Ann. Surg. 154:972, 1961.

Brayton, D., and Norris, W. J.: Further experience with the treatment of imperforate anus, Surg., Gynec. & Obst. 107:719, 1958.

Breen, J. L., and Weinberg, C. R.: Genito-urinary and intestinal duplication: Case report and survey of the literature, Obst. & Gynec. 26:804, 1965.

Brenner, E. C.: Congenital defects of the anus and rectum, Surg., Gynec. & Obst. 20:579, 1915.

Brenner, R. W., and Swenson, O.: Colostomy in infants and children, Surg., Gynec & Obst. 124:1239, 1967.

Brown, S. S., and Schoen, A. H.: Congenital ano-rectal stricture, J. Pediat. 36:746, 1950.

Browne, D.: Some congenital deformities of the rectum, anus, vagina and urethra, Ann. Roy. Coll. Surgeons England 8:173, 1951.

Browne, D.: Congenital deformities of the anus and rectum, Arch. Dis. Childhood 30:42, 1955.

Bruni, C.: Seltene anomalie der urogenital Organe doppelter Penis, Ztschr. Urol. 21:193, 1927.

Brunschwig, A.; Dargeon, H. W., and Russell, W. A.: Duplication of the entire colon and lower ileum with termination of one colon into vaginal anus, Surgery 24:1010, 1948.

Bryce, T. H.: Description of a foetus the subject of retroflexion of the trunk—ectopia viscerum and spina bifida, with a discussion as to the cause of these associated abnormalities, J. Anat. (London) 29:553, 1895.

Bryndorf, J., and Madsen, C. M.: Ectopic anus in the female, Acta. chir. scandinav. 118: 466, 1960.
Burnell: Cited in Matas, q.v.
Butcher, H. R.: Abdomino-perineal operation for high imperforate anus in the newborn, A.M.A. Arch. Surg. 66:637, 1953.
Byrd, W. A.: Verneuil's modification of Amussat's operation for the relief of imperforate anus, Med. & Surg. Reporter, X:649, 1882.
Cain, W. S., and Kiesewetter, W. B.: Infant colostomy: Its role and complications, Arch. Surg. 91:314, 1965.
Campbell, J. P.: In Bodenhammer's treatise, q.v.
Carter, R. F., and Lyall, D.: Congenital recto-vaginal defects. Operative repair, Surg., Gynec. & Obst. 71:89, 1940.
Cartledge, J. McP.: Personal communication, 1970.
Cave, H. W.: Method of closure of temporary external fecal fistula, Surg., Gynec. & Obst. 61:499, 1935.
Ceci: Rep. operazioni sul retto. Casi clinici e studi sperimentali. Genoa (1891). Quoted by Sicur, Arch. prov. chir., t.v. no. 9, 1896.
Chandler, L. R.: Congenital malformations of the rectum and anus: Their surgical treatment, California & West. Med. 51:84, 1939.
Chaput: Therapeutique chirurgicale des affections du rectum, Paris, 1896.
Chassaignac: Bull. et mém. Soc. chir. Feb. 20, 1856.
Chatterjee, S. K., and Talukder, B. C.: Double termination of the alimentary tract in female infants, J. Pediat. Surg. 4:237, 1969.
Chiarleoni, G.: Duplicita genitale esterna e mancanza di ano in bambina di 33 mesi, Ann. ostet. 16:469, 1894.
Chisholm, T. C.: Exstrophy of the urinary bladder, Am. J. Surg. 101:649, 1961.
Christensen, E. R.: Duplications in the gastrointestinal tract in children, Danish M. Bull. 6:281, 1959.
Cohen, S. J.: Diphallus with duplication of colon and bladder, Proc. Roy. Soc. Med. 61: 305, 1968.
Conant, W. S.: Boston Med. & Surg. J., March, 1893.
Cooke, J.: *Mellificium Chirurgiae: Or the Marrow of Chirurgery Much Enlarged,* p. 669 and 4th ed., p. 158 (London: Marshall, 1685).
Cozzi, F., and Wilkinson, A. W.: Congenital abnormalities of anus and rectum: Mortality and function, Brit. M. J. 1:144, 1968.
Cripps, H.: *Disease of the Rectum and Anus* (New York, The Macmillan Company, 1914).
Crowell, E. A., and Dulin, J. W.: Congenital anomalies of the anus and rectum, Surgery 7:529, 1940.
Cule, J. H.: John Pughe 1814–1874. A scholar surgeon's operation on the imperforate anus in 1854, Ann. Roy. Coll. Surgeons England 37:247, 1965.
Czerny, V.: Über sacrale Operationen, Verhandl. Deutsch. Gesellsch. chir. 2:34, 1893.
David, V. C.: The treatment of congenital openings of the rectum into the vagina – atresia ani vaginalis, Surgery 1:163, 1937.
Davis, D. A.: In *Diseases of Colon and Ano-rectum,* Turrell, R. (ed.), vol. 2 (Philadelphia: W. B. Saunders Company, 1959), p. 1031.
Delagenière, P.: Du traitement de l'imperforation de l'anus, Arch. prov. chir. 3:405, 1894.
Delbet, P., and Brechot: *Maladies de l'Anus et du Rectum* (Paris: J. B. Baillière et fils, 1916).
Del Duca, V.; Davies, E. V., and Barroway, J. N.: Congenital absence of sacrum and coccyx: Report of 2 cases, J. Bone & Joint Surg. 33-A:248, 1951.
Delens: Anus double; excision de la cloison, Bull. et mém. Soc. chir. 1:245, 1875.
Delens: Imperforation anale; énterotomie périnéale avec résection du coccyx; guérison avec prolapsus rectale, Bull. et mém. Soc. chir. 1:247, 1875.
Demarcquay: Suggestion cited by Mastin, Surg., Gynec. & Obst. 7:3, 1908.

Demelin: Rev. obst. Inf. Toulouse 1:209, 1895.

Dennison, W. M.: Congenital malformations of the rectum and anus, Glasgow M. J. 36: 283, 1955.

De Staercke, P.: Congenital malformations of the anus and rectum, Acta. chir. belg. 61: 174, 1962.

Dickinson, S. J.: Agenesis of the descending colon with imperforate anus. Correlation with modern concepts of the origin of intestinal atresia, Am. J. Surg. 113:279, 1967.

Dieffenbach, J. F.: In *Die Operative Chirurgie*, Band I. (Leipzig: F. A. Brockhaus, 1845). p. 670.

Dietrich: Über Bauch-Blasen–Genitalspaltung, Ztschr. Geburtsh. Gynäk. 19:299, 1904.

Dmytryk, E. T.: Congenital malformations of the anus and rectum, Arch. Surg. 50:253, 1945.

Donovan, E. J., and Stanley-Brown, E. G.: Imperforate anus, Ann. Surg. 147:203, 1958.

Drueck, C. J.: Malformations of the anus and rectum, Internat. Clin. 1:181, 1925.

Duboise: A pioneer of left iliac colostomy as an adjunct in the surgical treatment of imperforate anus; Cited by Matas, q.v.

Duhamel, B.: From the mermaid to anal imperforation. The syndrome of Caudal Regression, Arch. Dis. Childhood 36:152, 1961.

Duhamel, B.; Haegel, P., and Pages, R.: *Morphogenese Pathologique "Des Monstruosities aux Malformations"* (Paris [VI^{c}]: Masson & Cie, 1966), p. 151.

Duthie, H. L., and Gairns, F. W.: Sensory nerve endings and sensation in the anal region of man, Brit. J. Surg. 47:585, 1960.

Duthie, H. L., and Bennett, R. C.: The relation of sensation in the anal canal to functional anal sphincter: A possible factor in anal continence, Gut 4:179, 1963.

Duthie, H. L., and Watts, J. M.: Contribution of the external anal sphincter to the pressure zone in the anal canal, Gut 6:64, 1965.

Eckerle, W. J.: Congenital anomalies of anus, rectum and sigmoid colon and their surgical management, Am. J. Surg. 82:651, 1951.

Edwards, D. A., and Phillips, S. F.: A hypothesis of anal continence, Proc. Roy. Soc. Med. 58:790, 1965.

Ehrenpreis, T.: Important source of error in roentgen examination of anal atresia, Nord. med. Tidskr. 25:72, 1945.

Elliot, J. W.: Med. News, New York, Oct. 17, 1896.

Emrys-Roberts, E., and Paterson, A. M.: A case of ectopia viscerum, associated with spina bifida and other abnormalities, J. Anat. (London) 40:332, 1906.

Feggeter, S.: Imperforate anus in identical twins, Newcastle M. J. 19:20, 1939.

Fisher, J. H.: Management of ano-rectal anomalies, Am. J. Proctol. 12:52, 1961.

Fitchet, S. M.: Imperforate anus. Surgical treatment of cases of maldevelopment of terminal bowel and anus, Boston M. & Surg. J. 195:25, 1926.

Forshall, I.: Ano-rectal abnormalities, Brit. J. Clin. Pract. 11:842, 1957.

Forshall, I.: Prognosis for children undergoing operations during the first few weeks of life, Proc. Roy. Soc. Med. 53:954, 1960.

Fowler, R., Jr.: Landmarks and legends of the anal canal, Australian & New Zealand J. Surg. 27:1, 1957.

Fraser, J.: *Surgery of Childhood*, vol. 2 (New York: William Wood & Co., 1926).

Fraser, J. E.: *Manual of Embryology* (London: Baillière, Tindall & Cox, 1931), p. 433.

Freedman, B.: Congenital absence of sacrum and coccyx. Report of cases and review of literature, Brit. J. Surg. 37:299, 1950.

Freeman, N. V.: Congenital atresia and stenosis of the colon, Brit. J. Surg. 53:595, 1966.

Friedman, E.: Atresia of the esophagus and imperforate anus communicating with the bladder, J. Obst. & Gynaec. Brit. Emp. 51:546, 1944.

Gans, S. L., and Friedman, N. B.: Some new concepts in the embryology, anatomy, physiology and surgical correction of imperforate anus, Western J. Surg. 69:34, 1961.

Gans, S. L.; Friedman, N. B., and David, J. S: Congenital ano-rectal anomalies: Changing concepts in management, Clin. Pediat. 2:605, 1963.

Gans, S. L.: Personal communication, 1970.

Gaston, E. A.: The physiology of fecal continence, Surg., Gynec. & Obst. 87:280 and 669, 1948.

Gemmell, J. E., and Patterson, A. M.: Duplication of bladder, uterus, vagina and vulva, with successive full-time pregnancy and labour in each uterus, J. Obst. & Gynaec. Brit. Emp. 23:25, 1913.

Giordani, C.: Clinical aspects of congenital agenesis of sacrum, Minerva ortop. 8:83, 1957.

Gleiss: Doppelbildung der Unterleibsorgane, Arch. klin. Chir. 74:187, 1904.

Goligher, J. C., and Hughes, E. S. R.: Sensibility of the rectum and colon; its role in the mechanism of anal continence, Lancet 1:543, 1951.

Gough, M. H.: Ano-rectal agenesis with persistence of cloaca, Proc. Roy. Soc. Med. 52: 886, 1959.

Gray, A. W.: Triplication of the large intestine, Arch. Path. 30:1215, 1940.

Greig, D. M.: Processus vermiformis duplex, Edinburgh M. J. 41:277, 1934.

Grohé, B.: Duplicites intestini crassi cum utero et vagina dupl., Deutsche Ztschr. Chir. 57:425, 1900.

Gross, R. E.: *The Surgery of Infancy and Childhood* (Philadelphia: W. B. Saunders Company, 1953).

Haab, O.: Beitrage zu den angeborenen Fehlern des Auges, Albrecht von Graefes Arch. Ophth. 24:257, 1878.

Hadra: Berlin Klin. Wchnschr. No. 7, 1886.

Hall, E. G.; McCandless, A. E., and Rickham, P. P.: Vesico-intestinal fissure with diphallus, Brit. J. Urol. 25:219, 1953.

Hamilton, W. J.; Boyd, J. D., and Mossman, H. W.: *Human Embryology (Prenatal Development of Form and Function)* (3rd ed.; Cambridge: W. Heffer, 1962).

Hamm, F. C., and Harlin, H. C.: Imperforate anus associated with urinary tract fistulae, New York J. Med. 53:561, 1953.

Hanley, P. H.; Hines, M. O., and Stephenson, J. E.: Anal sphincter preserving operations for congenital low recto-vaginal and recto-perineal fistula, Am. J. Surg. 88:737, 1954.

Hanley, P. H.: Management of low recto-vaginal fistulas with imperforate anus, J. Dis. Colon & Rectum 8:119, 1965.

Harken, D. E.: Congenital malformation of the rectum and anus: Analysis of the embryological background, treatment, and results in 25 cases, Surgery 11:422, 1942.

Harris, L. D., and Pope, C. E., II: "Squeeze" vs. resistance: An evaluation of the mechanism of sphincter competence, J. Clin. Invest. 43:2272, 1964.

Harris, L. E.; Corbin, H. P. F., and Hill, J. R.: Anorectal rings in infancy: Incidence and significance, Pediatrics 13:59, 1954.

Hartl, H.: On surgery of high anal and rectal atresia, Wien. med. Wchnschr. 110:516, 1960.

Haynes: Am. J. M. Sc., July, 1884.

Hecker, W. C.: Zur Chirurgie der Anal und Rectumatresie mit Fistelbildung, Chir. Praxis, Heft 3:383, 1961.

Heinecke: München. med. Wchnschr., No. 37, 1888.

Helwig, F. C.: Imperforate anus with exit through prostatic urethra; report of 3 cases, Am. J. Dis. Child. 38:559, 1929.

Hiatt, R. B., and Santulli, T. V.: Important factors influencing the treatment of imperforate anus, Dis. Colon & Rectum 5:110, 1962.

Higgs, S. L.: Specimen of congenital absence of the sacrum, Proc. Roy. Soc. Med. 17:39 (part III), 1924.

Hinckle, W. A.: Case of double anus, vagina and uterus, J.A.M.A. 90:455, 1928.

Hutchinson, C.: Cited by Matas, q.v. 1897

Imdahl, H.; Koch, W., and Hermanns, A.: Thalidomid in der Frühschwangerschaft und enddarmmissbildungen, Bull. Soc. Int. Chir. 22:602, 1963.

Ives, E. J.: Thalidomide and anal abnormalities, Canad. M. A. J. 87:670, 1962.

Jaros, M.: Congenital aplasia of the sacrum; dyspygia, Acta chir. orthop. et traumatol. cechoslovaca 23:293, 1956.

Jeffreys and Maxwell: Quoted in Gaston, J. M., Congenital imperforation of rectum and anus, Internat. Clin. 3:217, 1919.

Johnston, J. H., and Penn, I. A.: Exstrophy of the cloaca, Brit. J. Urol. 38:302, 1966.

Johnston, T. B.: Extroversion of the bladder, complicated by the presence of intestinal openings on the surface of the extroverted area, J. Anat. (London) 48:89, 1913.

Jones, F. W.: The nature of malformations of the rectum and the urogenital passages, Brit. M.J. 2:1630, 1904.

Jones, F. W.: The delimitation of the rectum and its subdivisions, Proc. Roy. Soc. Med. 4: 85, 1911.

Jones, F. W.: Explanation of rectourethral anomaly and some points in normal anatomy, Lancet 2:860, 1915.

Judy, W. S., Jr.: Colon duplex, Northwest Med. 56:586, 1957.

Kaijser, K., and Malmström-Groth, A.: Ano-rectal abnormalities as a congenital familial incidence, Acta paediat. 46:199, 1957.

Katz, J. F.: Congenital absence of sacrum and coccyx, J. Bone & Joint Surg. 35-A:398, 1953.

Katzen, M.: Ano-rectal malformations: Their management and sequelae, South African M. J. 36:954, 1962.

Keen, W. W.: Therapeutic Gazette: Philadelphia, April, 1897.

Keibel, F., and Mall, F. P.: *Manual of Human Embryology,* vol. 2 (London: J. B. Lippincott Company, 1912), p. 322.

Keiller, V. H.: Imperforate anus with report of 3 cases, Texas J. Med. 20:278, 1924.

Keith, A.: Malformations of the hind end of the body, Arch. klin. Chir. 70:555, 1905.

Keith, A.: Three demonstrations on malformations of the hind end of the body. I. Specimens illustrating malformations of the rectum and anus, Brit. M. J. 2:1736, 1908.

Kelly, J. H.: Personal communication, 1968.

Kelly, J. H.: The radiographic anatomy of the normal and abnormal neonatal pelvis, J. Pediat. Surg. 4:432, 1969.

Kelly, J. H.: Cine radiography in anorectal malformations, J. Pediat. Surg. 4:538, 1969.

Kennedy, W.: Claim to have successfully operated on a male child with congenitally absent anus, cited by J. H. Cule, q.v.

Kiesewetter, W. B.: Imperforate anus, S. Clin. North America 36:1531, 1956.

Kiesewetter, W. B., and Turner, C. R.: Continence after surgery for imperforate anus: A critical analysis and preliminary experience with the sacro-perineal pull through, Ann. Surg. 158:498, 1963.

Kiesewetter, W. B.; Turner, C. R., and Sieber, W. K.: Imperforate anus. Review of a 16 year experience with 146 patients with imperforate anus, Am. J. Surg. 107:412, 1964.

Kiesewetter, W. B.; Sukarochana, K., and Sieber, W. K.: Frequency of aganglionosis associated with imperforate anus, Surgery 58:877, 1965.

Kiesewetter, W. B.: Imperforate anus: The role and results of the sacro-abdomino-perineal operation, Ann. Surg. 164:655, 1966.

Kiesewetter, W. B., and Nixon, H. H.: Imperforate anus. I. Its surgical anatomy, J. Pediat. Surg. 2:60, 1967.

Kiesewetter, W. B.: Imperforate anus. II. The rationale and technique of the sacro-abdomino-perineal operation, J. Pediat. Surg. 2:106, 1967.

Kirmisson: Quoted in Matas, q.v.

Kocher: Deutsch. Ztschr. Chir. Bd. XIII.

Koff, A. K.: Development of the vagina in the human fetus, Contr. Embryol. Carnegie Inst. 24:59, 1933.

Kottmeier, P. K.: A physiological approach to the problem of anal incontinence through use of the levator ani as a sling, Surgery 60:1262, 1966.

Kottmeier, P. K., and Dziadiw, R.: The complete release of the levator ani sling in fecal incontinence, J. Pediat. Surg. 2:111, 1967.

Kraske, P.: Extirpation of high rectal cancer, Vesh. deutsch. Gesellsch. Chir. 14:464, 1885.

Kratzer, G. L.; Dixon, C. F., and Bargen, J. A.: Duplication of the entire colon and terminal part of the ileum associated with parasitic twin, Proc. Staff Meet. Mayo Clin. 26:15, 1951.

Krönlein: Berlin klin. Wchnschr. 35:526, 1879.

Kurlander, G. J.: Roentgenology of imperforate anus, Am. J. Roentgenol. 100:190, 1967.

Ladd, W. E., and Gross, R. E.: Congenital malformations of anus and rectum, Am. J. Surg. 23:167, 1934.

Lannelongue: Bull. et mém. Soc. chir. 10:200, 1884.

Lawler, R. H.: Imperforate anus, Am. J. Proctol. 12:241, 1961.

Le Duc, E.: Congenital recto-urethral fistula: Report of case without rectal anomaly, J. Urol. 93:272, 1965.

Lee, M. J., Jr.: Congenital anomalies of the lower part of the rectum: Analysis of 16 cases, Am. J. Dis. Child. 68:182, 1944.

Leiserink, H.: Atresie ani, Fehlen des Rectum. Operation nach der Methode von Stromeyer, Deutsche Ztschr. chir. 1:494, 1872.

Leon-Diaz, F.: Cited by Ravitch, M. M., Ann. Surg. 137:588, 1953.

Lesbre, F. X.: *Traité de Tératologie* (Paris: Vigot Frères, 1927).

Littré: Quoted in Matas, q.v., 1897

Lloyd, J. R.: Ano-rectal anomalies, Harper Hosp. Bull. 22:63, 1964.

Loufti, A. H.: Personal communication, 1970.

Louw, J. H.: Congenital intestinal atresia and stenosis in the newborn. Observations in its pathogenesis and treatment, Ann. Roy. Coll. Surgeons England 25:209, 1959.

Louw, J. H.: Malformations of the anus and rectum: A report on 85 consecutive cases. South African M. J. 33:874, 1959.

Louw, J. H.: Investigations into the etiology of congenital atresia of the colon, Dis. Colon & Rectum 7:471, 1964.

Louw, J. H.: Congenital Abnormalities of the Rectum and Anus. *Current Problems in Surgery* (Chicago: Year Book Medical Publishers Inc., May, 1965).

Louw, J. H.: Colostomy in infants, South African J. Surg. 4:39, 1966.

Lowsley, O. S.: Persistent cloaca in female: Report of 2 cases corrected by operation, J. Urol. 59:692, 1948.

Lynn, H. B., and Arcari, F. A.: Anal atresia: Results of surgical treatment, Surgery 51: 691, 1962.

Magnus, R. V., and Stephens, F. D.: Imperforate anal membrane: The anatomy and function of the sphincters of the anal canal, Australian Paediat. J. 2:165, 1966.

Magnus, R. V.: The comparative anatomy of the levator ani and ano-rectal muscles, Victorian Vet. Proc. p. 41, 1967–68.

Magnus, R. V.: Rectal atresia as distinguished from rectal agenesis, J. Pediat. Surg. 3:593, 1968.

Magnus, R. V.: Ectopia cloacae – A misnomer, J. Pediat. Surg. 4:511, 1969.

Mahoney, P. J., and Chamberlain, J. W.: Hydrometrocolpos in infancy; congenital atresia of vagina with abnormally abundant cervical secretions, J. Pediat. 17:772, 1940.

Maitre, J.: Thèse de Lyon, June 1887.

Mantell, T.: Case of imperforated anus successfully treated, Med. Soc. London Mem. 3: 389, 1792.

Martin, Le Jeune: Société de Santé de Lyon: t.i.p. 180, 1798.

Mastin, W. M.: A resume of the surgical treatment of ano-rectal imperforation of the newborn, Surg., Gynec. & Obst. 7:316, 1908.

Matas, R.: The surgical treatment of congenital ano-rectal imperforation considered in the light of modern operative procedures, Tr. Am. Surg. A. 15:453, 1897.

Maylard: Cited in Matas, q.v., 1897

Mayo, C. W., and Rice, R. G.: Ano-rectal anomalies: A statistical study of 165 cases with

special reference to "distal loop trouble," Surgery 27:485, 1950.
Meckel, J. F.: *Handbuch der Pathologischen Anatomie* (Leipzig, Reclam), vol. 1, 1812, and vol. 2, 1816.
Menton, M. L., and Denny, H. E.: Duplication of the vermiform appendix, the large intestine and the urinary bladder; report of case, Arch. Path. 40:345, 1945.
Milligan, E. T. C., and Morgan, C. N.: Surgical anatomy of anal canal, with special reference to ano-rectal fistula, Lancet 2:1150, 1934.
Mishalany, H.: Personal communication, 1970.
Moore, T. C., and Lawrence, E. A.: Congenital malformations of the rectum and anus: Clinical features and surgical management in 120 cases, Surgery 32:352, 1952.
Moore, T. C., and Lawrence, E. A.: Congenital malformations of the rectum and anus: Associated anomalies in series of 120 cases, Surg., Gynec. & Obst. 95:281, 1952.
Morestin: Thèse des operations qui se pratiquent par la vole sacrée, Paris, 1894.
Murdoch, R. L.: A new operation for atresia ani vaginalis, Tr. Am. Proctol. Soc. 42:274, 1942.
Murugasu, J.: Personal communication, 1968.
Mysorekar, V. R.; Kolte, D. T., and Shirole, D. B.: A case of intestinal and urogenital duplication, J. Obst, & Gynaec. Brit. Commonwealth 74:596, 1967.
MacMahon, R. A.; Cohen, S. J., and Eckstein, H. B.: Colostomies in infancy and childhood, Arch. Dis. Childhood 38:114, 1963.
MacCormac, W.: On a case of imperforate anus, Lancet 2:12, 1886.
McDonald, A. L.: Imperforate anus. Tr. West S. A. 46:224, 1937.
McLeod, N.: Case of imperforate rectum with a suggestion for a new method of treatment, Brit. M. J. 2:657, 1880.
McPherson, A. G.: Congenital ano-rectal anomalies, Brit. J. Surg. 50:515, 1963.
Naidu, P. M., and Krishna, S.: Vestibular anus: A report of 2 cases, J. Obst. & Gynaec Brit. Commonwealth 68:851, 1961.
Neff, E. B.: Some observations on appendicitis, J. Oklahoma M. A. 33:14, 1940.
Nicolai, C. H.: Ano-rectal malformations and associated urinary fistulae. A report of 100 cases, J. Urol. 78:487, 1957.
Nicolai, I., and Rehbein, F.: Management of imperforate anus with recto-urethral fistula, Arch. Dis. Childhood 38:167, 1963.
Ninh, T. N., and Bohn, G. L.: Rectovestibular fistula in South Vietnam, Paediatric Surgery Congress, Melbourne, 1970.
Nixon, H. H.: Ano-rectal anomalies, Postgrad. M. J. 35:80, 1959.
Nixon, H. H.: *Imperforate Anus, British Surgical Practice* (Surgical Progress Volume, 1961) (London: Butterworth & Co., Ltd., 1961).
Nixon, H. H., and Callaghan, R. P.: Ano-rectal anomalies: Physiological considerations, Arch. Dis. Childhood 39:158, 1964.
Nixon, H. H., and Callaghan, R. P.: Defects in operations for imperforate anus, Dis. Colon & Rectum 7:459, 1964.
Nixon, H. H.: Personal communication, 1970.
Norris, W. J.; Brophy, T. W., III, and Brayton, D.: Imperforate anus: A case series and preliminary report of the one-stage abdomino-perineal operation, Surg., Gynec. & Obst. 88:623, 1949.
Oeconomopoulos, C. T.: Congenital anomalies of the rectum and anus. The technique of perineal proctoplasty, Am. J. Proctol. 12:363, 1961.
O'Hare, H. A.: Imperforate anus and tracheo-oesophageal fistula, Pennsylvania M. J. 40: 914, 1937.
Okamoto, E., and Ueda, T.: Embryogenesis of intramural ganglia of the gut and its relation to Hirschsprung's disease, J. Pediat. Surg. 2:437, 1967.
Ombredanne, L.: Une filette splanchnodyne, Mém. Acad. chir. 62:747, 1936.
Paine, J. R., and Nessa, C. B.: Observations on distribution and transport of gas in gastrointestinal tract of infants and young children, Surgery 11:281, 1942.

Palmer, J. A.: Congenital malformations of the anus, Canad. M. A. J. 74:882, 1956.

Paris, J., and Christiaens, L.: Megarectum caused by congenital stenosis of the anus with partial agenesis of the sacrum, Pediatrics 12:458, 1957.

Parkkulainen, K. V.: Sacrococcygeal and urological anomalies in connection with congenital malformations of anus and rectum; a preliminary report. Ann. paediat. Fenniae 3:51, 1957.

Parkkulainen, K. V.; Hjelt, L., and Sulamaa, M.: Anal atresia combined with aganglionic megacolon, Acta. chir. scandinav. 118:252, 1959.

Parks, A. G.; Porter, N. H., and Melzak, J.: Experimental study of reflex mechanism controlling muscles of the pelvic floor, Dis. Colon & Rectum 5:407, 1962.

Partridge, J. P., and Gough, M. H.: Congenital abnormalities of the anus and rectum, Brit. J. Surg. 49:37, 1961.

Patten, B. M.: *Human Embryology* (2d ed.; London: J. & A. Churchill, Ltd., 1953).

Patterson, N. G., and Maxwell, J. P.: A case of double vulva with hematometra on one side, J. Obst. & Gynaec. Brit. Emp. 46:71, 1939.

Patton, R. J.: Congenital ano-rectal atresia. Report of a case, Arch. Surg. 58:907, 1949.

Pegum, J. M.; Loly, P. C. M., and Falkiner, N. McI.: Development and classification of anorectal anomalies, Arch. Surg. 89:481, 1964.

Pellerin, D.: Congenital malformation of the anus and rectum: Anal imperforations, J. chir. 73:268, 1957.

Pellerin, D.: Communication sur le traitement des anus vulvaires, Ann. chir. infant. 4:15, 1963.

Pellerin, D., and Saied, H.: Contribution of histological examination to the choice of procedure for surgical cure of ano-rectal malformations in girls, Ann. chir. infant. 6:349, 1965.

Pennock, W. J., and Stark, W. J.: Persistence of cloaca, J. Urol. 16:93, 1926.

Peral Aranda, E.: Sobre un caso de agenesia sacrocoxígea subtotal, Arch. españ. urol. 9:12, 1953.

Perry, E. G.: Congenital median band of the anus, Australian & New Zealand J. Surg. 32: 292, 1962.

Piccoli, G.: Anomalia (un) de Sviluppo Fetale, Progr. med. Napoli 6:32, 1892.

Polaillon: Bull. Soc. chir., July 14, 1875.

Porter, N. H.: A physiological study of the pelvic floor in rectal prolapse, Ann. Roy. Coll. Surgeons England 31:379, 1962.

Poth, E. D.: (In discussion section of Thomson, I. M. and Hooks, C. A.) The urologic significance of imperforate anus, Am. Surgeon 22:1112, 1956.

Potts, W. J.; Riker, W. L., and DeBoer, A.: Imperforate anus with recto-vesical, recto-urethral, recto-vaginal and recto-perineal fistula, Ann. Surg. 140:381, 1954.

Potts, W. J.: *The Surgeon and the Child* (Philadelphia: W. B. Saunders Company, 1959).

Prasad, P. B.: Personal communication, 1970.

Prochiantz, A.: Imperforate anale, Ann. chir. Paris 11:C 373, 1957.

Ragius, H., and Van Prohaska, J.: Megarectum, Ann. Surg. 145:249, 1957.

Ramakrishnan, M. S.: Personal communication, 1970.

Ravitch, M. M.: Anal ileostomy with sphincter preservation in patients requiring total colectomy for benign conditions, Surgery 24:170, 1948.

Ravitch, M. M., and Handelsman, J. C.: One stage resection of entire colon and rectum for ulcerative colitis and polypoid adenomatosis, Bull. Johns Hopkins Hosp. 88:59, 1951.

Ravitch, M. M.: Hindgut duplication – doubling of colon and genital urinary tracts, Ann. Surg. 137:588, 1953.

Ravitch, M. M., and Scott, W. W.: Duplication of the entire colon, bladder and urethra, Surgery 34:843, 1953.

Ravitch, M. M.: Pseudo-Hirschsprung's disease, Ann. Surg. 147:781, 1958.

Rehbein, F., and Hüther, W.: Hirschsprung's disease without a narrow segment, Kinderärztl. Praxis 25:403, 1957.

Rehbein, F.: Operation for anal and rectal atresia with recto-urethral fistula, Chirurg. 30:417, 1959.

Rehbein, F.: Zur Operation der hohen Rectumatresie mit Recto-Urethral-Fistel. Abdomino-sacro-perinealer Durchzug, Ztschr. Kinderchir. 2:503, 1965.

Rehbein, F.: Imperforate anus: Experiences with abdomino-perineal and abdomino-sacro-perineal pull through procedures, J. Pediat. Surg. 2:99, 1967.

Rehbein, F.: Personal communication, 1970.

Rhoads, J. E.; Piper, R. L., and Randall, J. P.: A simultaneous abdominal and perineal approach in operations for imperforate anus with atresia of the rectum and rectosigmoid, Ann. Surg. 127:552, 1948.

Rhoads, J. E., and Koop, C. E.: Symposium on function and disease of anorectum and colon: Surgical management of imperforate anus, S. Clin. North America 35:1251, 1955.

Rhodes, R. L.: Further observations upon imperforate anus, Ann. Surg. 123:877, 1946.

Rickham, P. P.: Vesico-intestinal fissure, Arch. Dis. Childhood 35:97, 1960.

Riker, W. L.: Diagnosis and treatment of aganglionosis of the myenteric plexus, Arch. Surg. 75:362, 1957.

Rizzoli, F.: A new operative method executed in 4 cases of congenital atresia ani, with opening of the rectum into the vulva, Surg. Mem. 2:321, 1869.

Robertson, D. A. R.; Samuel, E., and MacLeod, W.: Radiological assessment of imperforate anus, Brit. J. Radiol. 38:444, 1965.

Robson, A. M.: A suggested method of operating on a uniform principle in the treatment of imperforate anus; with case. Tr. Clin. Soc. London 20:103, 1887.

Romualdi, P.: A new technique for surgical treatment of some rectal malformations, Arch. klin. Chir. 296:371, 1960.

Romualdi, P.: Treatment of some particularly difficult cases of anus prostaticus by means of abdomino-perineal intrarectal operation, Rev. chir. pediat. 3:27, 1961.

Rosenblatt, M. S., and May, A.: Malformations of the anus and rectum, Surg., Gynec. & Obst. 83:499, 1946.

Roux de Brignolles: Cited in Matas, q.v., 1897.

Russell, K. F.: Case of complicated exstrophy of bladder presenting many unusual features, Brit. J. Urol. 11:31, 1939.

Salzberg, A. M., and Martin, C. M.: Imperforate anus, South. M. J. 54:1101, 1961.

Santulli, T. V.: Treatment of imperforate anus and associated fistulas, Surg., Gynec. & Obst. 95:601, 1952.

Santulli, T. V.; Schullinger, J. N.; Amoury, R. A., and Berdon, W. E.: Malformations of the anus and rectum, S. Clin. North America 45:1253, 1965.

Santulli, T. V.: Congenital anomalies of the gastrointestinal tract, Pediat. Clin. North America 14:21, 1967.

Santulli, T. V.: In *Pediatric Surgery,* Mustard, Ravitch, Snyder, Welch and Benson (eds.) (2d ed.; Chicago: Year Book Medical Publishers Inc., 1969).

Santulli, T. V.: Personal communication, 1970.

Saphir, J. F.: Congenital anorectal malformations, Med. Rec. New York 156:22, 1943.

Sauvage, L. R., and Bill, A. H.: Imperforate anus repair through a buttock reflecting incision, Surgery 57:448, 1965.

Saviord: Cited by Crowell, E. A., and Duein, J. W., Surgery 7:529, 1940.

Schachenmann, G.; Schmid, W.; Frascaro, M.; Mannini, A.; Tiepolo, L.; Perona, G. P., and Sartori, E.: Chromosomes in coloboma and anal atresia, Lancet 2:290, 1965.

Schapiro, S.: Proctologic problems in children, Lancet 84:134, 1960.

Scharli, A. F., and Kiesewetter, W. B.: Imperforate anus: Anorectosigmoid pressure studies as a quantitative evaluation of post-operative continence, J. Pediat. Surg. 4:694, 1969.

Schnaufer, L.; Talbert, J. L.; Haller, J. A.; Reid, N. C. R.; Tobon, F., and Schuster, M. M.: Differential sphincter studies in the diagnosis of ano-rectal disorders of childhood, J. Pediat. Surg. 2:538, 1967.

Scott, J. E. S.: The anatomy of the pelvic autonomic nervous system in cases of high imperforate anus, Surgery 45:1013, 1959.

Scott, J. E. S., and Swenson, O.: Imperforate anus, results in 63 cases and some anatomical considerations, Ann. Surg. 150:477, 1959.

Scott, J. E. S.; Swenson, O., and Fisher, J. H.: Some comments on the surgical treatment of imperforate anus, Am. J. Surg. 99:137, 1960.

Scott, J. E. S.: The microscopic anatomy of the terminal intestinal canal in ectopic vulval anus, J. Pediat. Surg. 1:441, 1966.

Scultet: Cited in Matas, q.v., 1897.

Seitz, A., and Bautze, H. J.: Familiärer Anus vestibularis, Zentralbl. Gynäk. 73:1543, 1951.

Shahi, U. N., and Mishra, S. N.: Congenital anorectal anomalies. A study of 100 cases, Indian J. Pediat. 28:447, 1961.

Shepherd, R., and Kiesewetter, W. B.: Hyperchloraemic acidosis – a complication of imperforate anus with recto-urinary fistula, J. Pediat. Surg. 1:62, 1966.

Shopfner, C. E.: Roentgenologic demonstration of the "ectopic anus" associated with imperforate anus, Radiology 84:464, 1965.

Shopfner, C. E.: Roentgenologic evaluation of imperforate anus, South. M. J. 58:712, 1965.

Sieber, W. K., and Klein, R.: Cloaca with non-adrenal female pseudohermaphrodism, Pediatrics 22:472, 1958.

Sieur: Arch. Provincilaes chir., t. v. no. 9, 1896.

Sitkovskii, N. B.: Congenital fistula between the rectum and the vaginal vestibule in a normal anus, Akush. i ginek. 39:137, 1963.

Sitkovskii, N. B.: The treatment of atresia of the anus and rectum with fistulas into the genital system in girls, Khirurgie, Moskva 42:80, 1966.

Smith, B.: Esophageal atresia and imperforate anus, Am. J. Surg. 100:140, 1960.

Smith, E. D.: Congenital anomalies of the sacrum, Australian & New Zealand J. Surg. 29:165, 1959.

Smith, E. D.: *Spina Bifida and the Total Care of Spinal Myelomeningocele* (Springfield, Ill.: Charles C Thomas, Publisher, 1965).

Smith, E. D.: Management of the urinary tract in spinal myelomeningocele: The case for early surgical diversion of urine, Australian Paediat. J. 2:27, 1966.

Smith, E. D.: Urinary anomalies and complications in imperforate anus and rectum, J. Pediat. Surg. 3:337, 1968.

Smith, E. D.: Duplications of the anus and genitourinary tracts, Surgery 66:909, 1969.

Smith, E. I., and Gross, R. E.: The external anal sphincter in cases of imperforate anus: A pathological study, Surgery 49:807, 1961.

Smith, S., and Boulgakov, B.: A case of dicephalis dibrachius, dipus showing certain features of embryological interest, J. Anat. 61:94, 1926.

Snyder, W. H., Jr.: Imperforate anus, Am. J. Surg. 101:633, 1961.

Snyder, W. H., Jr.: Some unusual forms of imperforate anus in female patients, Am. J. Surg. 111:319, 1966.

Soave, F.: Hirschsprung's disease; a new surgical technique, Arch. Dis. Childhood 39: 116, 1964.

Soave, F.: Surgery of rectal anomalies with presentation of the relationship between the colonic mucosal sleeve and puborectalis muscle, J. Pediat. Surg. 4:705, 1969.

Solowiejczyk, M.: Suggested aids to the surgical treatment of imperforate anus and congenital malformations of rectum, J. Internat. Coll. Surgeons 35:371, 1961.

Sommerschild, H.; Knutrud, O., and Fretheim, B.: Ano-rectal anomalies, Acta. chir. scandinav. 127:536, 1964.

Soothill, J. F.: Congenital absence of sacrum and coccyx, Guy's Hosp. Rep. 103:87, 1954.

Soper, R. T., and Kilger, K.: Vesico-intestinal fissure, J. Urol. 92:490, 1964.

Spence, H. M.: Anomalies and complications of the urogenital tract associated with congenital imperforate anus, J. Urol. 71:453, 1954.

Spencer, R., and Geer, J. C.: Ileocaecal exstrophy with bifid intra-abdominal urinary bladder, J. Pediat. Surg. 2:69, 1967.

Spriggs, N. J.: Congenital intestinal occlusion. An account of twenty-four unpublished cases, with remarks based thereon and upon the literature of the subject, Guy's Hosp. Rep. 66:143, 1912.

Starlinger, F., and Richter, W.: Ummittelbare Erfolge und Fernergebnisse der Behandlung des angeborenen Enddarmverschlusses (Atresia ani et recti), Zentralbl. Chir. 60:2893, 1933.

Steinbuchel: Über Nabelschnurbruch und Blasen-Bauchspalte mit Cloakenbildung von Seiten des Dünndarmes, Arch. Gynäk. 60:465, 1900.

Stelzner, F.: The problems of continence in anorectal surgery, Chirurgia 28:155, 1957.

Stephens, F. D.: Congenital imperforate rectum, recto-urethral and rectovaginal fistulae, Australian & New Zealand J. Surg. 22:161, 1953 (a).

Stephens, F. D.: Malformations of the anus, Australian & New Zealand J. Surg. 23:9, 1953 (b).

Stephens, F. D.: Imperforate rectum. A new surgical technique, M. J. Australia 1:202, 1953.

Stephens, F. D.: Congenital malformations of rectum and anus in female children, Australian & New Zealand J. Surg. 31:90, 1961.

Stephens, F. D.: *Congenital Malformations of the Rectum, Anus and Genito-Urinary Tract* (Edinburgh and London: E. & S. Livingstone, Ltd., 1963).

Stephens, F. D.: Congenital rectal fistulae and their sphincters, Australian Paed. J. 1: 107, 1965.

Stephens, F. D.: Urethro-vaginal malformations, Australian & New Zealand J. Obst. & Gynaec. 5:64, 1966.

Stephens, F. D.: The female anus, perineum and vestibule: Embryogenesis and deformities, Australian & New Zealand J. Obst. & Gynaec. 8:55, 1968.

Stevenson, J. K., and Herron, P. W.: Hirschsprung's disease. A rare cause of constipation in patients following surgical correction of imperforate anus, Am. Surgeon 33:555, 1967.

Stieda, A.: Über Atresia Ani Congenita und die damit verbundenen Missbildungen, Arch. klin. Chir. 70:555, 1903.

Stone, H. B.: Imperforate anus with recto-vaginal cloaca, Ann. Surg. 104:651, 1936.

Storm-Mathison, A.: Myelodysplasia with absence of sacrum (one case), Acta psychiat. et neurol. scandinav. 29:145, 1954.

Stromeyer: *Handbuch der Chirurgie*, 2 vols. (Freiburg: 1844 and 1848).

Suckling, P. V.: Familial incidence of congenital abnormalities of anus and rectum, Arch. Dis. Childhood 24:75, 1949.

Suppiger, J.: Bildungsfehler der weiblichen Beckenorgane, Correspondenz-Blatt für Schweizer Ärzte 6:418, 1876.

Swain, V. A. J., and Tucker, S. M.: The results of operation in 46 cases of malformations of the anus and rectum, Gut 3:245, 1962.

Swan, H., and Christensen, S. P.: Exstrophy of cloaca, Pediatrics 12:645, 1953.

Swenson, O., and Grana, L.: Long term results of surgical treatment of imperforate anus, Dis. Colon & Rectum 5:13, 1962.

Swenson, O., and Donnellan, W. L.: Preservation of the puborectalis sling in imperforate anus repair, S. Clin. North America 47:173, 1967.

Swenson, O.: *Pediatric Surgery* (2d ed.; New York: Appleton-Century-Crofts, Inc., 1967).

Tank, E. S., and Watts, H.: Hyperchloraemic acidosis from urethro-rectal fistula and imperforate anus, Surgery 63:837, 1968.

Tench, E. M.: Development of the anus in the human embryo, Am. J. Anat. 59:333, 1936.

Thompson, I. M., and Hooks, C. A.: The urologic significance of imperforate anus, Am. Surgeon 22:1112, 1956.

Trusler, G. A.; Mestel, A. L., and Stephens, C. A.: Colon malformations with imperforate anus, Surgery 45:328, 1959.

Trusler, G. A., and Wilkinson, R. H.: Imperforate anus: A review of 147 cases, Canad. J. Surg. 5:269, 1962.

Valentin, B.: Agenesia sacro-coccygea (Anchipodia) (ein Übersichtsbericht), Zentralbl. allg. Path. 90:281, 1953.

Van Gelder, D. W., and Kloepfer, H. W.: Familial anorectal anomalies, Pediatrics 27:334, 1961.

Van Velzer, D. A.; Barrick, C. W., and Jenkinson, E. L.: Duplication of the colon: A case presentation, Am. J. Roentgenol. 75:349, 1956.

Van Zwalenburg, B. R.: Double colon: Differentiation of cases into two groups, Am. J. Roentgenol. 68:22, 1952.

Veal, J. R., and McFetridge, E. M.: Exstrophy of bladder (persistent cloaca) associated with intestinal fistulas with brief analysis of 36 cases of anal and rectal anomalies from records of Charity Hospital, New Orleans, J. Pediat. 4:95, 1934.

Verneuil, A.: De la resection du coccyx pour faciliter le formation d'un anus perineale dans l'imperforation du rectum, Bull. et mém. Soc. de chir. 2:288, 1873.

Vincent: Lyon med.: 408, 1887.

Volpe, M.: Dell 'asta Doppia, Il Policlin Roma 10:46, 1903.

Von Geldern, C. E.: The etiology of cloacal exstrophy and allied malformations, J. Urol. 82:134, 1959.

Waite, V. C.: Surgical treatment of anorectal anomalies, Postgrad. Med. 16:526, 1954.

Wallace, F. T.; Colvin, E. M., and Spartanburg, S. C.: Complications of imperforate anus repair, Surgery 24:832, 1948.

Walls, E. W.: Anorectal anomaly, Proc. Roy. Soc. Med. 51:425, 1958.

Wangensteen, O. H., and Rice, C. O.: Imperforate anus. A method of determining the surgical approach, Ann. Surg. 92:77, 1930.

Weber, H. M., and Dixon, C. F.: Duplication of entire large intestine (colon duplex): Report of case, Am. J. Roentgenol. 55:319, 1946.

Weinstein, E. D.: Sex linked imperforate anus, Pediatrics 35:715, 1965.

Wilkinson, A. W.: Imperforate anus: Some observations regarding diagnosis of the level of obstruction, Am. J. Dis. Child. 19:138, 1944.

Williams, D. I., and Nixon, H. H.: Agenesis of the sacrum, Surg., Gynec. & Obst. 105:84, 1957.

Williams, D. I.: *Urology in Childhood,* vol. XV (Berlin: Springer-Verlag, 1958).

Wilson, A. K.: Roentgen examination in congenital intestinal obstructive defects in infants: Its aid in planning suitable surgical approach and procedures for their correction, Am. J. Roentgenol. 54:498, 1945.

Wilson, P. M.: Anchoring mechanisms of the anorectal region, South African M. J. 41: 1127, 1967.

Winkel-Smith, C. C.: Seven cases of imperforate anus treated by the abdomino-perineal replacement of the rectum, Acta. chir. scandinav. 105:305, 1953.

Winslow, O.; Litt, R., and Altman, D.: Imperforate anus from a roentgenologic view point, Am. J. Roentgenol. 85:718, 1961.

Wolff, E.: *La Science des Monstres* (Paris: Gallimard, 1948).

Woolam, G. L.: Congenital anomalies of anus and rectum, Mayo Clin. Proc. 39:866, 1964.

Young, H. H.: Imperforate anus; bowel opening into urethra; hypospadias, presentation of new plastic methods, J.A.M.A. 107:1448, 1936.

Zaidi, Z. H.: Congenital absence of most of the colon; anomaly associated with imperforate anus, syndactylism and polydactylism, A.M.A. Am. J. Dis. Child. 98:385, 1959.

Zeligs, I. M.: Congenital absence of sacrum, Arch. Surg. 41:1220, 1940.

Zoehner: quoted in Matusovszki, A. Ein Fall von Anus Urethralis, Zentralbl. Gynäk. 52: 496, 1928.

Zwiren, G. T., and Patterson, J. H.: Exstrophy of the cloaca; report of a case treated surgically, Pediatrics 35:687, 1965.

APPENDIX A

Procedure for Identification and Management

Diagnosis and Management of Ano-Rectal Malformations in the Newborn

Male Malformations

Search carefully for bowel communication to external skin.

1. *If orifice found* (translevator, except rectal atresia).

   Anterior perineal anus (Z–10, Appendix C)—normal caliber orifice anteriorly: no treatment.

   Ano-cutaneous fistula (Z–11, Appendix C)—anterior fistula in the raphe, probe passes backwards: cutback.

   Anal stenosis (Z–7, 9 and 13, Appendix C)—various types, stenotic orifice, probing and digital examination: dilatation or incision.

   Rectal atresia (Z–4, Appendix C)—normal anus, but occlusion to digit: preliminary colostomy.

   Optional investigations: Fistulography and invertography.

2. *If orifice not found* cannot predict level, although most will be supralevator. Inspect urethral meatus for meconium or gas and collect and examine urine for meconium.

   (a) *Meconium not present in urine*—noncommunicating deformity. Inversion radiography and micturition cystourethrography required.

      Ano-rectal agenesis (Z–1, Appendix C), gas at or above P/C line, no fistula: preliminary colostomy.

      Anal agenesis (Z–5, Appendix C) (no fistula), gas at I point or between I point and P/C line: preliminary colostomy.

      Covered anus—complete (Z–8, Appendix C)—gas below I point: incision and dilatation.

      Imperforate anal membrane (Z–12, Appendix C), gas below I point and approximating skin marker: incision and dilatation.

(b) *Meconium present in urine*—communicating deformity. All patients with meconium in urine require preliminary colostomy, but inversion radiography and micturition cystourethrography highly desirable for exact identification.

Recto-vesical fistula (Z–2, Appendix C), gas above P/C line, fistula: preliminary colostomy.

Recto-urethral fistula (Z–3, Appendix C), gas at P/C line, fistula: preliminary colostomy.

Recto-bulbar fistula (Z–6, Appendix C), gas at I point, fistula: preliminary colostomy.

Optional investigations: Direct needle aspiration of meconium and injection of opaque medium.

Female Malformations

Determine whether the vulva is "open" or partially closed. If open, examine the orifices which open externally. If partially closed over, convert to open by midline incision and then inspect all the exposed orifices.

1. *If bowel orifice, meconium or gas found*—communicating deformity, i.e., orifice or fistula opens into cloaca, vagina, vestibule or perineum. Identification depends upon the number of orifices which open externally onto vestibule or perineum.

(a) *One orifice in vulva common to urethra, vagina and rectum.*

Recto-cloacal (Z–16, Appendix C) or recto-vesical fistula (Z–15, Appendix C): preliminary colostomy.

(b) *Two orifices, those of urethra and vagina in vulva.*

Recto-vaginal fistula (Z–17 and 20, Appendix C): preliminary colostomy.

Covered anus—complete (Z–23, Appendix C), hypertrophied raphe: incision and dilatation.

(c) *Three orifices, those of urethra, vagina and bowel.* Further identification depends upon site of bowel orifice, appearance of surrounding epithelium and probe tests.

(i) *Anus sited normally*

Perineal groove (Z–32, Appendix C), anterior mucosal ectropion: no treatment.

Perineal canal (Z–33, Appendix C), probe enters fistula from vestibule to anus: fistulectomy.

Imperforate anal membrane (Z–30, Appendix C), digital and probe examination: incision and dilatation.

Anal stenosis (Z–22, 24 and 31, Appendix C), various types, stenotic orifice, digital and probe examination: dilatation or incision.

Rectal atresia (Z–18, Appendix C), normal anus, but occlusion to probe: preliminary colostomy.

(ii) *Orifice at perineal site*

Anterior perineal anus (Z–25, Appendix C), normal caliber anus anteriorly: no treatment.

Ano-cutaneous fistula (Z–26, Appendix C), beveled anterior orifice, dry skin surrounding orifice, probe passes preferentially backwards: cutback.

(iii) *Orifice at vulvar site*

Vulvar anus (Z–27, Appendix C), normal anus in vestibule: no treatment.

Ano-vulvar fistula (Z–28, Appendix C), orifice in vestibule but dry skin posteriorly, probe passes backwards: cutback.

Ano-vestibular fistula (Z–29, Appendix C), narrow orifice in fossa navicularis, surrounded by wet mucosa, probe passes preferentially upwards with some backward play: dilatation or cutback.

Recto-vestibular fistula (Z–21, Appendix C), narrow orifice in fossa navicularis, probe passes strictly caudocranial, measure length of fistula with marked Foley catheter: colostomy.

Optional investigations: Fistulography, inversion radiography and vaginoscopy.

2. *If orifice not found*—non-communicating deformities, but rare in a female infant. Adopt inversion radiography and correlate findings with plan of remaining perineal orifices.

Ano-rectal agenesis (Z–14, Appendix C) (no fistula), gas at P/C line, no fistula: preliminary colostomy.

Anal agenesis (Z–19, Appendix C) (no fistula), gas at or cranial to I point, no fistula: preliminary colostomy.

Covered anus—complete (Z–23, Appendix C), gas below I point: incision and dilatation.

Imperforate anal membrane (Z–30, Appendix C), gas below I point and approximating skin marker: incision and dilatation.

Optional investigations: Direct needle aspiration of meconium and injection of opaque medium.

Other Essential Tests and Investigations

1. *Assessment of nerve supply to levator ani muscle*—by examining bladder, urethral sphincters and perineal skin, which are innervated by same sacral outflow.

(a) Bladder expressibility and control.

(i) Normal—regular and spontaneous micturition, normal control, not expressible: sacral outflow to nervi erigentes is intact.

(ii) Neurogenic disturbance—freely expressible bladder and leaking, or firm, large, nontender bladder, difficult to express: impaired sacral outflow.

(b) Perineal sensation—absence of appreciation of pinprick indicates impaired sacral outflow. This together with impaired urethral function means impaired sacral outflow and defective innervation of levator ani muscle: permanent colostomy for rectal deformities.

2. *Assessment of extent of formation of levator ani muscle* by radiograph of sacrum and lumbar spine (anteroposterior and lateral views). A normal spine portends a well-developed levator ani muscle. A defective spine presages imperfections of the levator ani muscle.

(a) Agenesis of sacral vertebrae incurs adaptions of posterior attachments of the levator ani; however, these muscles are otherwise well formed and adequately innervated if sacral outflow tests are normal, but rudimentary in formation and defective in innervation if sacral outflow tests show the impairments described.

(b) Spina bifida, which involves highest sacral vertebrae and perhaps lumbar vertebrae indicates meningocele or myelomeningocele. In such cases, levatores ani muscles are well formed; the central connections are intact if the sacral outflow tests are all normal (meningocele), but dysplastic if the tests show impairment (myelodysplasia of the cord): permanent colostomy required for rectal deformities if muscle grossly defective.

3. *Assessment of urinary tract abnormalities.*

(a) Micturition cystourethrography is desirable in conjunction with inversion radiography, or within a few days of treatment to document unsuspected fistulae and the presence of ureteric reflux.

(b) Microscopic examination of the urine (catheter or suprapubic aspiration), and blood urea estimation.

(i) If the urine is pus-free and sterile and the blood urea is normal, further investigations of the upper urinary tract may be delayed until soon after the more immediate and urgent operation on the bowel. At least intravenous pyelography should then be performed.

(ii) If the urine is infected or the blood urea is raised, it is important to fully estimate the extent of the abnormalities which may radically influence the management. This may require intravenous and retrograde pyelography, endoscopy and renography. In this way the plan of treatment of both the malformations of the bowel and the urinary tract can be mapped out to best advantage in advance. Serious urinary tract disease is a strong indication for less radical surgery for the rectal deformity; diversion colostomy, cleansing of the distal segment, the sorting out and consideration and management of the urinary lesions should precede the surgery of the rectum.

4. *Assessment of other visceral malformations,* e.g., cardiac, alimentary, etc. Pass a firm No. 10 rubber catheter down esophagus if symptoms suggest tracheo-esophageal fistula.

Postcolostomy Management

1. *Completion of other essential tests and investigations, as above.*
2. *Diligent clearance of the distal limb of the colostomy* to prevent urinary infection in the presence of a fistula. Check by cologram.
3. *Detailed analysis of level and anatomical type.*

Males

(i) *Noncommunicating:* Erect colography of distal limb of colostomy to confirm level of occlusion.

Ano-rectal agenesis (Z–1, Appendix C) (no fistula), occlusion at or above P/C line: sacro-abdomino-perineal rectoplasty.

Anal agenesis (Z–5, Appendix C) (no fistula), occlusion at I point, sacro-perineal proctoplasty.

(ii) *Communicating:* Colography as for (i) but combined with micturition cystourethrography and later urethroscopy.

Recto-vesical fistula (Z–2, Appendix C), fistula above P/C line: sacro-abdomino-perineal rectoplasty.

Recto-urethral fistula (Z–3, Appendix C), fistula at verumontanum at P/C line: sacro-abdomino-perineal rectoplasty.

Recto-bulbar fistula (Z–6, Appendix C), fistula at bulb at I point: sacro-perineal proctoplasty.

Females

(i) *Noncommunicating:* As in male.

(ii) *Communicating:* Colography and vaginography are not essential but may aid in diagnosis. Endoscopy of vagina and urethra is of more value to confirm location of rectal orifice and to determine the topography of the urinary and genital tracts: sacro-perineal or sacro-abdomino-perineal rectoplasty.

APPENDIX B

Summary of Factors Essential for Good Results

(A) *Preoperative Factors*

1. *Accurate assessment of level of deformity and anatomical type in relation to sphincters before any operation (Chapter 8):*
   Careful inspection of orifices.
   Detection of meconium in urine.
   Invertography, its validity and fallacies.
   Micturition cystourethrography of neonate.
   Dye studies of orifices and fistulae.
   Colography.
2. *Assessment of muscle and nerve integrity* (see Chapter 8):
   X-ray spine and sacrum.
   Clinical tests.
3. *Assessment of associated anomalies* (see Chapter 11).
4. *Diagnosis and treatment of urinary infection* (see Chapter 12):
   Diagnosis of urinary anomalies early.
   Postcolostomy prevention of urinary infection through fistula.
   Treatment of urinary anomalies.

(B) *Operative Factors*

1. *Colostomy technique and care:*
   Separation of limbs to prevent spill-over.
   Washing out of distal limb.
2. *Minor surgery for translevator anal deformities:*
   No deep dissection in perineum.
3. *Correct choice and technique of rectoplasty in rectal deformities* (supralevator and intermediate):
   Delayed until late infancy.
   Sacro-perineal or sacro-abdomino-perineal exposure with or without Rehbein procedure.
   Accurate placement of rectum through pubo-rectalis sling.

Preservation of pubo-rectalis sling by small tunnel, minimal stretching at operation.
Preservation of nerves.
Preservation of sensation.
Protection of urethra.
Avoidance of stricture.
Avoidance of exposed mucosa.

(C) *Postoperative Factors*

1. *Gentle dilatation of pubo-rectalis sling.*
2. *Prevention of anal strictures* by prolonged dilatation and by anoplasty.
3. *Prevention and treatment of constipation.*
4. *Treatment of excess mucosa.*
5. *Training and "toilet tricks."*
6. *Dietary stability.*
7. *Parental, social and emotional stability.*

Appendix C is in the pouch on the inside back cover.

Index

R

S

V

W